Serotonin and the CNS - New Developments in Pharmacology and Therapeutics

Edited by Berend Olivier

Published in London, United Kingdom

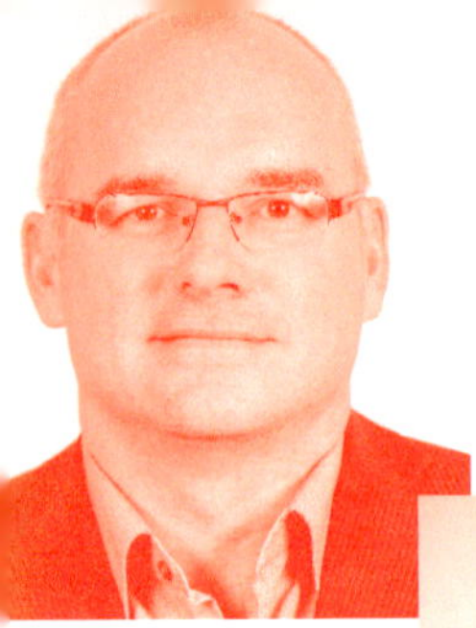
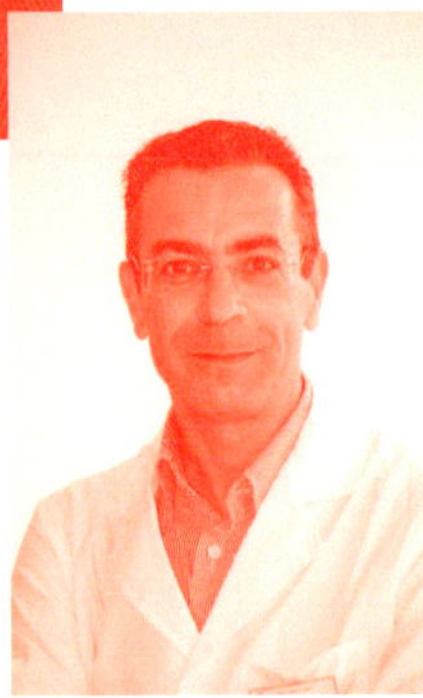
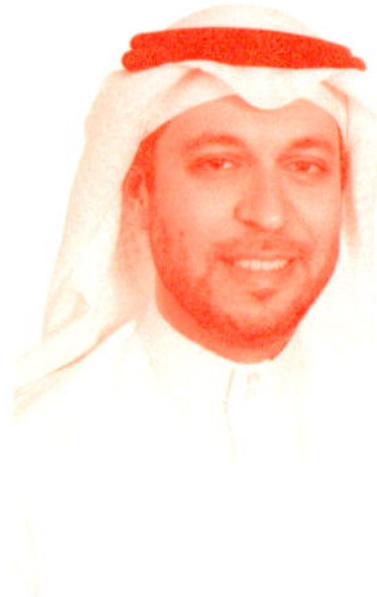
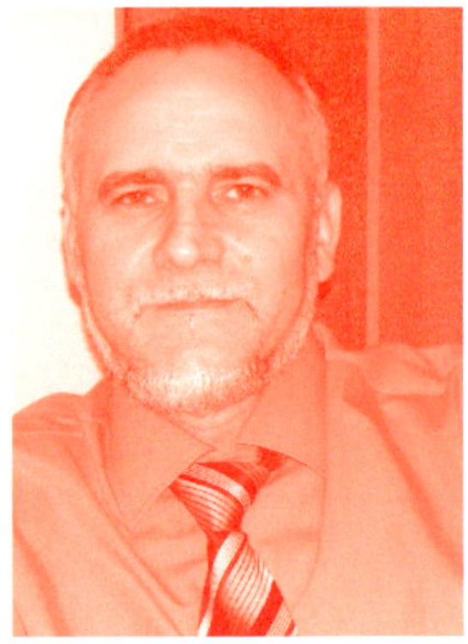
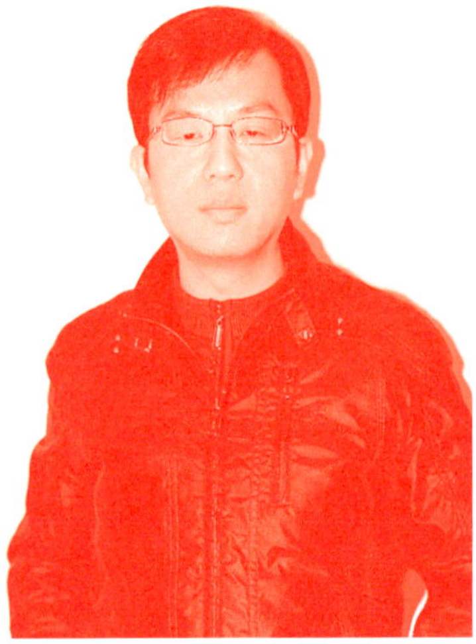
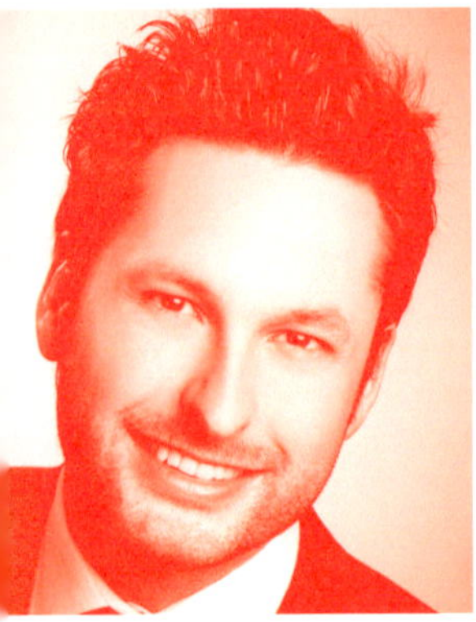
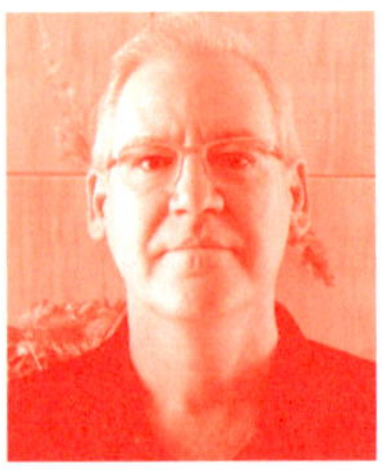

IntechOpen

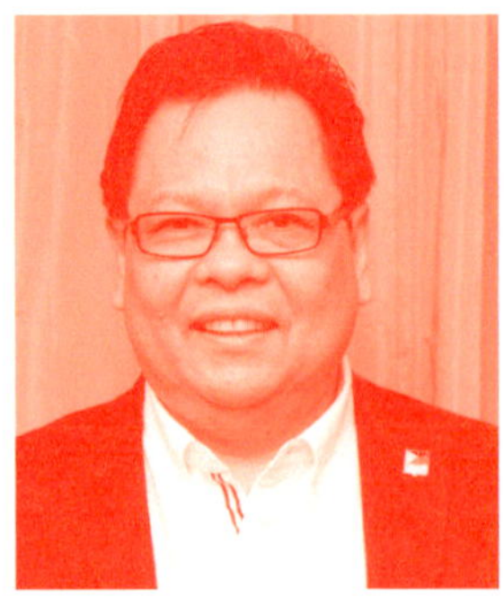
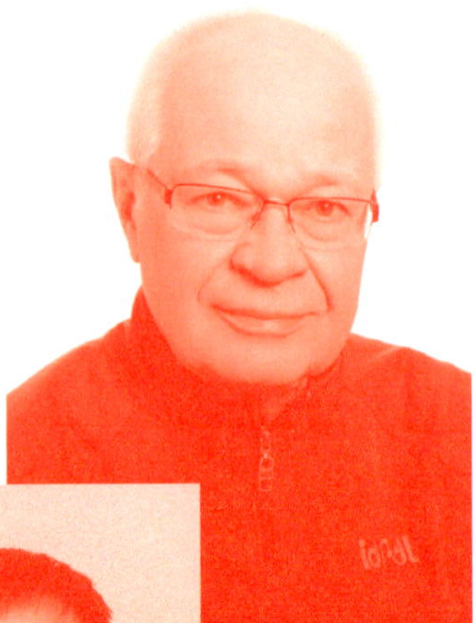
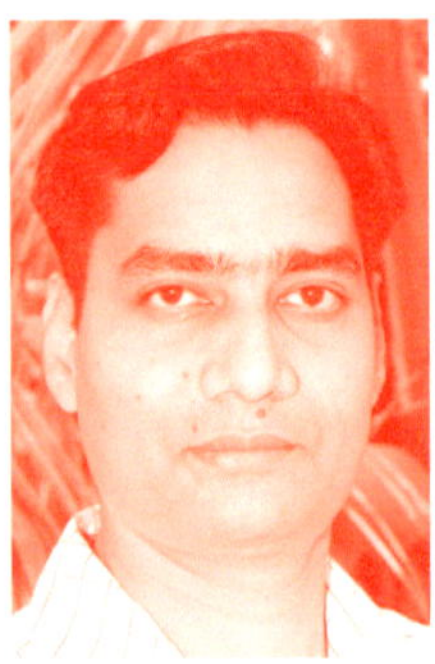
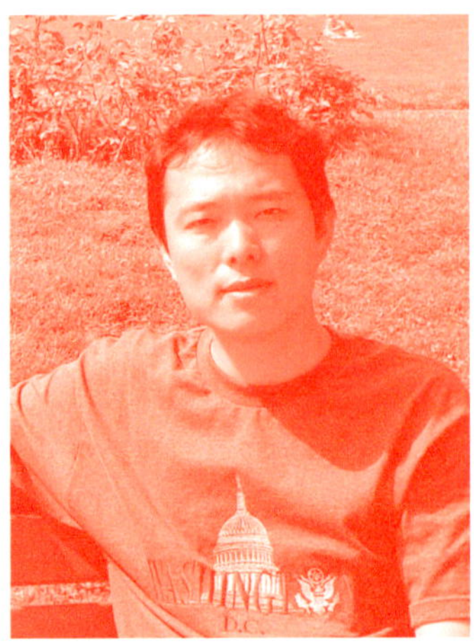
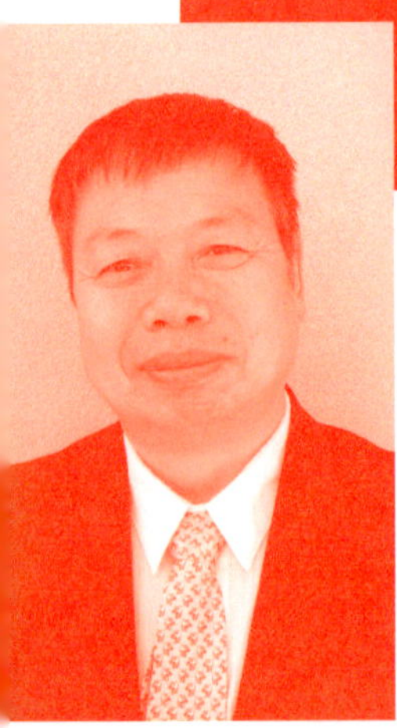
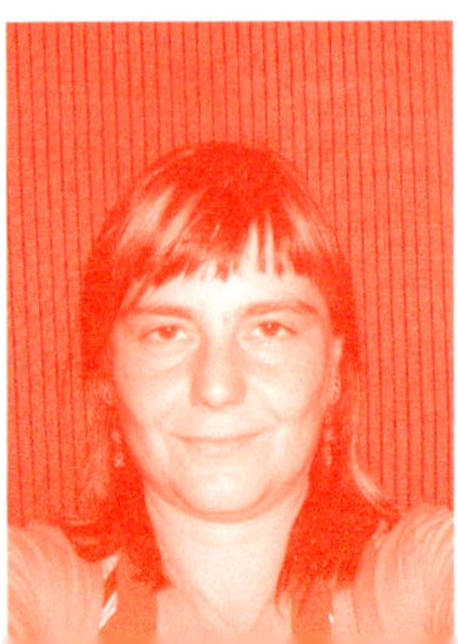

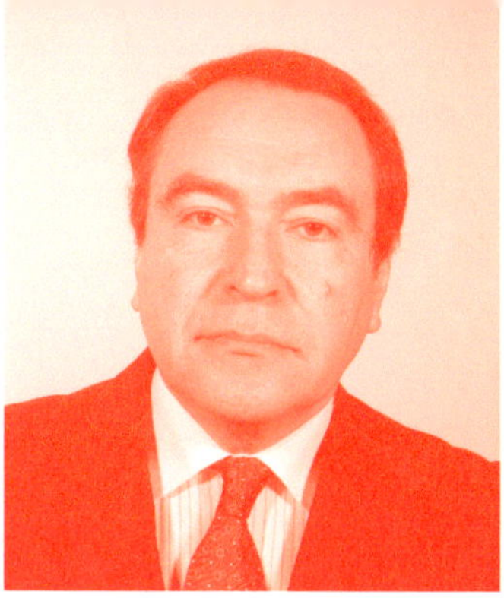
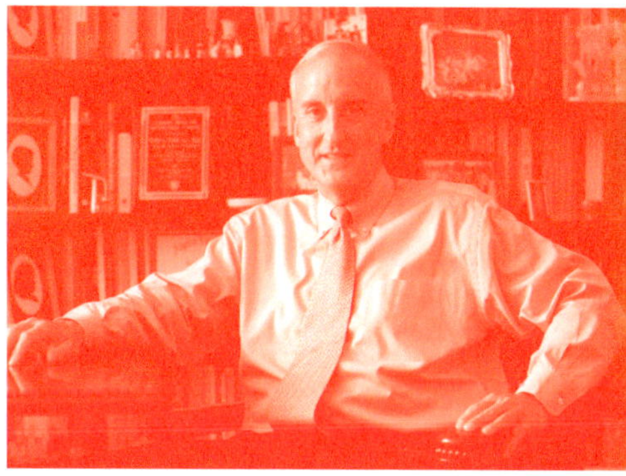
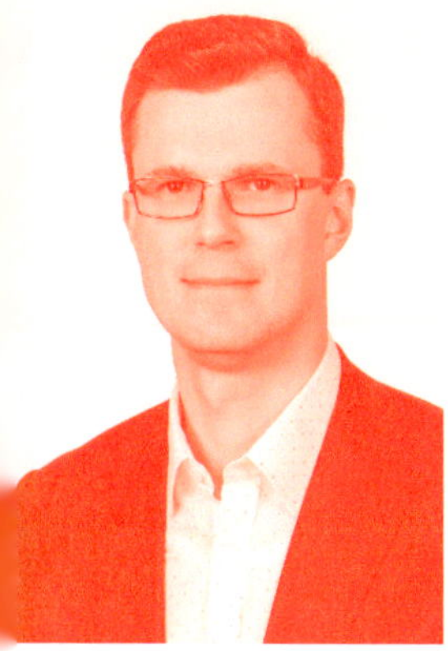
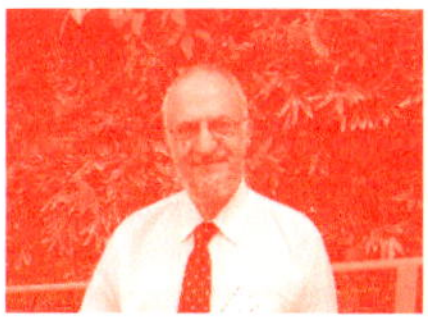
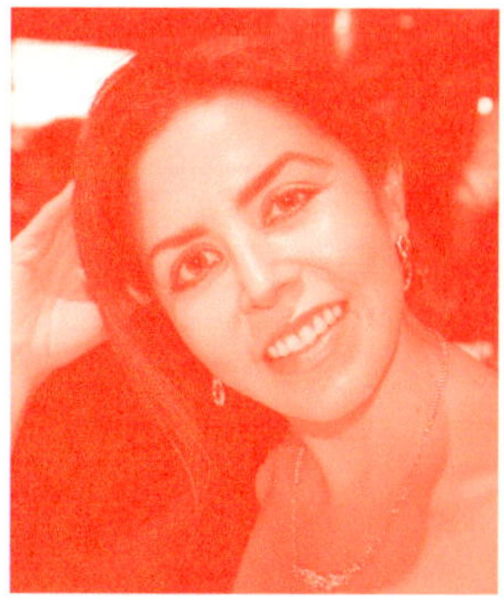

Supporting open minds since 2005

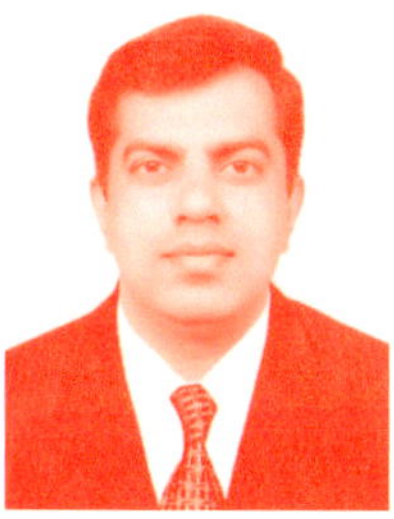
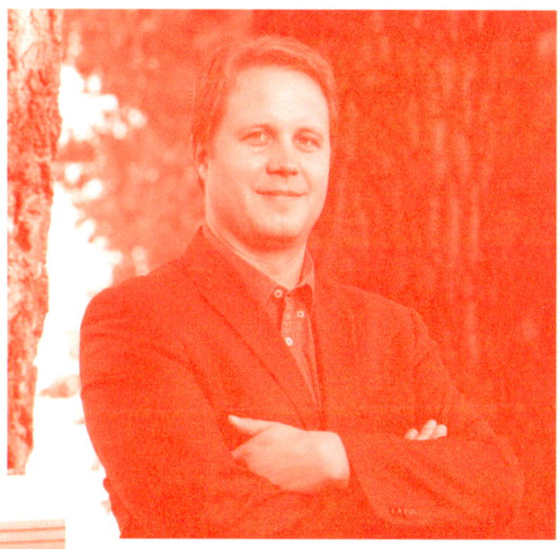
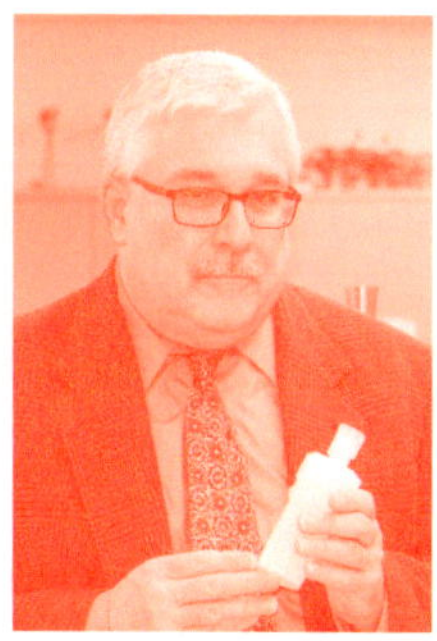
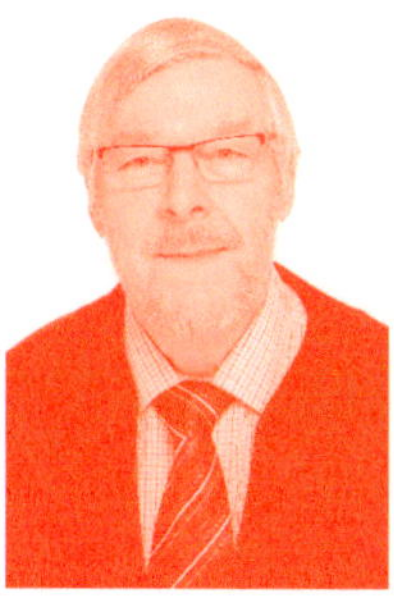
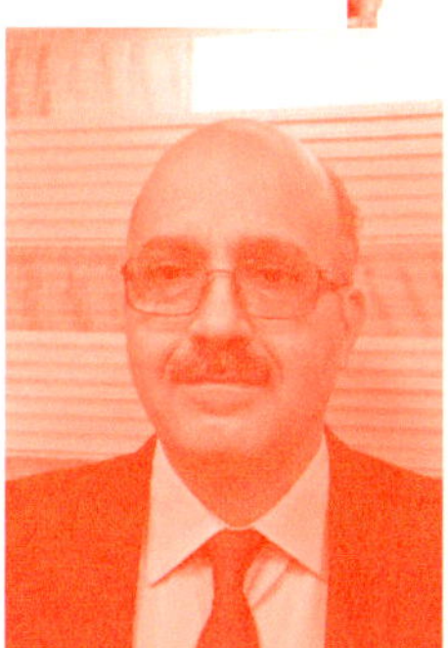
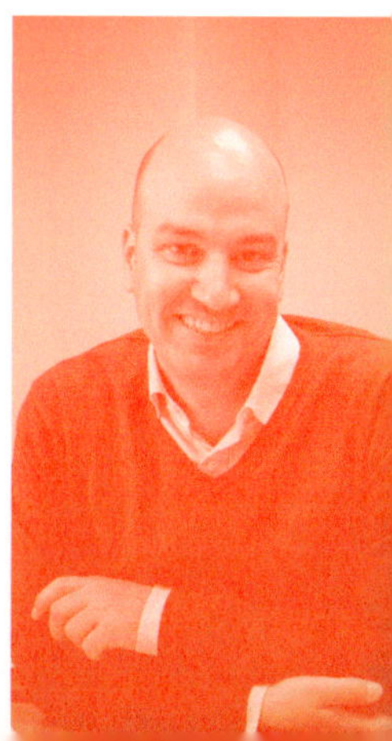
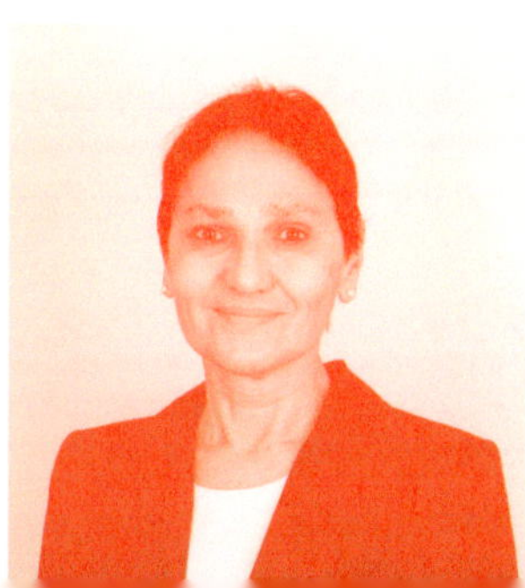

Serotonin and the CNS - New Developments in Pharmacology and Therapeutics
http://dx.doi.org/10.5772/intechopen.90962
Edited by Berend Olivier

Contributors
Anurag Kuhad, Priya Badyal, Jaspreet Kaur, Claudia Volpi, Giada Mondanelli, Vladimir M. Kovalzon, Rumen Nikolov, Kalina Koleva, Tania Vitalis, Catherine Verney, Janet Best, Michael C. Reed, Herman Frederik Nijhout, Parastoo Hashemi, Anna Marie Buchanan, Katrine M. Qvortrup, Charlotte Uldahl Jansen, Berend Olivier, Jocelien D.A. Olivier

First published in London, United Kingdom, 2022 by IntechOpen
IntechOpen is the global imprint of INTECHOPEN LIMITED, registered in England and Wales, registration number: 11086078, 5 Princes Gate Court, London, SW7 2QJ, United Kingdom
Printed in Croatia

British Library Cataloguing-in-Publication Data
A catalogue record for this book is available from the British Library

Additional hard and PDF copies can be obtained from orders@intechopen.com

Serotonin and the CNS - New Developments in Pharmacology and Therapeutics
Edited by Berend Olivier
p. cm.
Print ISBN 978-1-83969-199-7
Online ISBN 978-1-83969-200-0
eBook (PDF) ISBN 978-1-83969-201-7

For EU product safety concerns:
IN TECH d.o.o., Prolaz Marije Krucifikse Kozulić 3, 51000 Rijeka, Croatia, info@intechopen.com or visit our website at intechopen.com.

Meet the editor

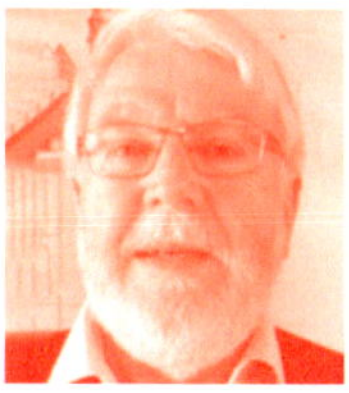

Berend Olivier obtained a Ph.D. in Neurobiology at Groningen University, Netherlands. He worked for twenty-two years at Solvay Pharmaceuticals leading research and development of antidepressants, antipsychotics, anxiolytics, and serenics. He was involved in the research and development of fluvoxamine, a marketed SSSR antidepressant, anxiolytic and anti-OCD medication. During the period from 1999 to 2001, he worked in New York to start a biotech company, PsychoGenics Inc., developing psychiatric and neurological (genetic) models to screen, find and develop new drugs. From 1992 to 2014 he was a professor of CNS Pharmacology at Utrecht University, Netherlands, performing research on animal models, brain mechanisms, and pharmacology of psychiatric disorders. Since 2014, he has been developing new animal models of male sexual disorders in the hopes of finding new medicines for premature and delayed ejaculation.

Contents

Preface

Although serotonin (5-HT) was discovered as a neurotransmitter less than 80 years ago, the successive decades have yielded a dramatic increase in our knowledge of serotonin, its receptors, enzymes, transporters and accessory proteins and its associated functions. Serotonin constitutes one of the oldest neurotransmitter systems in nature; it is estimated to have originated about 800 million years ago. This enormous time span enabled the serotonergic complex to evolve into a highly important system involved in many important biological processes in the body, particularly in the central nervous, gastro-intestinal, cardiovascular and immune systems. It is remarkable that the neurotransmitter itself has not evolved during evolution, but the molecules with which it interacts have shown an amazing diversity, variability and extent and seem to vary according to species, organ, cell, gender and disease state. The complexity of the involvement of serotonin is illustrated in the chapters contributing to this volume.

In Chapter 1 investigators from various countries and backgrounds have collaborated on mathematical modeling of neurotransmitter metabolism, focusing on 5-HT and histamine, applying various techniques and trying to connect their findings to neuropsychiatric disorders, notably depression. By eloquently combining various advanced methods and techniques they present a new serotonin model of 5-HT synthesis, release, reuptake and autoreceptor control and make an intriguing connection to neuro-inflammation as a causative factor in major depression.

Chapter 2 deals with the interconnection between serotonin, sleep and depression. The involvement of 5-HT neurotransmission in sleep and wakefulness has been known since the sixties, but many questions have not been resolved. In this chapter a new hypothesis is formulated involving 5-HT and excessive long pre-morning periods of REM-sleep, leading to a complete stop of monoamine release. It is suggested that fragmentation of this sleep phase may have antidepressant effects.

Chapter 3 describes the putative role of the serotonergic system in post-traumatic stress disorder (PTSD), a troublesome condition that is increasing in prevalence worldwide. This review shows the involvement of the serotonergic system in the regulation of sensitivity to highly stressful events and how to cope with them.

Chapter 4 deals with the use of small molecule drugs for the treatment of Alzheimer's Disease which is developed on the basis of a mechanistic understanding of the Serotonin Receptors 4 and 6.

Chapter 5 deals with serotonergic brain mechanisms of aggression and sexual behavior, focusing on 5-HT1A- and 5-HT1B-receptors, as there is evidence for (partly) overlapping in CNS circuitry for aggression and sexual behavior. As 5-HT1B-receptors seem particularly involved in aggression and 5-HT1A-receptors in sexual behavior, their precise interrelationship is not clear and far from understood. This information is badly needed to develop anti-aggressive (serenic) and pro-sexual drugs for human applications.

Chapter 6 describes new ligands for 5-HT4- and 5-HT6-receptors that might create new treatments in the modulation of cognition and amyloid pathology. The chapter nicely describes recent progress in understanding how to modulate underlying systems by medicinal chemistry methods of advanced pharmacophores. This will hopefully lead to new pharmacological approaches and drugs to treat Alzheimer's disease.

Chapter 7 discusses the role of serotonin in cerebral edema after traumatic brain injury. Traumatic brain injury leads to very complex processes where many different mechanisms play a role. Serotonin is clearly involved in early cytotoxic edema after traumatic brain injury. Maintaining low serotonin levels in the brain immediately after an injury has neuroprotective effects and may contribute to a better outcome for the patient.

Chapter 8 is a nice overview of the role of 5-HT pathways in neuro-immuno communication and their role in autoimmune and inflammatory pathology in CNS diseases, including multiple sclerosis, Alzheimer's disease and mood disorders. The chapter also outlines the important role of the 'brain-gut axis' and shows the involvement of brain-gut communication in the pathogenesis and pathophysiology of several brain disorders.

This book excellently illustrates the broadness of research and therapy in the serotonergic field. It also indicates that new developments continuously occur in a 'seemingly old' system. It is evident that we still are only at the beginning of understanding the role of serotonin in health and disease.

Dr. Berend Olivier
Professor,
Professor Emeritus Pharmacology of the Central Nervous System,
Faculty of Sciences,
Department of Psychopharmacology,
Utrecht Institute for Pharmaceutical Sciences,
Utrecht University,
Utrecht, Netherlands

Adjunct Professor,
Department of Psychiatry,
Yale University School of Medicine,
New Haven, USA

Chapter 1

Mathematical Models of Serotonin, Histamine, and Depression

Janet Best, Anna Marie Buchanan, Herman Frederik Nijhout, Parastoo Hashemi and Michael C. Reed

Abstract

The coauthors have been working together for ten years on serotonin, dopamine, and histamine and their connection to neuropsychiatric illnesses. Hashemi has pioneered many new experimental techniques for measuring serotonin and histamine in real time in the extracellular space in the brain. Best, Reed, and Nijhout have been making mathematical models of brain metabolism to help them interpret Hashemi's data. Hashemi demonstrated that brain histamine inhibits serotonin release, giving a direct mechanism by which inflammation can cause a decrease in brain serotonin and therefore depression. Many new biological phenomena have come out of their joint research including 1) there are two different reuptake mechanisms for serotonin; 2) the effect of the serotonin autoreceptors is not instantaneous and is long-lasting even when the extracellular concentrations have returned to normal; 3) that mathematical models of serotonin metabolism and histamine metabolism can explain Hashemi's experimental data; 4) that variation in serotonin autoreceptors may be one of the causes of serotonin-linked mood disorders. Here we review our work in recent years for biological audiences, medical audiences, and researchers who work on mathematical modeling of biological problems. We discuss the experimental techniques, the creation and investigation of mathematical models, and the consequences for neuropsychiatric diseases.

Keywords: serotonin, histamine, depression, mathematical model

1. Introduction

It is worthwhile to begin by reminding ourselves that the question of depression and the brain is so difficult because the brain consists of many different systems that interact with each other. First is the **electrophysiology** of the brain including the biophysics of individual neurons and the behavior of neural networks. Second is the **biochemistry** of the brain, not just cell biochemistry and the structure and function of receptors, but also the fact that many brain neurons do not do one-to-one signaling with other neurons. These neurons, like the serotonin (5-HT) neurons of the dorsal raphe nucleus (DRN) have dense projections to other brain regions in which their axons have myriad varicosities that release the transmitter when the neuron fires, thus changing the concentration of the transmitter in the extracellular space of the projection region. In a sense, these neurons project changes in biochemistry over long distances in the brain. Example are the 5-HT projections from the DRN to the striatum and the dopamine projection from the substantia nigra to the striatum. Third is the **genomics** of the brain, not just the genotypes of individuals but also how gene expression levels vary depending on electrophysiology, biochemistry, and the other systems below. Fourth is the **endocrine** system. The brain is an endocrine organ itself but is also influenced by other endocrine organs such as the ovaries and the adrenal glands. Fifth, the brain is affected by the current status of the **immune system** that affects the release of histamine from mast cells. Sixth, the brain creates **behavior** but behavior affects the endocrine and biochemical systems. And, these six systems operate on a wide range of spatial and temporal scales.

There are four additional difficulties. The brain is not fixed like a machine, but is dynamically changing on short and long time scales based on its challenges and history of challenges. Secondly, direct *in vivo* experimentation on humans is unethical, so one is left with remote sensing (imaging, drug responses, etc.) and extrapolation from animal experiments often performed on tissue slices. Third, there is an exceptional amount of individual variation. For example, it is known that gene expression levels vary by about 25% from person to person [1–3] and of course vary in time; so what does it mean to speak of "the brain?" Finally, not surprisingly, a myriad of homeostatic mechanisms (such as 5-HT_{1B} autoreceptors on 5-HT varicosities) have evolved so that the brain can keep functioning "normally", despite changing inputs, gene polymorphisms, and enormous biological variation. These mechanisms, whether gene regulatory networks or biochemical regulatory motifs, operate over limited scales and are almost always nonlinear, and this makes guessing the likely results of interventions very difficult.

In this situation where the system is complex and experimentation is difficult, mathematical modeling can provide a useful tool. A model gives voice to our assumptions about how something works. Every biological experiment is designed within the context of a conceptual model and its results cause us to confirm, reject, or alter that model. Conceptual models are always incomplete because biological systems are very complex and incompletely understood. Moreover, and as a purely practical matter, experiments tend to be guided by small conceptual models of only a very small part of a system, with the assumption (or hope) that the remaining details and context do not matter or can be adequately controlled. Mathematical models are formal statements of conceptual models. Like conceptual models, they are typically incomplete and tend to simplify some details of the system. But what they do have, which experimental systems do not, is that they are completely explicit about what is in the model, and what is not. Having a completely defined system has the virtue of allowing one to test whether the assumptions and structure of the model are sufficient to explain the observed results. The purpose of mathematical models is not just to match extant experimental or clinical data, but to provide an *in silico* platform for experimentation and investigation of system behavior. Such experiments are quick and inexpensive and so are particularly useful for testing hypotheses. Of course, to be useful, mathematical models should be based as much as possible on the underlying physiology.

Janet Best is a mathematician at Ohio State, Michael Reed is a mathematician at Duke University and H. Frederik Nijhout is a biologist at Duke. They have been working together on brain metabolism since 2008. They began by creating a large mathematical model of dopamine (DA) synthesis, storage in vesicles, catabolism, release, reuptake and control in synapses and varicosities [4] and a similar model for serotonin [5]. They used these models (and simpler ones) to study many phenomena, including passive and active stabilization of DA in the striatum [6], the role of 5-HT in the striatum [7], and the interaction of DA and 5-HT in the striatum in levodopa therapy for Parkinson's disease [8, 9]. Their papers on brain metabolism are available on the website sites.duke.edu/metabolism.

Parastoo Hashemi is an electrochemist and biomedical engineer at Imperial College London and the University of South Carolina. She was the first experimentalist to be able to measure the time course of 5-HT concentration and histamine concentration in the extracellular space of the brain *in vivo* [10]. In 2013, she contacted Best, Reed, and Nijhout and asked for help interpreting the results of her experiments, and the four us have been actively collaborating since then. All of our joint papers are available on the above website. Our collaboration always begins by active discussion of new experimental results that often change our previous understanding and therefore require changing previous models. The new models then often suggest new experiments to test new hypotheses that come from model experimentation. In this review, there will be many examples of this back and forth between experiment and modeling that we have found to be very productive. Anna Marie Buchanan is a graduate student in the Department of Chemistry and Biochemistry at the University of South Carolina.

In Section 2 we discuss the importance of homeostatic mechanisms in the brain. In Section 3 we discuss our first modeling paper with the Hashemi Lab [11]. That paper changed our understanding of 5-HT_{1b} autoreceptors and showed that the way we modeled autoreceptors in 2010 [5] was wrong. Section 4 describes our 2017 paper [12] creating a mathematical model for histamine dynamics in the brain and Section 5 discusses our 2020 paper [13] revising and expanding our original 5-HT model. In Section 6 we briefly describe the techniques for measuring 5-HT and histamine in the extracellular space and in Section 7 we describe our ideas and speculations about depression. Lastly, in Section 8 we discuss future work.

2. Homeostatic mechanisms

The extracellular space occupies a significant portion of brain volume and is extremely important. Not only is it the medium by which nutrients in the plasma are delivered to brain cells but it is all one important medium for communication between cells. Thus, it is not surprising that a variety of mechanisms have evolved to control the extracellular concentrations of neurotransmitters in different brain regions within fairly narrow limits. For example, DA is synthesized from tyrosine by tyrosine hydroxylase (TH) and TH shows substrate inhibition as does tryptophan hydroxylase (TPH) that synthesizes 5-HT from tryptophan. And, the concentration of DA in the extracellular space inhibits both synthesis and release of DA via the DA autoreceptors, a kind of end product inhibition. Similar mechanisms exist for 5-HT via the 5-HT autoreceptors. We will discuss the 5-HT autoreceptors in detail later. Our purpose here is to show what this homeostasis looks like and what the consequences are for DA.

The main determinants of the DA concentration in the extracellular space are rate of release from synapses and varicosities and rate of reuptake by the dopamine transporters (DATs). Release is dependent on the rate of synthesis via TH. **Figure 1** shows the concentration of DA in the extracellular space as a function of TH activity and DAT activity, computed by our 2009 mathematical model [4]. The normal steady state of the model is indicated by the large white dot that corresponds to 100% TH and DAT activity. The genes for TH and DAT have many common polymorphisms in the human population. The steady state extracellular DA concentration for combinations of these polymorphisms are shown by the small white circles on the surface. It's quite amazing, but all these points are on the homeostatic (approximately flat) part of the surface. Even though these polymorphisms are

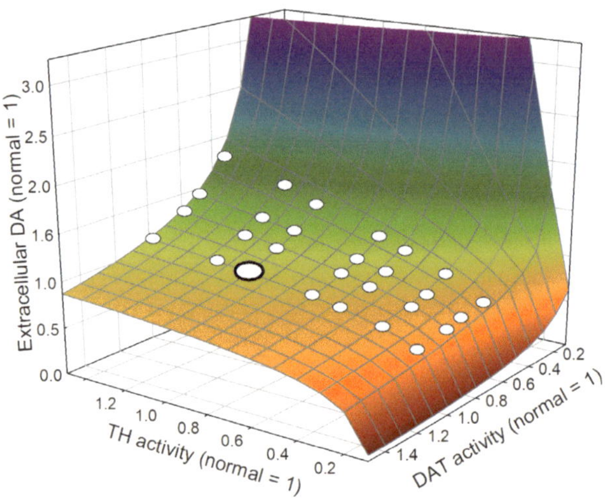

Figure 1.
Dependence of extracellular DA on TH and DAT activity. The large white dot shows the extracellular DA concentration when TH and DAT have normal activity, where, for each variable, normal is scaled to 1. The normal steady state is in the middle of a large relatively flat plateau, extracellular DA does not change much as TH and DAT activity vary. The small white dots show the steady states for different combinations of TH and DAT polymorphisms common in the human population. Though these polymorphisms are functional, in that they have large effects on activity, they do not affect extracellular DA very much. This homeostatic effect is created by the dopamine autoreceptors.

functional, that is they have big effects on the activities of TH and DAT, they do not affect the extracellular concentration of DA very much. This homeostasis is created by the above two mechanisms, substrate inhibition and the autoreceptors. From an evolutionary point of view maybe the fact that the steady states for the polymorphisms are on the flat part of the surface is not surprising. If a polymorphism pushed the steady up the blue cliff in the back (as in cocaine addiction) or off the orange cliff in the right front (as in Parkinson's disease) then that polymorphism would not likely be common in the human population. It's interesting to consider the row of polymorphism steady states nearest the orange cliff. They are on the homeostatic part of the surface, but barely. One could think of them as "predisposed" to low DA diseases. In fact, individuals with this low TH activity polymorphism often show muscle dystonia and other symptoms of low DA [14]. The surface in **Figure 1** was computed assuming variation in TH and DAT, but there are many other variables in the system, for example monoamine oxidase (MAO), and variations in those variables could change the locations of the white dots.

The point is that the existence of homeostatic mechanisms make linear arguments that assume that a large change in one variable automatically results in large changes in downstream variables both simplistic and often wrong. Therefore, it is important to investigate and understand homeostatic mechanisms in the brain and their consequences.

3. Revised understanding of serotonin dynamics

Efforts to understand the serotonergic system and in particular the clearance dynamics of serotonin date back decades, but results were limited by experimental technology. Only recently has the Hashemi Lab been able to measure serotonin concentrations in the extracellular space *in vivo*. With early fast scan cyclic voltammetry (FSCV, see Section 6) experiments, the Wightman lab was able to measure release and clearance of serotonin in electrically stimulated rat brain slices

[15]. The data were fit to a simple model for release and Michaelis–Menten reuptake of serotonin. Further experimental innovation enabled Hashemi to evoke the release of serotonin upon stimulation of the medial forebrain bundle (MFB), and measure the release and clearance *in vivo* in rat substantia nigra pars reticulata (SNr). In an early paper, average release and clearance data for five mice was fit with the Wightman model for release and reuptake [10].

Subsequent efforts in mice to elucidate the serotonergic system with its response to antidepressants and autoreceptor antagonists revealed that serotonin responses are actually heterogeneous, and that averaging the responses obscures potentially important phenomena [11]. Furthermore, some of the data could not be fit well with the Wightman model, as the K_m value appeared to change during the thirty second experiment. These data were the impetus for Hashemi to contact modelers Best, Reed, and Nijhout to suggest collaboration.

The mouse SNr data showed three distinct serotonin responses to a standard MFB stimulation, primarily differentiated by the clearance slopes, motivating our adoption of the terminology fast, slow, and hybrid. All three responses have a rapid rise. Fast responses are characterized by a rapid return to baseline, while slow responses show a more gradual, linear, return to baseline. Hybrid responses have both fast and slow attributes, descending rapidly for a short time and then switching to a slower decay. See **Figure 2**.

Our model, shown below, employs release and Michaelis–Menten clearance kinetics similar to the Wightman model. However, our model additionally incorporates a second reuptake mechanism, a basal concentration of serotonin, and autoreceptor effects. $[S(t)]$ denotes the concentration of serotonin in the SNr extracellular space. We assume that $[S(t)]$ satisfies the differential equation:

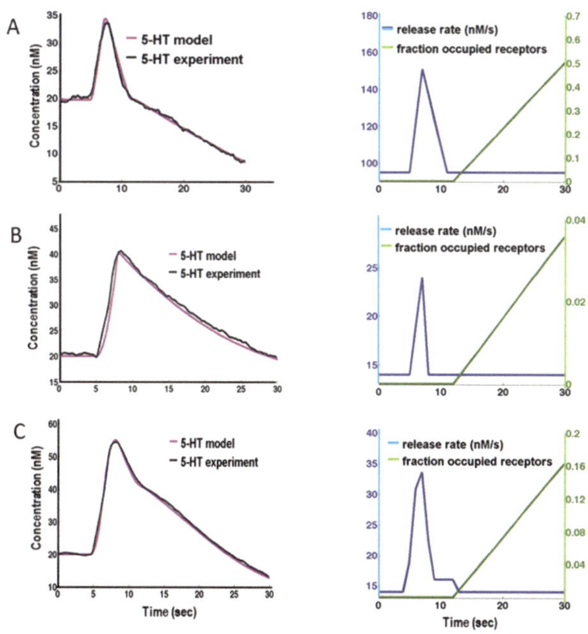

Figure 2.
Fast, slow, and hybrid responses. The three panels on the left show fast (A), slow (B), and hybrid (C) responses measured in the SNr after stimulation of the MFB [11]. The blue curves are experimental data and the red curves come from a simple mathematical model in which the auto receptor effect was changed as a function of time (green curves in the right panels). The data and the modeling provided the first in vivo evidence of two distinct reuptake mechanisms for 5-HT and also showed that autoreceptor effects are long lasting and continue after 5-HT concentrations have returned to baseline.

$$\frac{dS[(t)]}{dt} = R(t)(1 - A(t)) - \alpha \frac{V_{max1}[S(t)]}{K_{m1} + [S(t)]} - \beta \frac{V_{max2}[S(t)]}{K_{m2} + [S(t)]} \tag{1}$$

where $R(t)$ is the rate of release and $A(t)$ is the fraction of stimulated autoreceptors. $R(t)$ represents the neuronal firing in the DRN upon stimulation of the MFB and subsequent release of serotonin in the SNr. Firing rises and decays quickly (but not instantaneously) in response to the stimulation due to the non-instantaneous excitation/relaxation of the MFB-DRN-SNr circuitry. The two Michaelis–Menten reuptake mechanisms have different V_{max} and K_m values. V_{max1} and K_{m1} correspond to slow responses, while V_{max2} and K_{m2} correspond to fast responses. The constants α and β are the weights of the two reuptake mechanisms. For fast responses $\alpha = 0$ and $\beta = 1$, for slow responses $\alpha = 1$ and $\beta = 0$. For hybrid responses, α is taken as 1 at all times, while we incorporate β in a graded, concentration-dependent manner. When $[S(t)]$ is > 44 nM, β is 0.03 and then decays linearly to 0 as $[S(t)]$ decreases from 44 nM to 39 nM and $\beta = 0$ when $[S(t)]$ is < 39 nM, meaning that the reuptake associated with β is low affinity and so loses effectiveness at low concentrations. Thus hybrid responses have contributions from both reuptake mechanisms.

Figure 2 shows the model curves (magenta) superimposed onto the three experimental serotonin response types (black). We found that the following V_{max} and K_m values fit well to the experimental data: V_{max1} = 17.5 nM s^{-1}, $K_{m1} = 5$ nM and V_{max2} =780 nM s^{-1}, and $K_{m2} = 170$ nM, respectively. These values were fixed for all simulations while the choices of α, β differed as indicated above. These K_m and V_{max} values agree remarkably well with high affinity, low efficiency (Uptake 1) and low affinity, high efficiency (Uptake 2) as had been suggested by Snyder and colleagues [16]. Daws and colleagues verified pharmacologically that Uptake 1 is likely to occur primarily via serotonin transporters (SERTs) on serotonergic neurons and Uptake 2 includes other transporters on other cells including the dopamine transporter, the norepinephrine transporter, and the organic cation transporter [17, 18]. Our dataset, reviewed here, was the first endogenous, *in vivo* data to support the concept of these two distinct uptake mechanisms for serotonin. We remark that the Uptake 2 parameters that worked well for us are exactly the parameters used by Shaskan and Wightman to match their experimental data. Note that the Uptake 1 parts of the response curves are quite linear, which shows that the SERTs are saturated.

The $R(t)$ and $A(t)$ functions for each response are shown in **Figure 2**. We assume that in each case the baseline concentration of 5-HT in the extracellular space is 20 nM. For all three response types, we found that the model fit well with the autoreceptor effect increasing linearly after 12 sec and continuing through the end of the 30 sec experiment. To test our model's suggestion of autoreceptor control experimentally, we treated mice with methiothepin, a non-selective serotonin receptor antagonist with highest affinity for the serotonin autoreceptors [19]. We were able to fit the data with the hybrid model, setting the autoreceptor function $A(t)$ to zero. In our previous model [5], the autoreceptor effect was an instantaneous response to the current extracellular serotonin concentration. Modeling this data revealed that the autoreceptor response differs from our earlier model in two important ways: it is not instantaneous, and it lasts well beyond when the extracellular serotonin concentration returns to baseline; see **Figure 2**. These observations motivated us to improve our autoreceptor model, see Sections 4 and 5, although we would also learn that the autoreceptors were not solely responsible for these effects in the data. Note that in Panels A and C the concentration is well below baseline at $t = 30$ and still decreasing. We will come back to this issue in Section 5.

4. A model for histamine with new autoreceptors

Histamine is a small molecule that plays an important role in the immune system [20]. In the brain, histamine is stored in mast cells and other non-neuronal cells (containing roughly half of brain histamine [21, 22]), but it also occurs as a neurotransmitter [23]. The neuronal cell bodies are in the tuberomammillary nucleus of the hypothalamus and these neurons send projections throughout the CNS, in particular to the cerebral cortex, amygdala, basal ganglia, hippocampus, thalamus, retina, and spinal cord [20]. Histamine neurons make few synapses, but release histamine from the cell bodies and from varicosities when the neurons fire. Thus the histamine neural system modulates and controls the histamine concentration in projection regions [23].

Understanding the control of histamine in the extracellular space is important because we have shown that the release of histamine inhibits 5-HT release in the hypothalamus [24]. We stimulated the MFB and measured histamine and 5-HT simultaneously in the extracellular space of the hypothalamus *in vivo* in mice; see **Figure 3**. In Panel (a), the blue curve shows the average histamine curve in the extracellular space for 5 animals. The curve peaks shortly after the 2 second

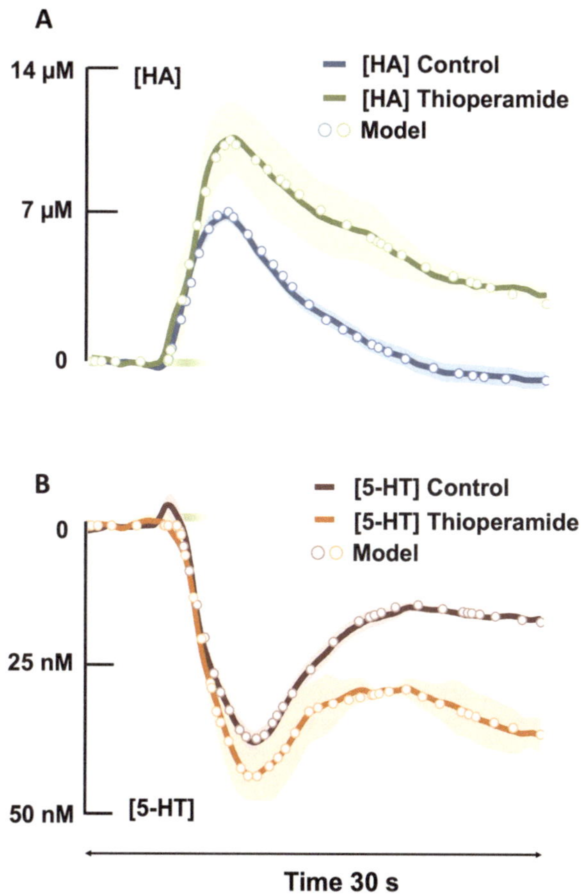

Figure 3.
Histamine inhibits 5-HT. Stimulation of the MFB releases histamine but not 5-HT in the hypothalamus. The blue curve in (A) shows extracellular histamine as a function of time and the maroon curve in (B) shows the corresponding inhibition of 5-HT release. 5-HT does not return to baseline even after histamine has returned to baseline because of the long-lasting effect of the H_3 histamine receptors on 5-HT varicosities. The green and orange curves show the histamine and 5-HT responses in the presence of thioperamide, a potent H_3 antagonist. Error bars showing SEM (n = 5 ±SEM) are lighter versions of the respective colors. Horizontal bars at 0 μM and 0 nM indicate the timing of the stimulus. Predictions of a simple mathematical model are shown by the dots.

stimulation from t = 5 sec to t = 7 sec, and then descends to slightly below baseline by t = 30 sec. Clearance of histamine from the extracellular space is likely due to its recycling via transport back into the cytosol. While such a histamine transporter has not been identified, our unpublished experimental data shows that it is hard to deplete vesicular stores, strongly suggesting that extracellular histamine must be reuptaken into the cytosol. As we will see, the descent below baseline is caused by H_3 receptors on the histamine varicosities that inhibit histamine release. Simultaneous average measurement of 5-HT in the extracellular space is shown by the maroon curve in Panel (b). As the histamine curve peaks in Panel (a), the 5-HT curve plunges in Panel (b). As the histamine recovers to baseline in Panel (a), the 5-HT curve in Panel (b) rebounds partway towards baseline and then levels off below baseline. It is known that there are histamine H_3 receptors on 5-HT neurons that inhibit 5-HT release [25, 26]. These curves show that the effect is long-lasting. In order to test these ideas, we redid the experiments in the presence of thioperamide, a potent H_3 receptor antagonist [27]. Now the histamine curve (green) in Panel (a) goes up higher and descends more slowly. The corresponding orange 5-HT curve in Panel (b) descends even further and rebounds less. Its complicated behavior probably results from two competing influences: histamine concentration is higher but thioperamide also partially blocks the H_3 receptors on the 5-HT varicosity. The white dots come from a simple mathematical model in which we adjusted the strengths of H_3 receptor effects on both of the varicosities by hand. The fact that we could match these curves by doing that provided further confirmation that the results of the experiments were due to H_3 receptors. We note that the scales in Panels (a) and (b) are very different, μM and nM.

These experiments and their interpretation provide a likely mechanism by which the neuroinflammation that occurs in a variety of disorders could cause depression. We therefore concluded that it was important to construct a full model of the synthesis, vesicular storage, release and reuptake of histamine, and control in the extracellular space by histamine autoreceptors [12]. Overall, this model is similar to the model that we constructed for serotonin [5]. In the case of both neurotransmitters, autoreceptors on the surfaces of varicosities inhibit release when the extracellular concentration is high and diminish the inhibition when the extracellular concentration is low; this is clearly a mechanism to stabilize the extracellular concentration. In our original serotonin paper [5], we modeled this inhibition to be instantaneous as a phenomenological response to the current concentration of neurotransmitter in the extracellular space. However, as described in the previous section, our FSCV data and modeling [11] showed that autoreceptor effects are long-lasting and persist even when the concentration in the extracellular space has returned to normal. This is almost certainly because the cellular machinery that creates the inhibition and the decay of that machinery take time. Therefore, in our histamine model we introduced a minimal mathematical model of signal transduction at the G-protein coupled autoreceptor consisting of a G-protein subunit and a regulator of G-protein signaling (RGS) protein.

Figure 4 shows a schematic of the model. The pink boxes indicate substrates that are variables in the model and the gray ovals contain the acronyms of enzymes and transporters. Histidine in the blood (*bHT*) is transported into the varicosity by the histidine transporter (*HTL*) where it becomes cytosolic histidine (*cHT*) or goes into the histidine pool (*HTpool*). Most of the histidine that enters the cell is used for other processes than making histamine and that is what the *HTpool* represents. *cHT* is converted to cytosolic histamine, *cHA*, by the enzyme histidine decarboxylase, *HTDC*. Some *cHA* is catabolized by the enzyme histamine methyltransferase, *HNMT*, some is transported into the vesicles by the monoamine transporter, *MAT*, and becomes vesicular histamine, *vHA*, and some leaks out of the cytosol into the

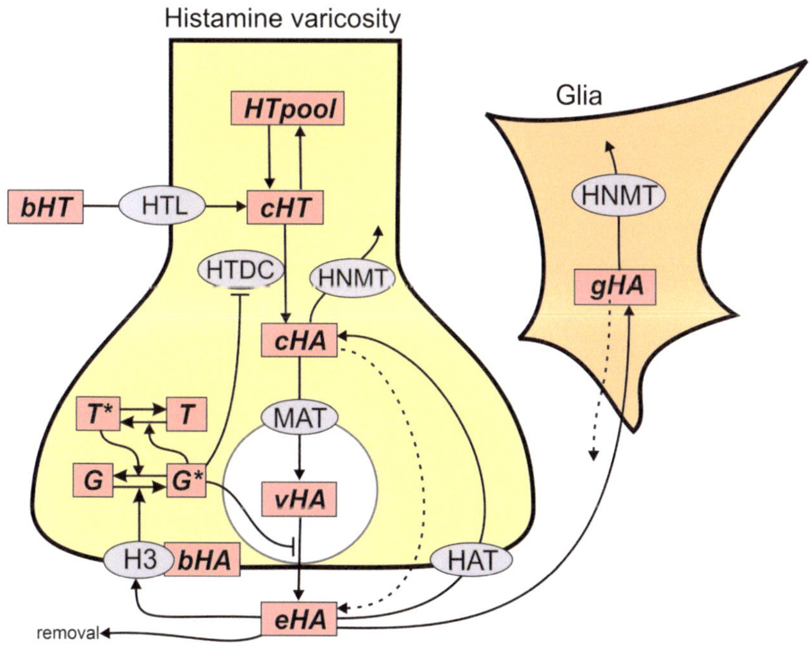

Figure 4.
Schematic of the mathematical model for histamine. bHT and cHT *represent blood histidine and cytosolic histidine, respectively.* cHA, vHA, eHT, $H_3 - bHA$, *and* gHA *represent cytosolic histamine, vesicular histamine, extracellular histamine, histamine bound to autoreceptors, and glial histamine, respectively.* G^* and G *represent activated and inactivated autoreceptor G-proteins and* T^* *and* T *represent activated and inactivated regulators of G-proteins. Names of enzymes and transporters are as follows: HTL, the histidine transporter; HTDC, histidine decarboxylase; HNMT, histamine methyltransferase; HAT, the putative histamine transporter;* H_3*, histamine autoreceptor; HTpool, the histidine pool.*

extracellular space (indicated by the dashed line). vHA is released into the extracellular space, at a rate proportional to neuronal firing, where it becomes extracellular histamine, eHA. In the extracellular space, eHA has several fates. It can be transported back into the cytosol by a putative histamine transporter, HAT. It can diffuse away (removal). It can be transported into glial cells where it becomes glial histamine, gHA, which then leaks out or is catabolized by $HNMT$. Finally, eHA can bind to the H_3 histamine autoreceptor. The concentration of histamine bound to the autoreceptor, bHA, stimulates the conversion of the G-protein subunit, G, to its activated state, G^*. And, G^* stimulates the conversion of the RGS protein, T, to its activated state, T^*, in which it facilitates the conversion of G^* back to G. It is the activated G-protein subunit, G^*, that inhibits release and synthesis of histamine. We remark that we only track T^* and G^* since total G-protein, $G + G^*$, is assumed constant, as is $T + T^*$.

The H_3 histamine receptor (the autoreceptor in this case) is in the rhodopsin family of G-protein coupled receptors [28]. The binding of an extracellular histamine molecule to the autoreceptor causes the release of a G-protein subunit that stimulates a signaling cascade that results in inhibition of release and synthesis. Most G-protein signals are limited by RGS molecules that stimulate the G-protein subunit to rebind [29]. In our minimal model, G represents $G_\alpha - GDP$ (the inactive G-protein subunit) and G^* represents $G_\alpha - GTP$ (the signaling G-protein unit). Similarly, T represents the inactive RGS protein and T^* represents the active RGS protein.

In our model, b_0 is the total concentration of autoreceptors and bHA is the concentration of receptors bound to eHA. Normally, G and G^* are in equilibrium and their sum is constant (g_0). The concentration of bound autoreceptors (bHA)

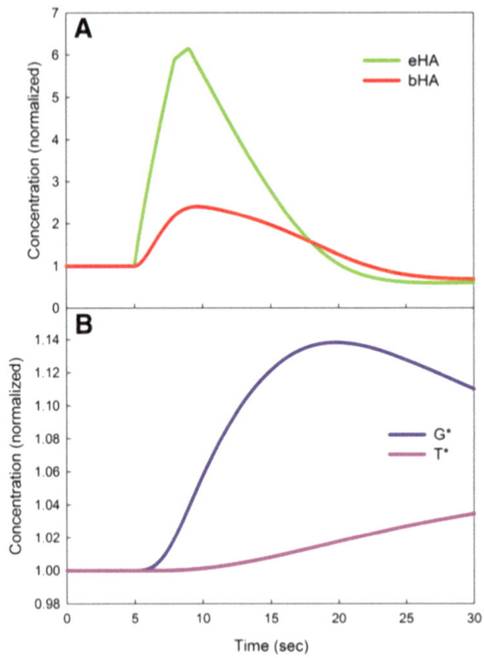

Figure 5.
Autoreceptor variable dynamics in the model after stimulation. Release of histamine causes extracellular histamine to rise and then descend as histamine is transported back into the cytosol and into glial cells (green curve in A). The rise in eHA causes the concentration of bound autoreceptors to rise (red curve in Panel A). The rise in bHA causes activation of G-proteins that inhibit release and synthesis of histamine (blue curve in Panel B). The rise in G^* activates the G-protein regulator, T^* *(pink curve in Panel B) and* T^* *starts to deactivate* G^*. *It is this dynamics that causes the* H_3 *receptor effect to be long-lasting.*

drives the equilibrium towards G^*. Similarly, T and T^* are at equilibrium and their sum is a constant (t_0). G^* drives the equilibrium towards T^*. T^*, in turn, drives the equilibrium between G and G^* back towards G. The concentration of G^* affects the release of histamine from the vesicular compartment through the function $inhib(G^*) = 2.4015 - (2.45)G^*$, and this same function appears in the formula for the velocity of the synthesis reaction (HTDC). Since $G^* = .6945$ at equilibrium, tonically the inhibition is 0.7. As $G^*(t)$ rises the inhibition gets stronger and if $G^*(t)$ decreases the inhibition becomes weaker.

The shape of the model prediction for eHA reflects the dynamics of bHA, G^*, and T^*. These curves are depicted in **Figure 5** along with the graph of eHA. As one can see, eHA goes up first, followed by an increase in bHA, the concentration of bound autoreceptors. This causes a rise in G^* that in turn causes a rise in T^* that makes G^* start to decline. The inhibition of release given by the function $inhib(G^*)$ depends on G^* as described above. This is the long-lasting autoreceptor effect. The dynamics of G^* and T^* plays out over the full 30 seconds and drives the eHA concentration below baseline. This autoreceptor model will be used for H_3 receptors on serotonin varicosities in Section 5. Full details of this histamine model can be found in [12].

5. The new serotonin model

In 2010, three of the authors (JB, HFN, MCR) created a mathematical model of serotonin synthesis in varicosities, storage in vesicles, release into the extracellular space, reuptake by serotonin transporters (SERTs), and control by serotonin autoreceptors [5]. In subsequent years, they used the model to study and evaluate various hypotheses about serotonergic function including connections with dopaminergic signaling [8, 30], bursts in the DRN [31], the effects of serotonin on levodopa therapy [9], and serotonin dynamics in the basal ganglia [7]. In 2013, they began the collaboration with Parastoo Hashemi, which led to new insights into serotonergic function [11, 24, 32]. As discussed in Section 3, the experimental results in [11] and later papers revealed that various aspects of the 2010 model were naive and too simplistic. So, in 2020, the authors and collaborators expanded and revised the original model to take account of the new findings that we had learned [13]. Here we will briefly discuss the changes and some of the new results. A schematic diagram of the new model is in **Figure 6**.

In the experiments in the Hashemi Lab, the MFB is stimulated for 2 seconds and the antidromic spikes excite the DRN. The DRN sends bursts of action potentials to projection regions such as the SNr, the pre-frontal cortex (PFC), and the hippocampus. Serotonin rises rapidly in the extracellular space in the projection regions and then typically plunges substantially below basal levels within 30 seconds [11, 13, 33–35]. This almost certainly is because inhibition of release by the autoreceptors continues well after the serotonin concentration in the extracellular space has returned to basal levels. In our 2010 model, extracellular serotonin instantaneously affected release, and the Hashemi experiments showed that this is wrong. Therefore, in our new model [13] we include a biochemical model of the

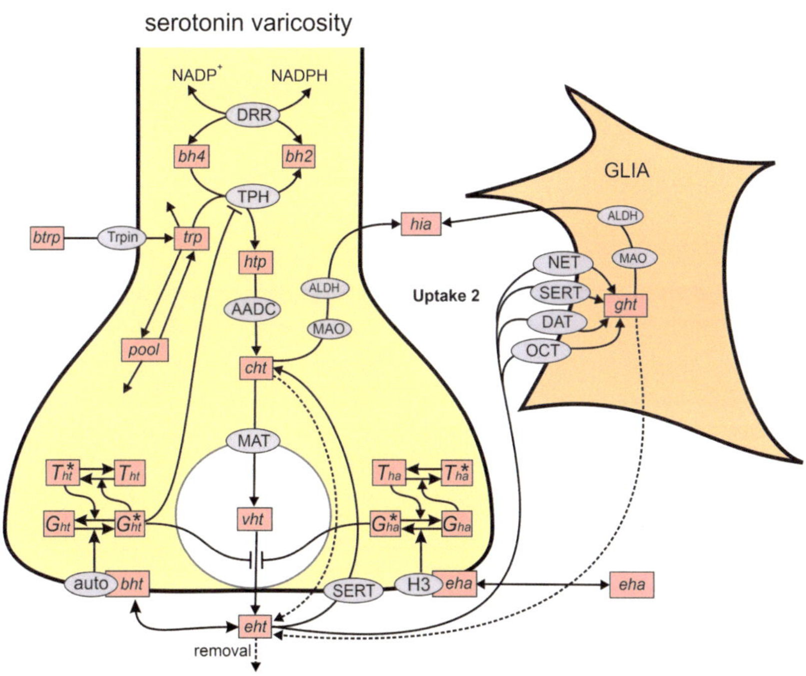

Figure 6.
Schematic diagram of the model. The rectangular boxes indicate substrates and blue ellipses contain the acronyms of enzymes or transporters. The names of the most important substrates are: Btrp, blood tryptophan; trp, cytosolic tryptophan; htp, 5-hydroxytryptamine; cht, cytosolic serotonin; vht, vesicular serotonin; eht, extracellular serotonin; hia, 5-hydroxyindoleacetic acid; ght, glial serotonin; eha, extracellular histamine. Names of enzymes and transporters are as follows: Trpin, neutral amino acid transporter; DRR, dihydrobiopterin reductase; TPH, tryptophan hydroxylase; AADC, aromatic amino acid decarboxylase; MAT, vesicular monoamine transporter; SERT, 5-HT reuptake transporter; auto, 5-HT$_{1B}$ autoreceptors; MAO monoamine oxidase; ALDH, aldehyde dehydrogenase; NET, norepinephrine transporter; DAT, dopamine transporter; OCT, organic cation transporter. Removal means uptake by capillaries or diffusion out of the system.

cellular dynamics caused by serotonin binding to the autoreceptor, including activated receptor G-proteins and activated regulators of G-proteins. This autoreceptor model is similar to the histamine autoreceptor model discussed in Section 4. In addition, we showed in [24, 36] that histamine in the extracellular space inhibits the release of serotonin from serotonin varicosities. Therefore, in the new model, we also include a biochemical model of a histamine H_3 receptor on the serotonin varicosity that changes the dynamics of serotonin release. Both of these biochemical models for receptors are indicated schematically in **Figure 6**. As described in Section 3, in [11] we also showed that there are two different serotonin uptake mechanisms, SERTs that pump serotonin back into the varicosities and another uptake, which we call Uptake 2, that pumps serotonin into glial cells [16, 18, 37]. The kinetics of the two uptakes are quite different and both are included in our new model. We also include the effects of serotonin binding protein (SBP) that binds serotonin tightly in vesicles but releases it quickly when the vesicles open to the extracellular space. We also include leakage of 5-HT from the cytosol of neurons and glial cells into the extracellular space (dashed lines). All details of these changes and the full mathematical model can be found in [13]. We discuss below our new model for release from the vesicles. We also made a systems population model from our deterministic model and will show below how we used it to investigate certain aspects of the serotonin system.

In our model there is a constant basal rate of serotonin release at steady state. The question is how should we model release during the Hashemi Lab experiments where the MFB is stimulated for two seconds? In our previous work using the 2010 model we simply increased the firing rate for the two seconds of stimulation and then dropped it back to the basal rate. This issue is complicated by the existence of serotonin binding protein (SBP) that is attached to the inner wall of vesicles and binds serotonin tightly [38, 39]. We will assume that the dissociation is a first order reaction

$$SBP - serotonin \xrightarrow{b} SBP + serotonin. \tag{2}$$

If we start with one unit (nM) of SBP-serotonin being released into the extracellular space at time zero, then $SBP(t) = e^{-bt}$ and $serotonin(t) = 1 - e^{-bt}$. The rate of release of serotonin is the derivative, be^{-bt}. However, we are stimulating for two seconds, so SBP-serotonin complexes are continuously released into the extracellular space between $t = 0$ and $t = 2$ seconds. Assume that the rate of release is 1 nM/sec, so in two seconds, 2 nM of the complex are released. What is the rate of appearance, $R(t)$, of free serotonin for $t \leq 2$ and $t > 2$?

$$R(t) = \int_0^t \chi_{[s,2]} be^{-b(t-s)} ds \quad \text{for} \quad t \leq 2, \tag{3}$$

and

$$R(t) = \int_0^2 \chi_{[s,2]} be^{-b(t-s)} ds \quad \text{for} \quad t > 2. \tag{4}$$

Here $\chi_{[s,2]}$ is the function that is 1 on the interval $[s, 2]$ and zero otherwise. A straightforward calculation shows that:

$$R(t) = \begin{cases} 1 - e^{-bt} & \text{if t} \leq 2, \\ e^{-b(t-2)} - e^{-bt} & \text{if t} > 2. \end{cases} \tag{5}$$

Thus, for a two second stimulation, the rate of release will be proportional to $fire(t) = \text{basal rate} + r \cdot R(t)$ where r is the strength of the stimulation. Unfortunately, the dissociation constant b (inverse seconds) is not known, but we think it is in the range $0.5 \leq b \leq 2$ from our simulations of the Hashemi data, so we take $b = 1$ as our baseline case. The release of serotonin into the extracellular space will also be proportional to vht and it will also depend on the inhibition from the serotonin autoreceptors and the histamine H_3 receptor. Thus, overall release as a function of time will be

$$inhib_{ht}\left(G_{ht}^{*}\right) \cdot inhib_{ha}\left(G_{ha}^{*}\right) \cdot (\text{basal rate} + r \cdot R(t)) \cdot vht. \qquad (6)$$

One of the first things that we did with our new model was to return to the 2014 data [11] that we discussed in Section 3 to see if our new serotonin model could easily match the average curves of fast, slow, and hybrid in the SNr, with relatively few, understandable changes of parameters. The experimental curves for fast, slow, and hybrid (**Figure 2**) do not look like typical response curves measured in the Hashemi Lab. For example, **Figure** 7 shows an average of 17 male responses in the CA2 region of the hippocampus. Typical response curves peak, descend towards baseline, drop below baseline, and then curve back towards baseline, whereas the experimental curves in **Figure 2** keep descending. In thinking about this, we remembered that when the MFB is stimulated not only is 5-HT released in the SNr but histamine is also released. So we were in a good position to see if our new serotonin model, with its H_3 receptor, would allow us to match the 2014 SNr data. Unfortunately, we do not have the time course of histamine in the SNr in those experiments, because in 2014 the Hashemi Lab had not yet optimized the techniques to simultaneously measure 5-HT and histamine *in vivo* [24, 36]. So we will take our histamine time course in the extracellular space, *eha*, from the control and model curves in **Figure 5** of [12]. Note how complicated the dynamics of *eht* are. When one stimulates the MFB, serotonin is released into the extracellular space stimulating dynamical changes in the 5-HT_{1B} autoreceptor variables, B_{ht}, G_{ht}^{*}, T_{ht}^{*}. However, histamine also increases in the extracellular space stimulating dynamical changes in the H_3 receptor variables, B_{ha}, G_{ha}^{*}, T_{ha}^{*}. Both of the activated G-proteins, G_{ht}^{*} and G_{ha}^{*} inhibit serotonin release via the functions $inhib\left(G_{ht}^{*}\right)$ and $inhib_{ha}\left(G_{ht}^{*}\right)$.

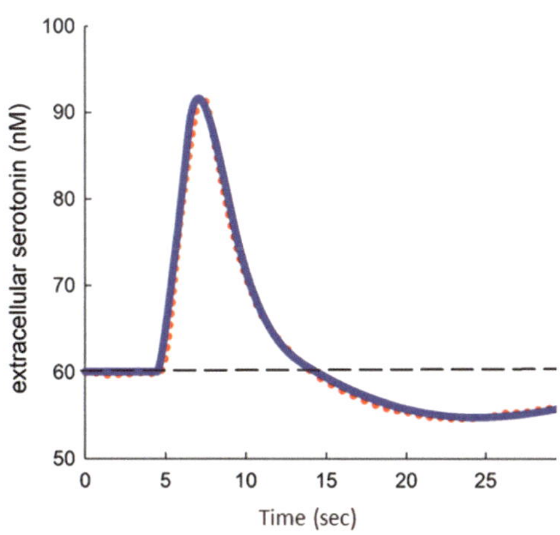

Figure 7.
Typical 5-HT response curves. The red dots show the average response of 23 male mice in the CA2 after stimulation of the MFB. The blue curve shows the average response predicted by the new 5-HT model. 5-HT rises rapidly and then descends rapidly as it is taken up by SERTs and Uptake 2. The concentration descend below baseline and then curve back towards baseline. This is the long-lasting autoreceptor effect. The average curve is simple and easy to interpret, but the individual curves show great variation; see ***Figure 8****.*

Furthermore, Uptake 2 is rapid but it probably also depends on the distance of glial cells from the electrodes in the three cases. Nevertheless, it was surprisingly easy to give adjustments for a small number of parameters that distinguish between fast, slow, and hybrid responses (see Figure 5 and Table 5 in [13]). The parameters that we had to change were the V_{max} of Uptake 2, the cutoff for Uptake 2, the strength of the inhibition by the 5-HT_{1B} and H_3 receptors, and the strength of firing during stimulation (r). It is completely reasonable that these parameters would be different for different electrode placements and different densities of receptors on the neuron. No other parameters were changed.

The model we have been discussing is a differential equations model (ODE); there is one differential equation for each of the pink boxed variables in **Figure 6**. All individuals, whether mouse or human, are different, and the variation is important for understanding experimental results and for precision medicine. We investigate this biological variation by creating a systems population model of the deterministic model given above. It is known that the expression levels of most enzymes can vary by about 25% or more between individuals [1–3]. Therefore, to create a systems population model, we choose new V_{max} values for each (or a subset) of the enzymes and transporters in **Figure 6** by selecting independently from a uniform distribution between 75% and 125% of the normal value. We then run the model to steady state and record all the concentrations and velocities. That is one virtual person (or mouse). If we do this 1000 times, we obtain a database of virtual individuals that we can analyze using the usual statistical tools. The difference is that all of these individuals have the same set of differential equations; only the coefficients are different. So we can experiment with the model to find the mechanistic reasons for particular statistical phenomena. We will give several examples that show why this approach is useful.

The steady state of *eht* in the ODE model is 60 nM; this should be thought of as the steady state for an average mouse (or an "average" person). We allowed the V_{max} values of TRPin, TPH, AADC, MAT, MAO, Uptake 2, and SERT to vary by 25% above and below their normal values independently. In addition, we allowed $fire(t)$ to vary 25% above and below its normal value and we vary the strength of the 5-HT_{1B} autoreceptors similarly. Distributions of *eht* in various cases are shown in **Figure 9**. The green bars in Panel B show the distribution of *eht* values with normal tryptophan in the blood. The green bars are similar to distributions measured in the Hashemi Lab. The whole distribution moves left (the yellow bars in Panel B) if blood tryptophan is lowered from its normal values of 96μM to 50μM. In Panel A, we show what the distribution of *eht* would look like with no autoreceptors (orange bars) or autoreceptors that are twice strong. Thus, the systems population model allows one to see the effects of changes on a whole population, not just on an individual. Further, if the underlying ODE model is a good representation of the real physiology, then the variation in the population model should correspond to what is seen in the Lab. This gives another way of testing the validity of the underlying ODE model.

In [13] we used the ODE model to fit the average response curves for male and female mice in the hippocampus. Here we want to discuss the variation in the response curves. Panel A of **Figure 8** shows the responses of the 17 male mice. The experimental responses are measured and graphed for each mouse relative to the baseline level of *eht* that is represented in Panel A by $eht = 0$. One can see how large the variation is. The curves peak at different times and at different heights. Most, but not all, of the curves descend below baseline and their shapes are quite different; some continue descending while others reach a minimum and then rebound towards zero. The thick red curve is the mean and the thick black curve is the standard deviation, which is substantial even between 15 seconds and 30 seconds although the stimulation was only between t = 5 sec and t = 7 sec.

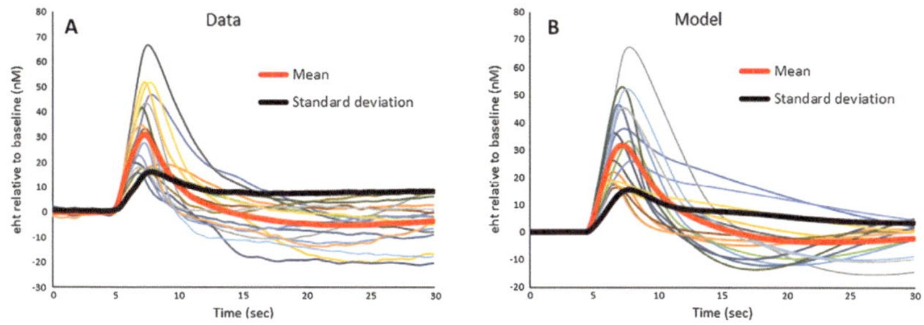

Figure 8.
Individual response curves. Panel A shows the time courses of eht in the hippocampus of 17 male mice after two seconds of stimulation at t = 5 seconds (Hashemi lab). The thick red and black curves are the time courses of the mean and standard deviation, respectively. The response curve are diverse and have different heights, peaks and shapes. Panel B shows 17 randomly selected response curves in a systems population model of 1000 individuals. The red and black curves are the time courses of the mean and the standard deviation of the 1000 model individuals, respectively. In both the experiments and the model, most (but not all) curves descend below baseline after peaking and then curve up towards the baseline. The mean curves and standard deviation curves are similar in the experiments and in the system population model.

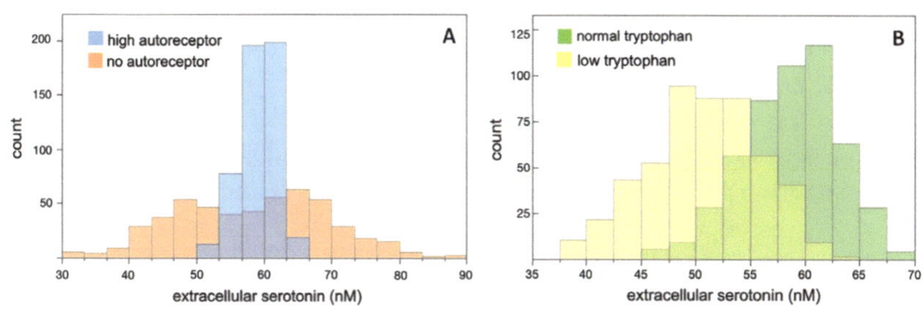

Figure 9.
Distributions of extracellular serotonin. Panel A shows the distribution of eht if there is no autoreceptor effect (pink bars) or if the autoreceptor effect is twice as strong as normal (blue bars). The green bars in panel B show the distribution of eht if the autoreceptor effect is "normal". The green bars are similar to distributions measured in the Hashemi lab. The yellow bars in panel B show the distribution of eht if blood tryptophan is lowered from its normal value of 96μM to 50μM. the distribution of eht moves substantially lower.

We investigated what variation in the main parameters of the model would be necessary to obtain the variation seen in the experiments. To do this we created a virtual population of 1000 individuals. The following parameters were varied uniformly from 40% below to 40% above their normal values: the V_{max} values for V_{AADC}, V_{CATAB}, V_{MAT}, V_{SERT}, V_{TPH}, V_{U2}; the slope of *inhib* and *inhibsyn*; *eha*, the concentration of histamine in the extracellular space, and β that controls the speed of the autoreceptors. In addition, we varied the parameter r in $fire(t)$ by 25% and the time of the peak by 20%. Panel B of **Figure 8** shows a random sample of 17 of the 1000 model male curves. The thick red curve is the mean of the 1000 model curves and the thick black curve is the standard deviation. The mean curve matches the experimental mean curve very well. The model standard deviation curve is very close to the experimental standard deviation except that at long times (20 second to 30 seconds) it descends slightly while the experimental standard deviation remains constant. Overall, one can see visually that the 17 model curves and the 17 experimental curves look similar as groups of curves. For each of the 1000 individuals, we record their steady state values as well as the values of all of their parameters so we can use multi-linear regression to find which parameters contributed most to the variation in the response curves. At $t = 7\,sec$ (roughly the time of the peak), the three variables that contributed most, in order, were the strength of fire(t), the timing of the peak in fire(t), and the V_{max} of the SERTs. At $t = 15\,sec$ (when most of

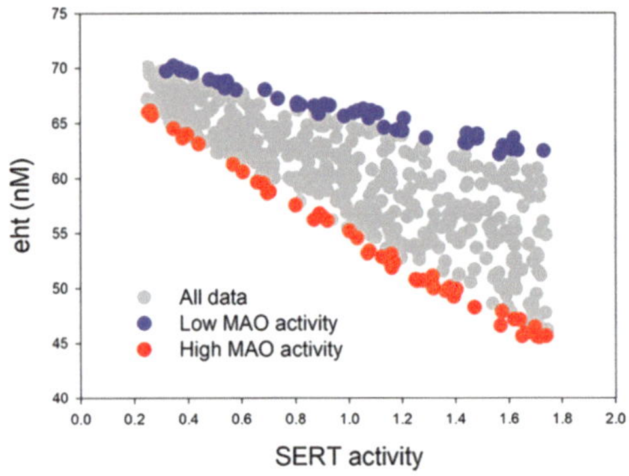

Figure 10.
Variation of SERT and MAO activity. In the population model, we varied only SERT activity and MAO activity. Each dot is one virtual individual, and the coordinates of each point are the activity of SERT (normal = 1) and the steady state concentration of eHT. The blue dots are individuals that have very low MAO activity and the red dots have very high MAO activity. Blocking the SERTs (changing the activity) has a much greater effect on high MAO activity individuals than on low MAO activity individuals.

the curves have returned to near baseline), the three parameters that contributed most to the variation in response were the V_{max} of TPH, the speed of the autoreceptors, and the V_{max} of MAT.

The population model allows us to approach a quite difficult mathematical question that would be very useful for understanding the biology and possible treatments. Suppose one has two populations of mice, for example male and female or obese and not obese or depressed and not depressed. Each of the two populations will produce a large family of experimental responses and those families of curves may be quite different. How can one estimate which parameters in the model cause the difference in the families? This is a way of using the response *eht* curves to probe the differences inside the neurons.

The expression levels of most enzymes can vary by about 25% or more between individuals [1–3]. This means that the V_{max} values of all the enzymes and transporters in our model vary by at least 25% and that any population of individuals will express this diversity. This poses large issues for drug discovery and treatment because it means that different individuals will react very differently to drugs, as is well-known [40–42]. Here, we present a simple example that shows how to use variation in a small number of variables to investigate questions about drug efficacy. In **Figure 10** we show results from our systems population model where we varied only two constants, the expression level (V_{max}) of SERT and the expression level of MAO, from 25–175% of normal. Each dot is an individual in a population of 500. The y-axis is the concentration of *eht*, extracellular serotonin, and the x-axis is the expression level of SERT. The blue dots are the individuals with low MAO activity and the red dots are individuals with high MAO activity. The conclusion is clear. Blocking SERTs with an SSRI (equivalent to lowering the expression level) will have a much greater effect on individuals with high MAO activity than on individuals with low MAO activity. Therefore, the systems population model suggests that it is high MAO individuals that will benefit the most from an SSRI. This shows how population models can be used to target specific questions.

6. Real-time *in vivo* neurotransmitter measurement techniques

To better answer physiological questions of the brain, especially about mental illness, it is critical to measure brain chemistry, specifically neurotransmitters.

Measuring neurochemistry is very challenging because neurotransmission is dynamic, and the brain tissue is very delicate. The earliest brain analysis methods utilized brain biopsies that were homogenized, separated and analyzed via HPLC [43]. These methods are offline and give an overview of whole tissue content, but not dynamic transmission. Microdialysis revolutionized brain analysis by utilizing a probe implanted into the brain, perfused with artificial cerebrospinal fluid [44, 45]. At the distal end of the probe is a semi-permeable membrane with a cut-off point such that analytes of interest can diffuse into the probe down a concentration gradient. The outcoming fluid, the dialysate, is collected and analyzed with a secondary method such as HPLC. The time resolution of this method is typically tens of minutes. Niche, electrochemical methods, such as fast scan cyclic voltammetry (FSCV) and fast scan-controlled adsorption voltammetry (FSCAV) can measure the subsecond temporal profile neurotransmission [33, 46, 47], outlined below.

6.1 Fast-scan cyclic voltammetry

Fast-Scan cyclic voltammetry is uniquely suited to measure neurotransmission *in vivo*. Its fast temporal dynamics allows for neurochemical detection on a subsecond timescale, approximately a thousand times faster than traditional cyclic voltammetry. Furthermore, FSCV measurements are performed at microelectrodes, typically carbon fiber microelectrodes (CFMEs). CFMEs have a small probe size (diameter 7 μm) and are biocompatible, creating minimal tissue damage and negligible immune response [48, 49]. Carbon electrodes also drive high sensitivity because their highly negative surface preconcentrates positively charged transmitters such as dopamine, serotonin, norepinephrine and histamine. These transmitters are then readily oxidized at the carbon surface, making it an ideal material for neurochemical measurements. Traditionally, FSCV has been utilized to measure dopamine [50–52]. However recent advances have allowed for the detection of other neurotransmitters, such as serotonin and histamine [24, 36, 53, 54].

Serotonin is measured using a CFME that has been modified by electropolymerization of a thin, uniform layer of Nafion. Nafion, a cation exchange polymer, increases the electrode sensitivity to serotonin while reducing the electrode poisoning effects of serotonin metabolites [54]. For *in vivo* experiments, this electrode is placed in the brain region of interest, such as the hippocampus, prefrontal cortex, or SNr. Because FSCV is a background subtracted technique, serotonin is evoked using an electrical stimulation placed in the MFB. Detection occurs by application of a waveform optimized for serotonin measurements. [12] This waveform has a resting potential of 0.2 V, scans up to 1.0 V, down to -0.1 V, and then back to the resting potential of 0.2 V at a scan rate of 1000 Vs^{-1}, applied at a frequency of 10 Hz. The signal is presented in the form of cyclic voltammograms (CVs) that qualify and quantify the substrate. **Figure 11** illustrates the FSCV experiment.

Histamine is particularly difficult to detect *in vivo* using FSCV because it lacks a clear, sharp oxidation peak. The Hashemi Lab developed a waveform that produces a unique electrochemical histamine signal. It has a resting potential of -0.5 V, scans to -0.7 V, up to 1.1 V, and then returns to the resting potential of -0.5 V at a scan rate of 600 Vs^{-1}. This waveform simultaneously detects serotonin and histamine release *in vivo* [24, 36].

6.2 Fast-scan controlled adsorption voltammetry

One limitation of FSCV is that because of the large capacitive current generated by the fast scan rate, it is a background subtracted technique [55]. This means that a

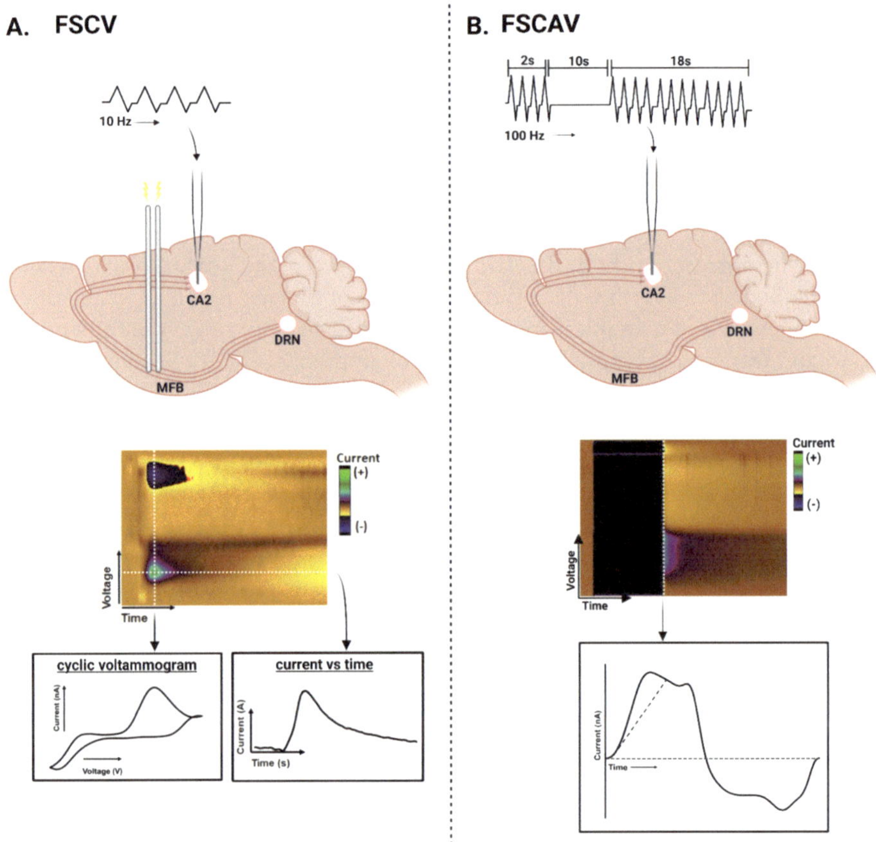

Figure 11.
Illustrative representation of an FSCV vs. FSCAV experiment described in-text. A. Shows the stimulation of the MFB to induce the release of serotonin in the CA2 and application of the serotonin waveform [53] to detect the evoked change in serotonin concentrations in the extracellular space over time. B. Depicts the modified waveform application for serotonin FSCAV [33] that negates the need for electrical stimulation to detect ambient concentrations of serotonin in the extracellular space each minute. This figure was created with Biorender.com.

change must be evoked, often electrically or pharmacologically. To address this issue, Atcherly et al. developed the method of fast-scan controlled adsorption voltammetry (FSCAV) to measure ambient concentrations of dopamine [56, 57]. This technique, illustrated in **Figure 11B**, was later adapted to measure serotonin [33]. FSCAV occurs at the same microelectrodes as FSCV. Serotonin FSCAV is performed in three steps: 1) The minimized adsorption step is implemented by applying the waveform at 100 Hz for 2 seconds. 2) The potential is held at +0.2 V for 10 sec for a period of controlled adsorption. 3) The waveform is reapplied at 100 Hz for 18 seconds. The CVs taken in the 3rd step are subtracted from the 1st step and thus serve as the ambient measurement.

7. The chemical basis of neuroinflammation

The vast majority of mental illnesses are associated with inflammation, especially depression which is highly comorbid with inflammation [58]. Increased levels of proinflammatory cytokines in the interleukin-1 and tumor necrosis factor families are linked to neuroinflammation [59, 60] across many different brain disorders. Chronic neuroinflammatory states have been implicated in neurodegenerative disorders such as Parkinson's Disease [61, 62], Alzheimer's Disease [63–65], and multiple sclerosis [66, 67], in addition to depression [58, 68] and bipolar disorder [69]. While these associations are clear, what is not known is the mechanism by which inflammation affects neurotransmission. We began to address this question by focusing on serotonin with FSCV and FSCAV. Serotonin is implicated in depression because the vast majority of antidepressants target the serotonin system [70]. Serotonin was first measured *in vivo* using FSCV in 1995 by Jackson et al. [53]. The authors detected serotonin in the rat striatum by forcing dopaminergic terminals to release serotonin following loading with 5-Hydroxytryptophan and dopamine depletion with α-methyl-p-tyrosine. More recently, using the same waveform we measured endogenous electrically evoked serotonin in the rat SNr [54]. Studies have since expanded to characterizing serotonin in different brain regions, studying differences in male and female mice, looking at serotonin and histamine co-modulation and observing the effects of inflammation on this co-modulation. We discuss our key findings below.

7.1 Serotonin dynamics in different brain regions

We first characterized evoked serotonin release and reuptake in the rat SNr following electrical MFB stimulation [54]. The SNr is of interest for serotonin detection as this area has the most dense serotonergic innervation in the brain and thus serotonin is the primary neurotransmitter released following electrical stimulation [71]. The signals obtained *in vivo* were pharmacologically verified using acute administration of the DAT inhibitor, GBR 12909, and the SSRI citalopram. The signals did not respond to DAT inhibition; however, following SERT inhibition, an increase in max amplitude and a slowing of the reuptake was observed. Serotonin response to varying doses of acute SSRI (1 mg kg^{-1}, 10 mg kg^{-1}, and 100 mg kg^{-1}) was examined [72], with uptake $t_{1/2}$ values increasing with dose concentration. However, no dose dependent trend was observed for max amplitude values. Further investigations of serotonin reuptake mechanisms [11] were performed by mathematical modeling through the development of a Michaelis–Menten kinetic model as previously described in Section 3. The presented model establishes a two uptake mechanism for serotonin, a notion that was described back in the 70s as Uptake 1 and 2 [16]. Uptake 1 refers to the high affinity, low efficiency system characterized by the serotonin transporters (SERTs) and Uptake 2 is serotonin clearance by the low affinity, high efficiency mechanism afforded by the dopamine, norepinephrine, organic cation, and plasma membrane transporters [16, 73].

While FSCV continues to provide insight into fast serotonin release and reuptake dynamics, it is limited by its inability to measure steady-state or ambient concentrations. To address this limitation, FSCAV was developed to detect absolute concentrations of both dopamine [57] and serotonin [33] *in vivo*. This technique (described above) yields fast, selective, and sensitive absolute concentrations of serotonin. Using FSCAV we reported serotonin concentrations of 64.9 ± 2.3 nM in the CA2 [33]. **Figure 12** shows ambient serotonin response to the monoamine oxidase B inhibitor, pargyline, in comparison to the DAT inhibitor, GBR 12909. Ambient serotonin levels increase following pargyline administration, but not following GBR administration, confirming that the signal is serotonin.

We expanded FSCV measurements of serotonin to the medial prefrontal cortex (mPFC) [32], another region associated with depression. Here, we found an interesting phenomenon whereby a double peak response was elicited in layers 1–3 of the mPFC. **Figure 13** shows examples of a single peak response as well as a variety of double peak responses in this brain region. Interestingly, each discrete peak had its own specific reuptake profile, thus we hypothesized that distinct axonal bundles in

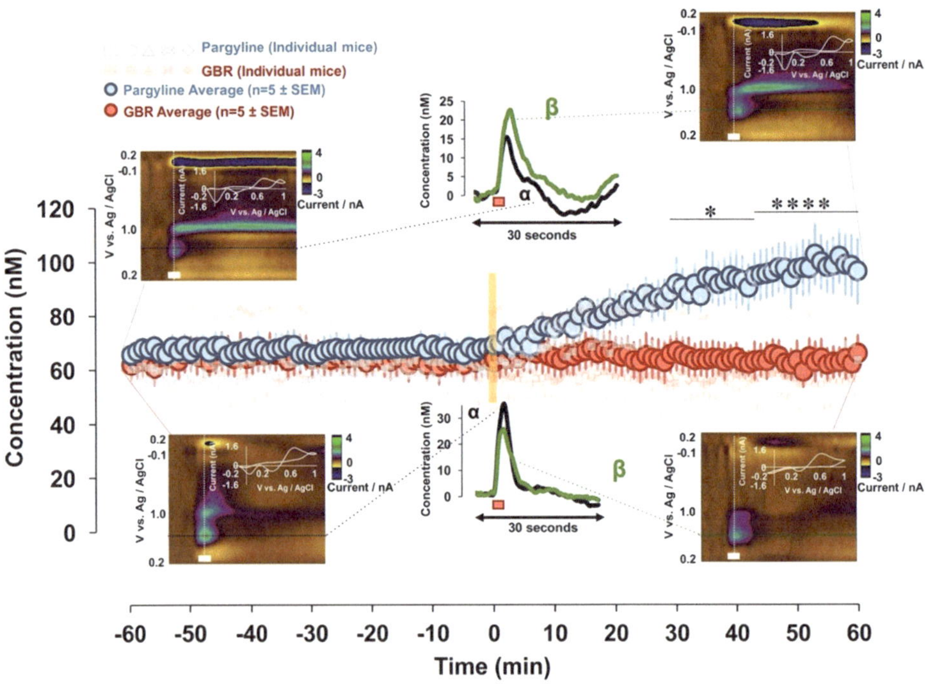

Figure 12.
*The dark blue markers represent the average response before and after pargyline (75 mg/kg, intra-peritoneal (i.p.)) administration and the dark red markers represent the average response before and after administration of GBR 12909 (15 mg/kg, i.p.). drug injection time is denoted by the yellow bar at 0 min. Representative colorplots, CVs, and concentration vs. time curves are inset (top, pargyline; bottom, GBR 12909, α = predrug and β = postdrug). (asterisks above blue markers indicate post hoc test: *p < 0.0001.) reprinted with permission from the American Chemical Society.*

the MFB terminate in layer-dependent mPFC domains with specific uptake transporters. A mathematical model confirmed that the double peaks could be explained by diffusion of neurotransmitter to the electrode from two different sources, one close and one further away.

Finally, in this part of our work, we compared the *in vivo* serotonin signals between the SNr, the CA2 region of the hippocampus, and the mPFC [35]. We found that the different responses could be modeled as a function of the percentage of Uptake 1/Uptake 2 transporters with the model predicting the largest concentration of serotonin transporters in the SNr. We verified this notion with confocal microscopy and concluded that FSCV could be a potentially useful tool for chemical imaging of local cytoarchitecture. Interestingly, and counterintuitively, the SNr, with the highest density of serotonin terminals and axons, had the lowest ambient levels of serotonin. We realized that this was because of the high affinity of SERTs (Uptake 1 transporters) in this region that serve to maintain steady state levels lower than the other two regions with fewer SERTs.

7.2 Serotonin dynamics between the sexes

The prevalence of depression differs between males and females, with women being more likely to suffer from the disorder than men [74–76]. As such, it is important to investigate neurochemical and pharmacodynamic disparities across the sexes. In the hippocampus, we observed no significant differences in the evoked serotonin maximum amplitude or the $t_{1/2}$ of clearance between male and female mice [34]. Furthermore, no differences were detected between the mean signal and

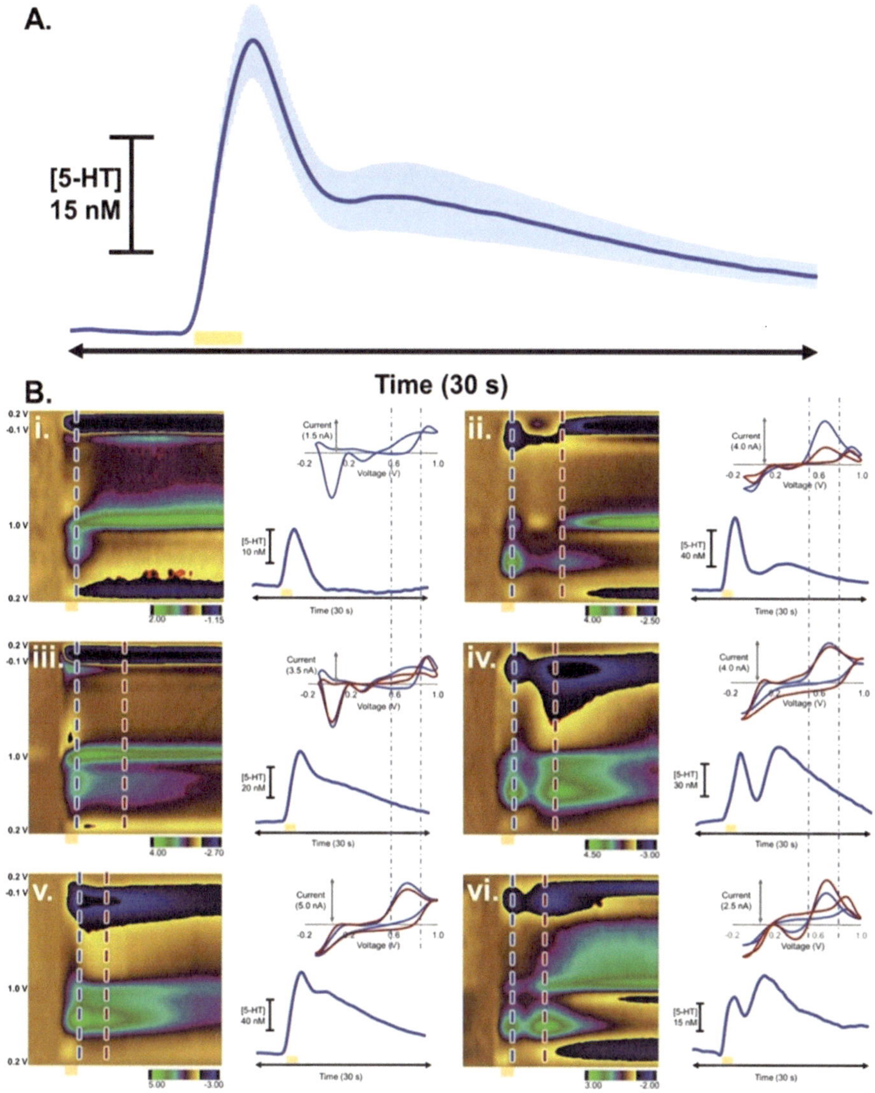

Figure 13.
Representation of single and double peaks reported by west et al. 2019 in the mPFC. The average serotonin response is depicted in (A). Varying signals are shown in (B) with a traditional single peak displayed in (i.) and five of the most common types of double peaks shown in (ii.-vi.). The inset contains the CVs of both peaks. The first peak is shown in blue and the second in red. Reprinted with permission from Elsevier.

the signal in different stages of the female mouse estrous cycle. This suggests that there are no major sex differences in the release or reuptake machinery in drug naive mice. Likewise, no significant differences were detected across sexes in ambient levels of serotonin using FSCAV. Differences in clinical efficacy have been observed following the administration of SSRIs, a class of commonly prescribed antidepressants [77]. Following acute administration of the SSRI, escitalopram, ambient serotonin concentrations increased significantly, however no differences were seen between male and female mice. On the other hand, differences were observed in the evoked serotonin reuptake decay curve. At all four doses given (1, 3, 10 and 30 mg/kg) the female mice had a lower percent change in reuptake compared to the males. We speculated that in female mice, compensatory mechanisms (likely via autoreceptors) exist to counteract hormone-mediated chemical fluxes that may affect serotonin.

7.3 Histaminergic transmission and modulation of serotonin

As outlined above, inflammation (peripheral and brain) is becoming synonymous with the pathophysiology of depression [58]. The monoamine histamine is a major inflammatory mediator in the body [77], associated with allergic reactions. However, less is known about histamine's role in the brain. While traditionally believed to be a neuromodulator in the CNS, recent studies have implicated histamine in neuroinflammatory processes as well [78, 79]. To study fast histaminergic dynamics, we optimized an FSCV waveform to simultaneously detect histamine and serotonin *in vivo* [24, 36]. Histamine oxidation was pharmacologically validated in the posterior hypothalamus following application of tacrine, a histamine N-methyltransferase inhibitor, and thioperamide, an H_3 receptor antagonist. Acute tacrine administration slowed the reuptake of histamine significantly, while thioperamide slowed the reuptake and increased the max amplitude. Upon electrochemical release of histamine, a rapid inhibition of serotonin is observed as shown in **Figure 3**. In this figure, release and reuptake of histamine (a) and serotonin (b) are shown before and after thioperamide (H_3 receptor antagonist) administration, where the dots are the result of a simple mathematical model where the receptor and autoreceptor strengths were changed dynamically by hand. Using the new full histamine and serotonin models (Sections 4 and 5) with the chemistry of the autoreceptors and the H_3 receptors, we were able to predict the experimental results just by using the release and reuptake curve for histamine in the extracellular space that we previously measured.

7.4 Serotonin and histamine in inflammation models

The inhibition of serotonin by histamine fueled our interest in the co-modulation of these analytes in inflammation models. In recent work, we found that upon acute lipopolysaccaride (LPS) induced inflammation, ambient serotonin levels rapidly decreased as a function of increased histamine. Escitalopram was much less capable of increasing the serotonin levels under this inflammation state. We found that this was because escitalopram (and other common antidepressants) inhibit histamine reuptake. This inhibition raises histamine, which depresses serotonin release, counteracting the effect of the antidepressant on the SERTs. Only with the dual strategy of inhibiting serotonin reuptake (by an SSRI) and inhibiting histamine synthesis were we able to return the serotonin to pre-inflammation control levels. We are now actively studying serotonin/histamine co-modulation in other inflammation/depression models in mice including chronic stress and neurodegeneration.

8. Future outlook

Our *in vivo* studies have allowed us to measure and compare and contrast serotonin in different brain regions, to study serotonin dynamics in male and female mice, to investigate serotonin and histamine co-modulation and to ask how this modulation changes under inflammation. This program has provided invaluable information about the dynamics of these two modulators in health and pathophysiology in mice. Our future goals are to apply our findings to *ex vivo* models that more closely mimic human inflammation as a path towards depression diagnosis and treatment. We are exploring a variety of stem cell models, derived from humans, as model systems for personalized diagnostic and drug screening platforms. The continuing, active collaboration and innovation between the experimentalists and the mathematical modelers, as has been the case in the last seven years, will drive novel discoveries in our future program.

Acknowledgements

The authors would like to thank Brenna Park for helpful edits and making **Figure 11**. Partial support for this research came from NIH through R01MH106563-01A1 (PH, JB, HFN, MCR) and 1R21MH109959-01A1 (PH, JB, HFN, MCR) and from the NSF through support for the Mathematical Biosciences Institute, DMS-1440386.

Abbreviations

5-HT	Serotonin
CFME	Carbon fiber microelectrode
CV	Cyclic voltammograms
DA	Dopamine
DAT	Dopamine transporter
DRN	Dorsal raphe nucleus
FSCV	Fast-scan cyclic voltammetry
FSCAV	Fast-scan controlled adsorption voltammetry
TH	Tyrosine hydroxylase
TPH	Tryptophan hydroxylase
MAO	Monoamine oxidase
MFB	Medial forebrain bundle
ODE	Ordinary differential equation
PFC	Prefrontal cortex
RGS	Regulator of G-protein signaling
SBP	Serotonin binding protein
SERT	Serotonin transporter
SNr	Substantia nigra pars reticulata [
SSRI	Selective serotonin reuptake inhibitor

Author details

Janet Best[1*†], Anna Marie Buchanan[2†], Herman Frederik Nijhout[3], Parastoo Hashemi[2,4] and Michael C. Reed[3]

1 The Ohio State University, Columbus, OH, USA

2 University of South Carolina, Columbia, SC, USA

3 Duke University, Durham, NC, USA

4 Imperial College, London, UK

*Address all correspondence to: best.82@osu.edu

† These authors contributed equally.

References

[1] Oleksiak, M., Churchgill, G., Crawford, D.: Variation in gene expression within and among natural populations. Nat. Genetics **32**, 261–266 (2002)

[2] Boeuf, S., Keijer, J., Hal, N., Klaus, S.: Individual variation of adipose gene expression and identification of covariated genes by cdna microarrays. Physiol. Genomics **11**, 31–36 (2002)

[3] Sigal, A., Milo, R., Chen, A., Gava-Zatorsky, N., Klein, Y., Liron, Y., Rosenfeld, N., Danon, T., Perzov, N., Alon, U.: Variability and memory of protein levels in human cells. Nature letters **444**, 643–646 (2006)

[4] Best, J.A., Nijhout, H.F., Reed, M.C.: Homeostatic mechanisms in dopamine synthesis and release: a mathematical model. Theor Biol Med Model **6**, 21 (2009)

[5] Best, J.A., Nijhout, H.F., Reed, M.C.: Serotonin synthesis, release and reuptake in terminals: a mathematical model. Theor Biol Med Model 7, 34 (2010)

[6] Reed, M.C., Best, J.A., Nijhout, H.F.: Passive and active stabilization of dopamine in the striatum. BioScience Hypotheses **2**, 240–244 (2009)

[7] Reed, M., Nijhout, H.F., Best, J.: Computational studies of the role of serotonin in the basal ganglia. Frontiers Integrative Neuroscience 7, 1–8 (2013)

[8] Best, J., Oakley, G., Reed, M., Nijhout, H.F.: Mathematical Models: Interactions between serotonin and dopamine in Parkinson's disease. In: Rana, A.Q. (ed.) Etiology and Pathophysiology of Parkinson's Disease. InTech, London, UK (2011)

[9] Reed, M., Nijhout, H.F., Best, J.: Mathematical insights into the effects of levodopa. Frontiers Integrative Neuroscience **6**, 1–24 (2012)

[10] Hashemi, P., Dankowski, E., Wood, K., Ambrose, R., Wightman, R.: In vivo electrochemical evidence for simultaneous 5-HT and histamine release in the rat substantia nigra pars reticulata following medial forebrain bundle stimulation. J. Neurochem. **118**, 749–759 (2011)

[11] Wood, K.M., Zeqja, A., Nijhout, H. F., Reed, M.C., Best, J.A., Hashemi, P.: Voltammetric and mathematical evidence for dual transport mediation of serotonin clearance in vivo. J. Neurochem. **130**, 351–359 (2014)

[12] Best, J., Nijhout, H.F., Samaranayake, S., Hashemi, P., Reed, M.: A mathematical model for histmine synthesis, release, and control in varicosities. Theoretical Biology and Medical Modelling **14**, 24 (2017)

[13] Best, J., Duncan, W., Sadre-Marandi, F., Nijhout, H.F., Reed, M.: Autoreceptor control of serotonin dynamics. BMC Neuroscience, 1–20 (2020)

[14] Knappskog, P., Flatmark, T., Mallet, J., Lüdecke, B., Bartholomé, K.: Recessively inherited L-DOPA-responsive dystonia caused by a point mutation (Q381K) in the tyrosine hydroxylase gene. Hum. Mol. Genet. **4**, 1209–1212 (1995)

[15] Bunin, M., Prioleau, C., Mailman, R., Wightman, R.: Release and uptake rates of 5-hydroxytryptamine in the dorsal raphe and substantia nigra of the rat brain. J Neurochem **70**, 1077–1087 (1998)

[16] Shaskan, E., Snyder, S.: Kinetics of serotonin accumulation into slices from rat brain: relationship to catecholamine uptake. J. Pharmacol. Exp. Ther. **175**, 404–418 (1970)

[17] Daws, L.C., Koek, W., Mitchell, N. C.: Revisiting serotonin reuptake inhibitors and the therapeutic effects of “uptake 2” in psychiatric disorders. ACS Chem. Neurosci. **4**, 16–21 (2013)

[18] Horton, R., Apple, E., Owens, W.: Decynium-22 enhances ssri-induced antidepressant-like effects in mice: uncovering novel targets to treat depression. J. Neurosci **33**, 10534–10543 (2013)

[19] Monachon, M.-A., Burkard, W.P., Jalfre, M., Haefely, W.: Blockade of central 5-hydroxytryptamine receptors by methiothepin. Naunyn-Schmiedeberg's Arch Pharmacol **274**, 192–197 (1972)

[20] Haas, H., Sergeeva, O., Selbach, O.: Histamine in the nervous system. Physiological Reviews **88**, 1183–1241 (2008)

[21] Schwartz, J.-C.: Histamine as a transmitter in brain. Life Sciences **17**, 503–518 (1974)

[22] Maeyama, K., Watanabe, T., Yamatodani, A., Taguchi, Y., Kambe, H., Wada, H.: Effect of alpha-fluoromethylhistidine on the histamine content of the brain of w/wv mice devoid of mast cells: turnover of brain histamine. J. Neurochem. **41**, 128–134 (1983)

[23] Feldman, R.S., Meyer, J.S., Quenzer, L.F.: Principles of Neuropharmacology. Sinauer Associates, Inc, Sunderland, MA. (1997)

[24] Samaranayake, S., Abdalla, A., Robke, R., Nijhout, H.F., Reed, M., Best, J., Hashemi, P.: A voltammetric and mathematical analysis of histaminergic modulation of serotonin in the mouse hypothalamus. J. Neurochem. **138**, 374–383 (2016)

[25] Annamalai, B., Varman, D.R., Horton, R.E., Daws, L.C., Jayanthi, L.D., Ramamoorthy, S.: Histamine receptors regulate the activity, surface expression, and phosphorulation of serotonin transporters. ACS Chem. Neurosci. **11**, 466–476 (2020)

[26] Spaethling, J.M., Piel, D., Dueck, H., Buckley, P.T., Morris, J.F., Fisher, S.A., Lee, J., Sul, J.-Y., Kim, J., Bartfai, T., Beck, S.G., Eberwine, J.H.: Serotonergic neuron regulation informed by *in vivo* single-cell transcriptomics. FASEB J **28**, 771–780 (2014)

[27] Bernaerts, P., Lamberty, Y., Tirelli, E.: Histamine H3 antagonist thioperamide dose-dependently enhances memory consolidation and reverses amnesia induced by dizocilpine or scopolamine in a one-trial inhibitory avoidance task in mice. Behav. Brain Res. **154**, 211–219 (2004)

[28] Nieto-Alamilla, G., Márquez-Gómez, R., Gárcia-Gálvez, A., Morales-Figueroa, G., Arias-Montaño, J.: The histamine H3 receptor: structure, pharmacology, and function. Mol Pharmacol **90**, 649–673 (2016)

[29] Willars, G.: Mammalian rgs proteins: multifunctional regulators of cellular signalling. Seminars in Cell and Developmental Biology **17**, 363–376 (2006)

[30] Best, J.A., Nijhout, H.F., Reed, M.C.: Models of dopaminergic and serotonergic signaling. Pharmacopsychiatry **43**(Supp. 1), 561–566 (2010)

[31] Best, J., Reed, M., Nijhout, H.F.: Bursts and the efficacy of selective serotonin reuptake inhibitors. Pharmacopsychiatry **44**(Supp1), 76–83 (2011)

[32] West, A., Best, J., Abdalla, A., Nijhout, H.F., Reed, M., Hashemi, P.: Voltammetric evidence for discrete serotonin circuits, linked to specific reuptake domains, in the mouse medial

prefrontal cortex. Neurochem. Inter. **123**, 50–58 (2019)

[33] Abdalla, A., Atcherley, C., Pathirathna, P., Samaranayake, S., Qiang, B., Pena, E., Morgan, S., Heien, M., Hashemi, P.: In vivo ambient serotonin measurements at carbon-fiber microelectrodes. Anal. Chem. **89**, 9703 (2017)

[34] Saylor, R., Hersey, M., West, A., Buchanan, A., Berger, S., Nijhout, H.F., Reed, M., Best, J., Hashemi, P.: In vivo hippocampal serotonin dynamics in male and female mice: Determining effects of acute escitalopram using fast scan cyclic voltammetry. Fronteirs Neurosci. **doi: 10.3389/fnins.2019.00362** (2019)

[35] Abdalla, A., West, A., Jin, Y., Saylor, R., Qiang, B., Pena, E., Linden, D., Nijhout, H.F., Reed, M., Best, J., Hashemi, P.: Fast serotonin voltammetry as a versatile tool for mapping dynamic tissue architecture: I. responses at carbon fibers describe local tissue physiology. J Neurochem **153**, 33–50 (2020)

[36] Samaranayake, S., Abdalla, A., Robke, R., Wood, K., Zeqja, A., Hashemi, P.: In vivo histamine voltammetry in the mouse premammillary nucleus. Analyst **140**, 3759–3765 (2015)

[37] Daws, L., Koek, W., N.Mitchell: Revisiting serotonin reuptake inhibitors and the therapeutic potential of "uptake-2" in psychiatric disorders. ACS Chem. Neurosci. **4**, 16–21 (2013)

[38] Gershon, M., Liu, K., Karpiak, S., Tamir, H.: Storage of serotonin in vivo as a complex with serotonin binding protein in central and peripheral serotonergic neurons. J. Neurosci **3**, 1901–1911 (1983)

[39] Liu, K.-P., Gershon, M., Tamir, H.: Identification, purification, and characterization of two forms of serotonin binding protein from rat brain. J. Neurochem. **44**, 1289–1301 (1985)

[40] Selim, K., Kaplowitz, N.: Hepatotoxicity of psychotropic drugs. Hepatology **29**, 1347–1351 (1999)

[41] J, W., Weale, M., Smith, A., Gatriz, F., Fletcher, B., Thomas, M., Bradman, N., Goldstein, D.: Population genetic structure of variable drug response. Nature Genetics **29**, 265–269 (2001)

[42] Cho, Y.-T., Yang, C.-W., Chu, C.-Y.: Drug reaction with eosinophilia and systemic symptoms (DRESS): An interplay among drugs, viruses, and immune system. Int. J. Molecular Sciences **18**, 1–21 (2017)

[43] Vanhala, A., Yamatodani, A., Panula, P.: Distribution of histamine-, 5-hydroxytryptamine-, and tyrosine hydroxylase-immunoreactive neurons and nerve fibers in developing rat brain. J Comp Neurol **347**(1), 101–114 (1994)

[44] Bito, L., Davson, H., Levin, E., Murray, M., Snider, N.: The concentrations of free amino acids and other electrolytes in cerebrospinal fluid, in vivo dialysate of brain, and blood plasma of the dog. J Neurochem **13**(11), 1057–1067 (1966)

[45] Delgado, J.M.R., DeFeudis, F.V., Roth, R.H., Ryugo, D.K., Mitruka, B.M.: Dialytrode for long term intracerebral perfusion in awake monkeys. Arch Int Pharmacodyn Ther **198**(1), 9–21 (1972)

[46] Robinson, D.L., Venton, J.M., Heien, M.L.A.V., Wightman, R.M.: Detecting subsecond dopamine release with fast-scan cyclic voltametry in vivo. Clinical Chemistry **49**, 1763–1773 (2003)

[47] Hersey, M., Berger, S.N., Holmes, J., West, A., Hashemi, P.: Recent developments in carbon sensors for at-

source electroanalysi. Anal. Chem. **91** (1), 27–43 (2019)

[48] Peters, J.L., Miner, L.H., Michael, A., Sesack, S.R.: Ultrastructure at carbon fiber microelectrode implantation sites after acute voltammetric measurements in the striatum of anesthetized rats. J Neurosci Meth **137**(1), 9–23 (2004)

[49] Jaquins-Gerstl, A., Michael, A.C.: Comparison of the brain penetration injury associated with microdialysis and voltammetry. J Neurosci Meth **183**(2), 127–135 (2009)

[50] Millar, J., Stamford, J.A., Kruk, Z.L., Wightman, R.M.: Electrochemical, pharmacological and electrophysiological evidence of rapid dopamine release and removal in the rat caudate nucleus following electrical stimulation of the median forebrain bundle. European Journal of Pharmacol **109**(3), 341–8 (1985)

[51] Stamford, J.A., Kruk, Z.L., Millar, J., Wightman, R.M.: Striatal dopamine uptake in the rat: In vivo analysis by fast cyclic voltammetry. Neurosci Lett **51**(1), 133–138 (1984)

[52] Yamamoto, B.K., Spanos, L.J.: The acute effects of methylenedioxymethamphetamine on dopamine release in the awake-behaving rat. Eur J Pharmacol **148**(2), 195–203 (1988)

[53] Jackson, B., Dietz, S., Wightman, R.: Fast-scan cyclic voltammetry of 5-hydroxytryptamine. Analytical Chemistry **67**, 1115–1120 (1995)

[54] Hashemi, P., Dankoski, E., Petrovic, J., Keithley, R., Wightman, R.: Voltammetric detection of 5-hydroxytryptamine release in the rat brain. Analytical Chemistry **81**, 9462 (2009)

[55] Howell, J.O., Kuhr, W.G., Ensman, R.E., Wightman, R.M.: Background subtraction for rapid scan voltammetry. J Electroanalytical Chemistry and Interfacial Electrochem **209**(1), 77–90 (1986)

[56] Atcherley, C.W., Laude, N.D., Parent, K.L., Heien, M.L.: Fast-scan controlled-adsorption voltammetry for the quantification of absolute concentrations and adsorption dynamics. Langmuir **29** (48), 14885–92 (2013)

[57] Atcherley, C.W., Wood, K.M., Parent, K.L., Hashemi, P., Heien, M.L.: The coaction of tonic and phasic dopamine dynamics. Chem. Commun. **51**, 2235–2238 (2015)

[58] Amodeo, G., Trusso, M., Fagiolini, A.: Depression and inflammation: Disentangling a clear yet complex and multifaceted link. Neuropsychiatry (London) **07**(4), 448–457 (2017)

[59] Singhal, G., Jaehne, E.J., Corrigan, F., Toben, C., Baune, B.T.: Inflammasomes in neuroinflammation and changes in brain function: a focused review. Front. Neurosci. **8**(315) (2014)

[60] Becher, B., Spath, S., Goverman, J.: Cytokine networks in neuroinflammation. Nature Reviews Immunology **17**(1), 49–59 (2017)

[61] McGeer, E.G., McGeer, P.L.: The role of anti-inflammatory agents in parkinson's disease. CNS Drugs **21**(10), 789–797 (2007)

[62] Nagatsu, T., Mogi, M., Ichinose, H., Togari, A.: Cytokines in Parkinson's disease. J Neural Transmission Suppl **58**, 143–151 (2000)

[63] Swardfager, W., Lanctot, K., Rothenburg, L., Wong, A., Cappell, J., Herrmann, N.: A meta-analysis of cytokines in Alzheimer's disease. Biol Psychiatry **68**(10), 930–941 (2010)

[64] Griffin, W.S., Stanley, L.C., Ling, C., White, L., MacLeod, V., Perrot, L.J.,

3rd, C.L.W., Araoz, C.: Brain interleukin 1 and S-100 immunoreactivity are elevated in Down syndrome and Alzheimer disease. PNAS **86**(19), 7611–7615 (1989)

[65] Strauss, S., Bauer, J., Ganter, U., Jonas, U., Berger, M., Volk, B.: Detection of interleukin-6 and alpha 2-macroglobulin immunoreactivity in cortex and hippocampus of Alzheimer's disease patients. Lab Invest **66**(2), 223–230 (1992)

[66] Palle, P., Monaghan, K.L., Milne, S. M., Wan, E.C.K.: Cytokine signaling in multiple sclerosis and its therapeutic applications. Medical Sciences (Basel, Switzerland) **5**(4), 23 (2017)

[67] Chang, J.R., Zaczynska, E., Katsetos, C.D., Platsoucas, C.D., Oleszak, E.L.: Differential expression of TGF-beta, IL-2, and other cytokines in the CNS of theiler's murine encephalomyelitis virus-infected susceptible and resistant strains of mice. Virology **278**(2), 346–360 (2000)

[68] Young, J.J., Bruno, D., Pomara, N.: A review of the relationship between proinflammatory cytokines and major depressive disorder. Journal of Affective Disorders **169**, 15–20 (2014)

[69] Fries, G.R., Walss-Bass, C., Bauer, M.E., Teixeira, A.L.: Revisiting inflammation in bipolar disorder. Pharmacology Biochemistry and Behavior **177**, 12–19 (2019)

[70] Mayo Clinic Staff: Selective Serotonin Reuptake Inhibitors (SSRIs). https://www.mayoclinic.org/diseases-conditions/depression/in-depth/ssris/art-20044825.

[71] Cragg, S.J., Hawkey, C.R., Greenfield, S.A.: Comparison of serotonin and dopamine release in substantia nigra and ventral tegmental area: region and species differences. J Neurochem **69**(6), 2378–86 (1997)

[72] Wood, K.M., Hashemi, P.: Fast-scan cyclic voltammetry analysis of dynamic serotonin reponses to acute escitalopram. ACS Chem. Neurosci. **4**(5), 715–720 (2013)

[73] Daws, L., Montenez, S., Owens, W., Gould, G., Frazer, A., Toney, G., Gerhardt, G.: Transport mechanisms governing serotonin clearance in vivo revealed by high speed chronoamperometry. J Neurosci Meth **143**, 49–62 (2005)

[74] Weissman, M.M., Klerman, G.L.: Sex differences and the epidemiology of depression. Archives of General Psychiatry **34**(1), 98–111 (1977)

[75] Kessler, R.C., McGonagle, K.A., Swartz, M., Blazer, D.G., Nelson, C.B.: Sex and depression in the National Comorbidity Survey I: Lifetime prevalence, chronicity and recurrence. J Affective Disorders **29**(2), 85–96 (1993)

[76] Grigoriadis, S., Robinson, G.E.: Gender issues in depression. Ann Clin Psychiatry **19**(4), 247–255 (2007)

[77] Branco, A.C.C.C., Yoshikawa, F.S. Y., Pietrobon, A.J., Sato, M.N.: Role of histamine in modulating the immune response and inflammation. Mediators of Inflammation **2018**, 9524075 (2018)

[78] Rocha, S.M., Pires, J., Esteves, M., G.Baltazar, Bernardino, L.: Histamine: a new immunomodulatory player in the neuron-glia crosstalk. Frontiers in Cellular Neuroscience **8**(120) (2014)

[79] Rocha, S.M., Saraiva, T., Cristovao, A.C., Ferreira, R., Santos, T., Esteves, M., Saraiva, C., Je, G., Cortes, L., Valero, J., Alves, G., Klibanov, A., Kim, Y.-S., Bernardino, L.: Histamine induces microglia activation and dopaminergic neuronal toxicity via H1 receptor activation. Journal of Neuroinflammation **13**(1), 137 (2016)

Chapter 2

Serotonin, Sleep and Depression: A Hypothesis

Vladimir M. Kovalzon

Abstract

For most cases of endogenous depression (major depression), the hypothesis of monoamine deficiency, despite a number of limitations it faces, is still considered the most acceptable explanation. The main difficulty faced by this hypothesis is the *reason* for the decrease in the level of cerebral monoamines (primarily serotonin) during depression. It is assumed either increased activity of the MAO enzyme, which metabolizes serotonin, or a mutation with the loss of function of the gene of the Tph-2 enzyme, which synthesizes serotonin, as possible causes. In this review, a third cause is proposed, which can explain a number of cases of «spontaneous» onset of depressive symptoms in apparently healthy people, as well as links the hypotheses of "monoamine deficiency" and "disturbances in circadian rhythms." It is assumed that the formation of endogenous depression is due to a combination of two factors: a reduced "basal" level of cerebral serotonin and excessively long pre-morning periods of REM sleep, during which the release of cerebral monoamines stops altogether. As a possible way to of non-drug treatment of depression, not deprivation, but fragmentation of this phase of sleep is suggested, that is much easier for patients to tolerate.

Keywords: serotonin, sleep, rem sleep, depression, monoamine hypothesis

1. Introduction

A hypothesis is put forward according to which two factors play an important role in the formation of a number of cases of so-called "endogenous" (major) depression. First, the initially lowered (but within the reaction norm) level of cerebral serotonin, reflecting the gene polymorphisms of the human population. Second, the excessively long pre-morning periods of REM sleep associated with the "pressure of civilization" on the natural structure of the human wakefulness-sleep cycle, during which the release of cerebral monoamines stops altogether. It is a combination of these two factors that can lead to the emotional imbalance seen in depression.

2. Serotonin and sleep

Serotonin (5-HT) is one of the oldest and most important mediators in the central nervous system, participating in a wide range of behavioral, physiological and pathological processes. The history of its study goes back about 70 years, nevertheless, serotonin remains one of the most mysterious neurotransmitters.

As is known, the largest accumulation of serotonergic neurons in the brain is observed in the dorsal raphe nuclei (DRN) and the pons varolii (zones B6 and B7 according to Dahlström & Fuxe [1]). The total number of such cells in human brain is relatively small - about one hundred thousand. The serotonergic system has two characteristics: first, the unusually numerous ramifications of its axons (up to a million bifurcations of a single axon). Secondly, the extraordinary variety of types (at least 7) and subtypes (at least 14; some researchers even count more than 20) of their receptors, among which there are both membrane depolarizing (subtypes 5-HT2A-C, 5-HT3, 5-HT6, 5-HT7) and hyperpolarizing it (5-HT1A,B). Due to the abundant "treelike" branching, several hundred thousands of serotonergic neurons of the brain stem innervate tens of billions of other neurons in the human brain: practically all the nerve cells of the neocortex, hippocampus, striatum, and hypothalamus, other parts of the brain as well as motor neurons of the spinal cord [1, 2]. Only the upper olive complex (part of the auditory system) and the optic chiasm are devoid of serotonin afferents [3]. And due to the receptor diversity, ligands of serotonin receptors can effect both activating and inhibitory processes on the brain and behavior in general.

The role of serotonin transmission in the regulation of wakefulness and sleep was first identified by the work of Michel Jouvet and his laboratory in Lyon, France. In these experiments of the classic of world somnology, performed on cats using primitive technologies of the 60s - early 70s of the last century, the following was shown. Intracerebral administration of serotonin, or electro-stimulation of the DRN or the median raphe nucleus (MnRN), where most 5-HT neurons in the brain are located, induces a short period of paradoxical (REM) sleep, followed by prolonged deep slow-wave sleep (NREM). If, on the contrary, the level of cerebral serotonin is reduced by systemic administration of parachlorophenylalanine (PCPA), which blocks serotonin synthesis, or by destruction of the MnRN, both phases of sleep are sharply reduced. This insomnia lasts at least 10 days. In this case, effect of PCPA is eliminated by the administration of the precursor of serotonin - 5-hydroxytryptophan. These and other early experiments served as the basis for Michel Jouvet's hypothesis about serotonin as "somnotonin" (as it was then called by the Swiss somnologist Werner Koella), the main factor in slow wave sleep [4]. However, further experiments performed in the same laboratory of Jouvet with electrical stimulation and reversible shutdown of DRN neurons caused by local tissue cooling to 10 °C, pointed, on the contrary, to serotonin as a factor of wakefulness. Eventually, it was proved that this hypothesis of Jouvet was wrong - in particular, insomnia caused by suppression of serotonergic neurotransmission was associated with a disorder of thermoregulation, a drop in body temperature, which led to an increase in the motor activity of cats to warm up [5]. And the insomnia that occurs in experimental rats and cats as a result of the administration of PCPA, as it turned out, is the result of a sharp increase in sensitivity to the surrounding animal stimuli, and not a disorder of the regulation of the wakefulness-sleep cycle [6].

Summing up the results of many years of research, a disciple of Michel Jouvet, Raymond Cespuglio, suggested that serotonin may be involved in the regulation of the wakefulness-sleep cycle in two different ways: in wakefulness serotonin is realized on the presynaptic membrane of the 5-HT neurons and promotes the formation and accumulation in target cells hypnogenic neuropeptides: vasointestinal polypeptide (VIP), corticotropin-like intermediate lobe peptide (CLIP), substance P (SP); in the subsequent period of sleep, under the influence of these peptides, dendritic (nonsynaptic) realization of serotonin in the nuclei of the raphe occurs and its binding to the 5-HT1B autoreceptors, as a result of which the synaptic release of serotonin is weakened and stopped [3]. However, this hypothesis also has not received convincing experimental confirmation [6].

Experiments with extracellular registration have shown that most serotonergic neurons are very active in the waking state, and during the transition to sleep and further into deep NREM sleep, they progressively slow down their activity and completely "silence" immediately before the transition to REM sleep. Thorough studies of the activity of not only large and medium-sized, but also small cells of the dorsal raphe of the model mouse brain in the wake–sleep cycle, carried out by Jouvet's disciple Kazuya Sakai, revealed a high anatomical, neurochemical and functional heterogeneity of these neurons. The majority of neurons in this area (52%) are indeed serotonergic (5-HT/DR), and almost all of them (48%) are active only in wakefulness, but a significant part (25% of all cells) are active in sleep, and judging by the spike shape, 19% of them are GABAergic, and only 6% are serotonergic [7]. Apparently, serotonin neurons are mainly responsible for maintaining calm (relaxed) wakefulness; thus, according to some data, they are most active during food consumption and reduce the frequency of impulses with increased behavioral activation [5].

Agonists of all serotonin receptors stimulate wakefulness and suppress NREM and REM sleep when administered systemically or intraventricularly. In this case, the activation of wakefulness occurs by depolarizing the histaminergic tuberomammillary neurons of the posterior hypothalamus, as well as GABA/parvalbumin-containing neurons of the basal forebrain region, which project into the hippocampus and neocortex. Suppression of NREM is carried out mainly by inhibition of neurons in the "sleep center" VLPO, mediated by the 5-HT1A receptor [5]. And the suppression of REM sleep occurs due to inhibition of cholinergic REM-on neurons of the pons [5].

With direct microinjection of inhibitory receptor 5-HT1A agonists into the dorsal raphe nuclei, an increase in REM sleep occurs, whereas similar injections of inhibitory autoreceptor 5-HT1B agonists and activating 5-HT2A/C, 5-HT3 and 5-HT7 receptors suppress REM sleep, which is consistent with the concept of the need for inhibition of 5-HT neurons to trigger REM sleep [8]. Systemic administration of non-selective antagonists of the 5-HT2A/C receptors, selective antagonists or reversible agonists of the 5-HT2A receptor in laboratory rats and mice, healthy subjects and patients with primary or comorbid insomnia causes an increase in NREM sleep, which, again, is consistent with the idea of the participation of 5-HT neurons in maintaining wakefulness [6].

Thus, according to the results of neural and pharmacological studies, serotonin seemed finally established as the status of a wakefulness mediator along with other monoamines (norepinephrine, dopamine, histamine), as well as acetylcholine and glutamate. The main source of serotonin - the DRN – were introduced on diagrams as one of the clusters of the reticular ascending activating system [9, 10]. It has also been shown to play an important role in the negative regulation of REM sleep: without turning off serotonin transmission, neither initiation nor maintenance of REM sleep is possible [6].

In this case, selective shutdown of serotonergic transmission should suppress wakefulness by increasing NREM sleep. Such a methodological opportunity appeared with the introduction of molecular genetic and other newest innovative techniques into neurophysiology. It was found that the brain has its own special isoform of the enzyme tryptophan hydroxylase - Tph2, which converts the amino acid tryptophan, which is supplied to the body with protein food, into 5-hydroxytryptophan, a precursor of serotonin, and encoded by a separate gene. This discovery made it possible to create knockout mice for this gene, in which the content of cerebral serotonin does not exceed 4% of its content in the brain of control mice (that is, practically absent). Figuratively describing the phenotype of such mice, which grew up "without serotonin in their brain", can be named as "evil dwarfs."

They are fertile and females have milk, but they do not care for their offspring, and therefore half of their offspring dies [11, 12]. Disorders of the wakefulness-sleep cycle in these mutants are limited, judging by the results of registration of locomotor activity, to a slight increase in sleep and suppression of wakefulness in daylight (daytime), which seems to correspond with the above hypothesis [13].

At the same time, in another study on genetically modified mice with the homozygous Tph2 mutation (intact neurons, but complete absence of serotonin in the central nervous system) and polysomnographic registration, the following was found. A small (but statistically significant) decrease in the duration of NREM sleep and a corresponding increase in active wakefulness in mutant animals compared with control occurred only when the light was turned on and off. Apparently, the absence of serotonin increases the reactivity of the animal to light stimulation. It was also shown that the sleep of the mutants was less fragmented. No further disturbances in the wake–sleep cycle were identified. In this series of experiments, the absence of serotonin caused only very small changes, not confirming the original hypothesis [14].

However, Tph2 knockout mice cannot serve as an adequate model for studying the role of serotonin in the regulation of the wakefulness-sleep cycle, since it is unclear whether the revealed phenotypic changes are the result of abnormal development, compensation for the lack of serotonin by other transmitters, or, indeed, impaired neurotransmission in adults. To solve this problem, a method was developed to turn off the expression of the Tph2 gene by microinjection of its blocker directly into the tissue of the raphe nuclei of the midbrain and pons in the genetically created mouse strain [15]. By visual analysis of video recordings, it was possible to reveal an increased level of motor activity, especially noticeable in the night (active) phase of the nychthemeron, when in the second half of the night the control individuals experienced a period of decreased activity, called by the authors "siesta". In mice with blocked serotonergic transmission, such periods were absent altogether; they ran almost continuously all night [15]. Thus, according to the results of this study, serotonin itself behaves more like "sleep factor" than "wake factor".

Since 5-HT containing neurons also secrete glutamate and various neuropeptides, the effect of their destruction may be quite different from that of the elimination of serotonin itself. In the work of Japanese authors [16], carried out using polysomnographic recording, neurotoxic destruction of serotonin-containing DR neurons in special genetically engineered mice led to a decrease in REM sleep at night, when its representation is already low. In addition, according to the data of the same authors, in the experimental mice, in comparison with the control ones, the response to the new environment was weakened and the power of the theta rhythm in wakefulness was increased. However, all these effects were so small that they were detected only with the help of statistical tricks. This, however, did not prevent the authors from concluding that their data support the main hypothesis about the role of serotonin as a factor of wakefulness (positive) and REM sleep (negative), presented above.

Finally, in a recently published study led by renowned Boston somnologist Patrick Fuller using a novel method of highly selective chemogenetic activation of serotonergic neurons in the DRN in combination with polysomnography and behavioral tests, no unambiguous results were obtained either [17]. A "compensatory" restoration of NREM sleep, slightly suppressed by the 5-HT neuron activator injection procedure, was shown to return to baseline levels. This effect can hardly be called somnogenic, but it is definitely not activating. In addition, a change in behavior in the open field was found, which the authors interpret as a decrease in the level of anxiety under the influence of the activation of serotonergic neurons in the DRN.

However, testing in a cruciform elevated maze revealed no changes. The authors refer to a recent study that revealed the existence of two mutually intertwining serotonergic subsystems in the DRN that innervate the orbital frontal cortex and the central amygdala differently. One of these subsystems supports anxiogenic and the other anxiolytic functions. It is possible that the simultaneous activation of both subsystems is associated with the uncertainty of the results obtained in such experiments [17].

As mentioned above, most serotonin-secreting neurons are "silent" during the entire period of REM sleep until the moment of its completion (by awakening or re-entering NREM sleep), and in fact not one single serotonin molecule is released from the presynaptic membrane during this time.

As can be seen from the **Table 1**, the intercellular fluid in wakefulness is saturated mainly with the mediators with depolarizing action on the postsynaptic membrane. During the transition to NREM sleep, all these molecules quickly disappear from the intercellular environment being replaced by the main inhibitory mediator of the brain, GABA, that concentration increases with the deepening of NREM sleep, and the peptide galanin colocolized with GABA. The cerebral biochemical environment in REM sleep is special. High levels of acetylcholine, glutamate and galanin are combined with a complete absence of orexin (hypocretin) and monoamines — serotonin, norepinephrine and histamine, with the exception of dopamine, the concentration of which may sometimes even exceed that in wakefulness. A new mediator appears, the MCH peptide, which mediates the hypothalamo-pontine level of REM sleep regulation. The release of GABA in general is significantly reduced, but remains high in areas of the orexinergic (LHA), histaminergic (TMN), serotonergic (DR) and noradrenergic (LC) neurons localization. In these systems, GABAergic neurons play the role of a "lock" preventing depolarization of these cells during the entire period of REM sleep.

Neurotransmitters	Localization	W	NREM sleep	REM sleep
5-HT	DR	↑↑	↓→↓↓	↔
Norepinephrine	LC	↑↑	↓→↓↓	↔
Histamine	TMN	↑↑	↓→↓↓	↔
Dopamine	VTA/SNpc/vPAG	↑↑	↓	↑
Acetylcholine	LDT/PPT/BF	↑↑	↓→↓↓	↑↑
Glutamate	PC/PB/BF	↑↑	↓→↓↓	↑↑
GABA	Total brain	↑/↓	↑↑	↑/↓
Orexin/Hypocretin	LHA	↑↑	↔	↔
Galanin	VLPO/MnPO	↓	↑↑	↑↑
MCH	LHA/PH	↓	↓	↑↑

Abbreviations: W – wake; NREM sleep – non rapid eye movement sleep; REM sleep - rapid eye movement sleep; 5-HT – serotonin; GABA – γ-aminobutyric acid; MCH – melanin-concentrating hormone; LC – locus coeruleus; DR – dorsal raphe; TMN – tubero-mammillar nucleus; VTA – ventral tegmental area; SNpc – substantia nigra/pars compacta; vPAG – ventral periaquetuctul gray matter; LDT/PPT – latero-dorsal tegmentum/pedunculo-pontine tegmentum; BF – basal forebrain; PC/PB – preceoruleus/parabrachialis nuclei; LHA – lateral hypothalamic area; VLPO – ventro-lateral preoptic area; MnPO – median preoptic area; PH – posterior hypothalamus; ↑ – increase in release; ↓ -decrease in release; ↑ ↑ - substantial increase in release; ↓ ↓ - substantial decrease in release; ↑ / ↓ - increase or decrease in release dependently of the site of cerebral localization; → – gradual decrease in release; ↔ – release ceased.

Table 1.
A simplified scheme for the secretion of cerebral neurotransmitters in the sleep–wake cycle (data from animal studies).

Obviously, the level of serotonin (as well as norepinephrine and histamine) at the sites of projection of aminergic neurons (and, possibly, in the brain as a whole) can decrease during this time. However, the periods of REM sleep in all animals are short, and in some species (small rodents, birds, etc.) they are extremely short (from a few seconds to 1 min) [18, 19]. So this decrease cannot be significant, and in the subsequent period of wakefulness, the normal, "basal" level of serotonergic transmission is quickly restored.

The situation is different in humans. In adults, unlike animals, sleep is of a continuous, so-called "monophasic" or "consolidated" nature. This means that an adult living in modern urban conditions is waking all day (16 hours), and the entire daily "quota" of sleep, usually 5 cycles 1.5 hour each, is realized at night "at a time." In this case, the first half of the night sharply differs from the second - and this is another important difference between human sleep and animal sleep (**Figure 1**, upper graph). In the first half of the night, a person implements mainly the need for deep slow wave sleep (NREM), which has accumulated over a long period of wakefulness (stage 3; according to the old classification - stages 3 + 4, "delta sleep" is apparently a state that is critical for the survival of the organism). In the second half of the night, the need for REM sleep is realized, which alternates with periods of superficial NREM sleep (stage 2). At the same time, individual periods of REM

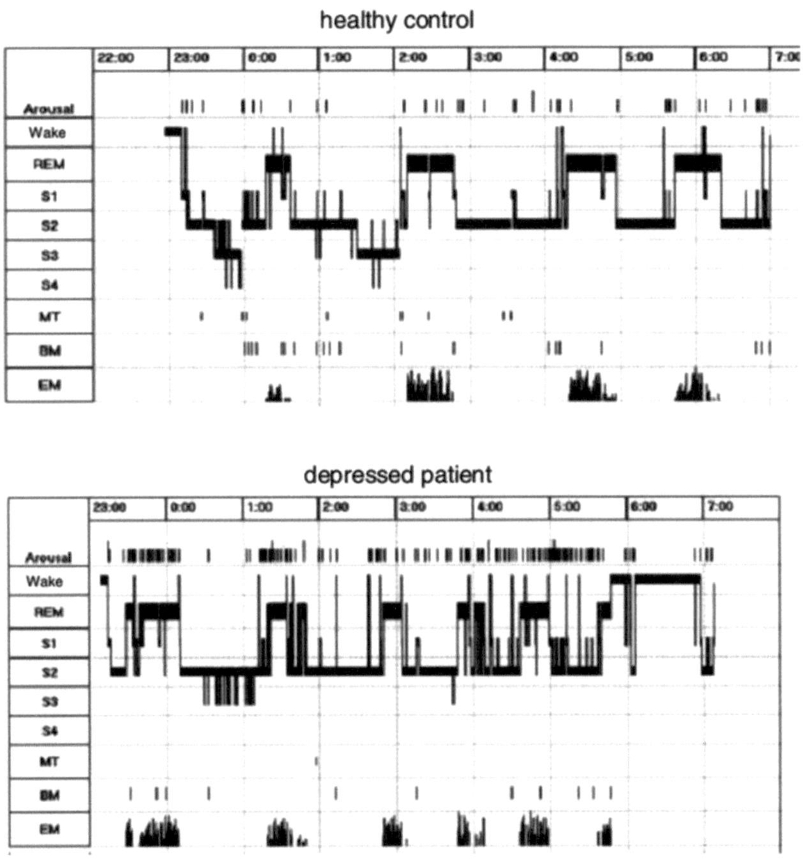

Figure 1.
A hypnogram of a healthy human subject (top) and a depressed patient (bottom) [20]. W - wakefulness, REM - REM sleep, S1-S4 - stages of NREM sleep, MT and BM - various types of movements during sleep, EM - rapid eye movements. It can be seen that the patient has fragmented sleep, REM sleep is disinhibited, and deep NREM sleep (stages 3 and 4; according to the new classification, they combined into one), on the contrary, is suppressed.

sleep, which in a healthy person occupies about 2 night hours, can last 20, 30, and even 40 minutes in the last sleep cycles [20]. Naturally, such long periods of inactivity of the "serotonin factory" of the brain cannot pass without leaving a trace.

What determines these differences in the structure of human sleep? A newborn baby sleeps around the clock with short sucking breaks, total about 16 hours, 8 of which is occupied by the so-called "activated sleep", which is considered as the precursor of adult REM sleep. A one-year-old child has two periods of daytime sleep, and a four-year-old is allowed to sleep only once a day, after lunch. An eight-year-old is already attending school and cannot sleep during the day, and this daily rhythm (without daytime sleep) is maintained by the majority of the modern urban population for life. Psychophysiological studies of the wakefulness-sleep rhythm carried out at one time in healthy subjects who were transferred to a 24-hour bed rest when isolated from the external environment [21], as well as some observations of ethnographers on the nature of sleep in primitive tribes living in isolation from civilization [22], allow to make the following assumption. By nature, a person has a sleep–wake rhythm with two periods of short naps. With this mode, the duration of night sleep is significantly shortened; a person can get up at dawn (in summer). Sleep becomes less consolidated, sleep cycles can be interspersed with more or less prolonged episodes of wakefulness. The differences between the first and second half of the night are smoothed out. In general, human sleep begins to resemble more animal sleep [21–23]. The monophasic nature of sleep of a modern person, apparently, is associated not so much with biological, genetic factors, as with the "pressure of civilization", distorting, disrupting the natural alternation of wakefulness and sleep. During a 16-hour daytime period of continuous wakefulness, a modern person experiences repeated "intrusions" of sleep mechanisms, realized in the form of episodes of local sleep, microsleep and an increase in the delta index in the EEG [24]. A monophasic diurnal rhythm (without daytime sleep) is acquired by the majority of the modern urban population in childhood and retained for the rest of their lives [25].

Thus, the circadian rhythm of a modern urban person is 16 hours of sleep deprivation, followed by 8 hours of sleep. And the law of "rebound" is as follows: first, delta sleep is restored (stage 3), then REM sleep [26]. On the other hand, superficial sleep is considered an "optional" state, which "can be dispensed with." Consequently, the unusually long pre-morning periods of REM sleep, in which serotonergic transmission can be severely depleted, are mainly due to "civilization pressure" disrupting natural circadian dynamics.

3. Serotonin and depression

Although the role of serotonin in the regulation of the wakefulness-sleep cycle remains not completely defined, its participation in emotional reactions is well known. In popular literature, serotonin is often referred to as the "happiness hormone". Excessive activation of serotonergic transmission in the brain causes movement disorders – part of the so-called "serotonin syndrome", and insufficient activation seems associated with diseases such as depression, schizophrenia, anxiety disorders, etc. [27, 28]. In the 50–60s of the last century, the so-called "catecholaminergic" hypothesis became widespread, linking the occurrence of depression with a lack of noradrenergic transmission. It was replaced by the "serotonin" hypothesis of endogenous depression, which was first published in the Lancet magazine in an article by a psychopharmacologist from Leningrad (USSR, now St. Petersburg, Russia) Izyaslav (Slava) Lapin and his graduate student Gregory Oxenkrug: "Intensification of the central serotoninergic processes as a possible determinant of the thymoleptic effect" [29]. The article had about 350 citations in the first 18 years (to date, according to Google searches, about 800). This led Eugene Garfield to include it in the "This Week's Citation Classic" section of the Current Contents and to publish a note by Oxenkrug on how the article was created [30].

Lapin and Oxenkrug were the first to link emotional disorders and sleep disturbances in depression with a common causative factor - impaired serotonin transmission due to changes in the turnover of cerebral serotonin. Reducing serotonergic transmission in the brain through the hypothalamus-pituitary–adrenal cortex axis disinhibits the release of cortisol. Cortisol activates the enzyme tryptophan dioxygenase (TDO), which "shunts" the normal turnover of serotonin and converts it (in the presence of the pro-inflammatory cytokine γ-interferon, which appears in response to stress) into kynurenine. As a result, serotonin is released less and less. Neuroactive kynurenines, in turn, increase anxiety and impair cognitive performance. Subsequently Lapin showed that the metabolism of kynurenine in the absence of vitamin B6 leads to the appearance of diabetogenic derivatives [31]. The impact of Lapin's ideas on the further development of world psychiatry and psychopharmacology was described in detailed reviews by Oxenkrug [32, 33].

Later, other authors developed a "new serotonin hypothesis" [34], according to which an increased level of glucorticoids, systemic inflammatory processes, and neuroimmune activation of microglia stimulate the synthesis of enzymes tryptophan dioxygenase and indoleamine dioxygenase (TDO/IDO) and finally shift the breakdown of tryptophan to the kynurenine pathway. Finally, the initial development of Lapin recently received a new generalization in the form of the so-called "serotonin-kynurenine-inflammatory" hypothesis of the onset of depression (see **Figure 2**) [35, 36]. Based on the latest biochemical and molecular biology studies, these authors show that the metabolites of kynurenine - oxidized kynurenine, quinolinic acid and the cation NAD+ (nicotinamide-adenine-dinucleotide), which have exito- and neurotoxic properties, cause an excessive increase in glutamatergic neurotransmission, suppressing neurogenesis in the *fascia dentata* of the hippocampus, apoptosis and neurodegeneration. The kynurenine pathway of serotonin metabolism occurs in microglia, and the proliferation of microglia has been found in a number of studies using neuroscanning of depressed patients. So, despite the fact that modern theories of the origin of depression concentrate more on neuroinflammatory and neurodegenerative processes [36–39], Lapin's serotonin idea, put forward more than half a century ago has not lost its relevance.

Back in 1960, a reduced (almost 3 times) level of serotonin in the cerebrospinal fluid of depressed patients was confirmed [40]. And selective serotonin reuptake inhibitors (increasing 5-HT concentration in the synaptic cleft) have been widely and successfully used in clinical medicine as antidepressants for more than 30 years [2]. However, the generalizing works of the last two decades have given some authors the basis for a paradoxical conclusion that not suppression, but, on the contrary, the excess of serotonin neurotransmission is the cause (or at least one of the causes) endogenous depression (melancholy), or that serotonin is not involved at all in the pathogenesis of this disease [41–44].

In recent years, researchers have turned their attention not to cerebral serotonin itself, but to its carrier protein (5-HTT) and the gene for this protein. It turned out that people homo- or heterozygous for its short allele are less resistant to stress and are more at risk of developing insomnia and depression than carriers of the long allele [45]. The short allele is associated with a decrease in the number of 5-HTT binding regions on the surface of the presynaptic membrane and, accordingly, in the reuptake of excess serotonin. From this point of view, the disorder of serotonin transmission in some types of depression, in fact, may be associated more with an excess than a lack of serotonin in the synaptic cleft.

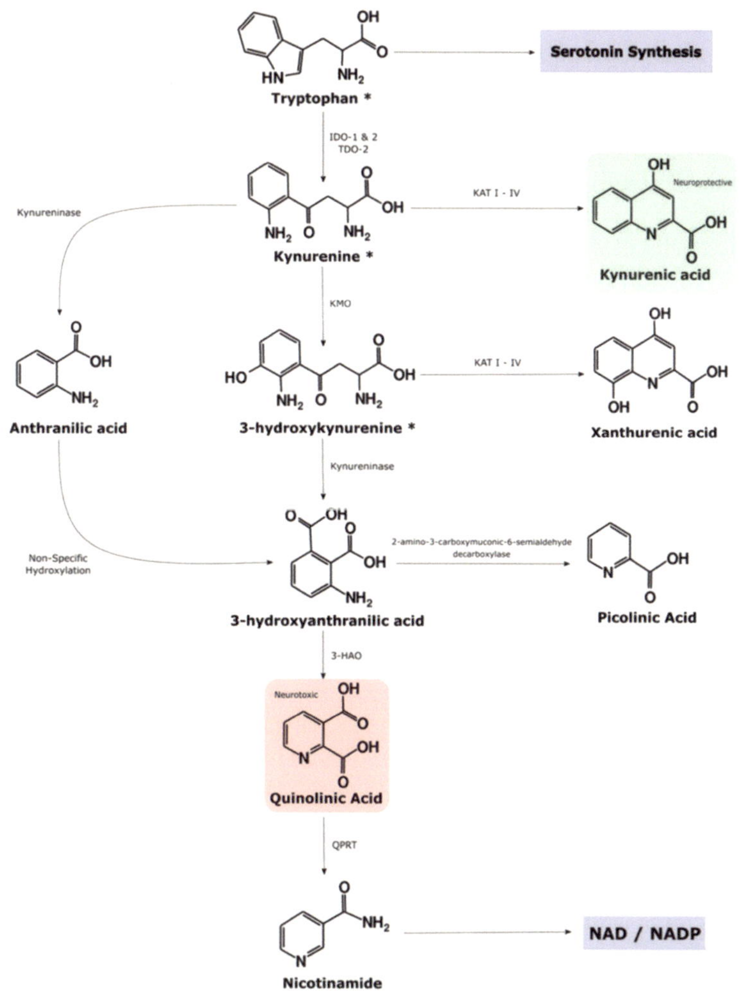

Figure 2.
Simplified illustration of the kynurenine pathway. Tryptophan (TRP) is predominantly converted into kynurenine (KYN) by the indoleamine 2,3-dioxygenase (IDO) isozymes and tryptophan dioxygenase (TDO). IDO-1 is expressed in various immune cells throughout the body, notably dendritic cells, monocytes, and macrophages. Less is known about the more recently discovered IDO-2 enzyme although it is more selectively expressed in dendritic cells, liver, kidney, and the brain and it does not appear to have a significant effect on peripheral kynurenine concentration. TDO-2 is an alternative nomenclature for TDO. KYN can be metabolized into kynurenic acid (KYNA), which is usually considered to be neuroprotective, by the KAT isozymes. Alternatively, it may be converted into anthranilic acid by kynureninase or 3-hydroxykynurenine (3HK) by kynurenine monooxygenase (KMO). Metabolism down the latter pathway increases under inflammatory conditions. 3HK is a free radical generator while quinolinic acid (QA) is a known neurotoxin and gliotoxin. Thus, metabolites in this pathway are usually considered to be neurotoxic. QA is the endogenous source of nicotinamide and nicotinamide adenine dinucleotide (NAD+) [35].

Apparently, under the general term “depression” there is several (and maybe even many) diseases of various etiologies [46]. At the same time, the majority of patients respond positively to the intake of selective serotonin reuptake inhibitors (SSRIs). Moreover, almost any drug that inhibits the reuptake of monoamines (primarily serotonin, but partly also norepinephrine and dopamine) has thymoleptic (antidepressant) properties [46]. However, a very long interval (calculated in weeks) from the start of antidepressant administration to the appearance of a therapeutic effect is an indirect indication that the lack of monoaminergic transmission is most likely a secondary, “downward” consequence of some still unknown primary disorders [46]. Nevertheless, for most cases of endogenous depression (major depression), the hypothesis of monoamine deficiency is still considered the most acceptable [46]. Apparently, the impairment of serotonergic neurotransmission is one of the links in a cascade of molecular biological events that ultimately lead to neuroinflammatory and neurodegenerative changes in certain parts of the brain, as mentioned above.

The main difficulty faced by this hypothesis is the *reason* for the decrease in serotonin levels in the brain during depression. Among the possible reasons, either an increased activity of the MAO enzyme, which metabolizes serotonin, or a mutation with loss of function of the gene of the Tph-2 enzyme, which synthesizes serotonin, is proposed. In this review, we propose a third reason that can explain a number of cases of "spontaneous" onset of depressive symptoms in apparently healthy people, as well as link the hypotheses of "monoamine deficiency" and "circadian rhythm disturbances" [46].

4. Sleep and depression

Depression is one of those relatively few diseases that are characterized by pronounced and rather specific sleep disorders. In addition, these disorders can occur much earlier than the main symptoms (mood disorders, etc.), and therefore serve as important predictors of the disease. Non-specific disorders in depression include difficulty falling asleep, frequent nighttime awakenings, and early morning awakenings. However, there is a more specific violation of the sleep structure: suppression of deep NREM sleep (stage 3) and disinhibition of REM sleep (see **Figure 1**, lower graph). The suppression of deep SWS manifests itself in the loss of stage 4 (according to the old classification), reduction and fragmentation of stage 3, a decrease in the EEG delta index, and lengthening of stage 2. The disinhibition of REM sleep is manifested both quantitatively and qualitatively. Quantitatively, by reducing the latency of the onset of the first REM period down to zero, when sleep can begin with a REM episode, which never happens in a healthy adult; lengthening the first REM period; an increase in the proportion of the total duration of REM sleep in all night sleep. Qualitatively, the disinhibition of REM sleep manifests itself in an increase in the generation of rapid eye movements already in the first REM sleep period. Although similar disorders of REM sleep are observed not in all patients with depression, but only in 50–70% (according to various sources), and similar phenomena of REM sleep "disinhibition" can sometimes be observed in other neuropsychiatric disorders (schizophrenia, manic psychosis), nevertheless for "major" depression, they are much more typical and more pronounced [37].

As noted above, suppression of neurogenesis in adult animals was shown in various experimental models of depression (mice, rats) [47]. Interestingly, in other models associated with an increase in REM sleep (some forms of stress), according to some data, neurogenesis in the hippocampus is also impaired. On the other hand, inhibition of neurogenesis is also observed in sleep deprivation [37].

One of the main arguments in favor of the hypothesis of a causal relationship (rather than just a correlation) between depression and REM sleep is the effects of antidepressants. It is well known that most antidepressants that prevent the natural breakdown of serotonin (and other brain amines): tricyclic drugs, selective serotonin reuptake inhibitors (SSRI), deeply inhibit REM sleep. Especially effective in this regard are MAO inhibitors, which can almost completely eliminate REM sleep for months and years [37–39]. Millions of patients around the world have taken and are taking these drugs. No cases of cognitive impairment were reported; instead, there is some evidence that MAO inhibitors even improve memory! On the contrary, the latest generation of benzodiazepines, used as hypnotics and practically do not disturb the duration and distribution of REM sleep, have a pronounced detrimental effect on memory due to the effect of these drugs on the GABA signaling system [48–51].

Now, imagine that in the human population, with its unusually wide gene diversity, there are subjects with initially lowered levels of cerebral serotonin. This may be due to some gene polymorphisms that cause, for example, the synthesis from dietary tryptophan, not serotonin, but kynurenines (as Lapin believed) [29, 31–33]), or a decrease in the formation of tryptophan hydroxylase-2, which synthesizes cerebral serotonin from its precursor, or an increased level of the MAO-A enzyme, which metabolizes serotonin, etc. For such people, long pre-morning periods of REM sleep become especially dangerous, since they can reduce the level of cerebral serotonin below a certain critical level, the threshold for disruption of general serotonergic transmission and the occurrence of emotional disorders. This approach is confirmed by the subjective reports of patients reporting the appearance of the first feelings of depression even during the experience of morning dreams and reaching their maximum severity immediately upon awakening. However, by the evening (as cerebral serotonin accumulates in the course of a vigorous state), the patient's condition gradually improves, depressive symptoms go away by themselves, and he/she feels completely healthy ... until a new period of sleep comes! [46]. It is clear that against the background of a low, near-threshold level of cerebral serotonin, even immersions in NREM sleep causing a decrease in serotonin release can re-launch pathological processes in the brain.

On the other hand, the release of cerebral serotonin is involved in the inhibition of the glutamatergic/cholinergic center of REM sleep triggering in the pons [5, 9, 10]. Then, the weakening of this inhibition may be associated with a well-studied increase in the "pressure" of REM sleep in depression, which manifests itself, in particular, in the shortening of the latent period of the first episode of this sleep phase, as mentioned above [37–39]. Moreover, according to some reports, even genetic relatives of such patients, who do not suffer from depression, but, assuringly might have the same gene polymorphism and, as a result, a lowered "basal" level of cerebral serotonin, also have excessively prolonged periods of REM sleep [37]. That is, one can assume that all people who initially have a lowered level of cerebral serotonin, due to this, have an increased "pressure" of REM sleep, which further lowers this level.

It becomes clear why it is not possible to create a more or less adequate experimental model of stress-induced anhedonia (depression) [52]. For this, apparently, it is necessary to adapt the experimental mice to "human conditions": a constant 16-hour sleep deprivation (in the dark period of the day) accompanied by its 8-hour "return" (in the light period). And it is necessary to influence chronic stress also in the dark period against the background of this artificial circadian rhythm. It is possible that in this case the applied impacts will be more effective.

5. Conclusion

Thus, according to the proposed hypothesis, the formation of depression is due to a combination of two factors - a reduced level of cerebral serotonin and the structure of human night sleep with extremely long pre-morning periods of REM sleep. It is known that total sleep deprivation (or selective REM sleep deprivation) is used as an effective but short-term thymoleptic action. According to the proposed approach, fragmentation of REM sleep can be just as effective. If it really turns out to be effective in alleviating depressive symptoms, then it can be relatively easily automated by giving the patient during REM sleep signals (for example, sound), selected so that they do not wake him up at all, but only wake him up, transferring from REM sleep to the 2nd or 1st stage of NREM sleep. Such a procedure, which is much more easily tolerated by patients, will also be suitable for chronic use.

Acknowledgements

This work was supported by the Russian Science Foundation (project No. 17-15-01433).

Author details

Vladimir M. Kovalzon
Severtsov Institute Ecology/Evolution, Russian Academy of Sciences, Moscow, Russia

*Address all correspondence to: kovalzon@sevin.ru

References

[1] Jacobs BL, Azmitia EC Structure and function of the brain serotonin system. Physiological Reviews. 1992;72(1):165-229.

[2] Müller CP, Cunningham KA., editors. Handbook of the Behavioral Neurobiology of Serotonin. 2nd ed. London: Elsevier; 2020.

[3] Cespuglio R. Serotonin: its place today in sleep preparation, triggering or maintenance. Sleep Medicine. 2018; 49:31e39. DOI: 10.1016/j.sleep.2018.05.034

[4] Jouvet M. Sleep and serotonin: an unfinished story. Neuropsychopharmacology. 1999;21:24S–27S.

[5] Brown RE, Basheer R, McKenna JT, Strecker RE, McCarley RW. Control of sleep and wakefulness. Physiol. Rev. 2012;92:1087-1187. DOI: 10.1152/physrev.00032.2011

[6] Monti JM. Serotonin control of sleep-wake behavior. Sleep Medicine Reviews. 2011;15:269-281. DOI: 10.1016/j.smrv.2010.11.003

[7] Sakai K. Sleep-waking discharge profiles of dorsal raphe nucleus neurons in mice. Neuroscience. 2011;197:200-224. DOI: 10.1016/j.neuroscience.2011.09.024

[8] Carr GV, Lucki I. The role of serotonin receptor subtypes in treating depression: a review of animal studies. Psychopharmacology. 2011;213:265-287. DOI 10.1007/s00213-010-2097-z

[9] Datta S, MacLean RR. Neurobiological mechanisms for the regulation of mammalian sleep–wake behavior: Reinterpretation of historical evidence and inclusion of contemporary cellular and molecular evidence. Neuroscience and Biobehavioral Reviews. 2007;31:775-824.

[10] Kovalzon VM. Ascending reticular activating system of the brain. Transl. Neurosci. Clin. 2016;2(4):275-285. DOI: 10.18679/CN11-6030/R.2016.034

[11] Mosienko V, Bader M, Alenina N. The serotonin-free brain: behavioral consequences of Tph2 deficiency in animal models. In: Müller CP, Cunningham KA, editors. Handbook of the Behavioral Neurobiology of Serotonin. 2nd ed. London: Elsevier; 2020, p.601-607. DOI: 10.1016/B978-0-444-64125-0.00035-9

[12] Mosienko V, Beis D, Pasqualetti M, Waider J, Matthes S, Qadri F, Bader M, Alenina N. Life without brain serotonin: Reevaluation of serotonin function with mice deficient in brain serotonin synthesis. Behavioural Brain Research. 2015;277:78-88. DOI: 10.1016/j.bbr.2014.06.005

[13] Alenina N, Kikic D, Todiras M, Mosienko V, Qadri F, Plehm R, Boye P, Vilianovitch L, Sohr R, Tenner K, Hortnagl H, Bader M. Growth retardation and altered autonomic control in mice lacking brain serotonin. PNAS. 2009;106(25):10332-10337. DOI: 10.1073/pnas.0810793106

[14] Solarewicz JZ, Angoa-Perez M, Kuhn DM, Mateika JH. The sleep-wake cycle and motor activity, but not temperature, are disrupted over the light-dark cycle in mice genetically depleted of serotonin. Am. J. Physiol. Regul. Integr. Comp. Physiol. 2015;308:R10–R17. DOI: 10.1152/ajpregu.00400.2014

[15] Whitney MS, Shemery AM, Yaw AM, Donovan LJ, Glass JD, Deneris ES. Adult brain serotonin deficiency causes hyperactivity, circadian disruption, and elimination of siestas. The Journal of Neuroscience. 2016;36(38):9828-9842. DOI: 10.1523/JNEUROSCI.1469-16.2016

[16] Iwasaki K, Komiya H, Kakizaki M, Miyoshi C, Abe M, Sakimura K, Funato H, Yanagisawa M. Ablation of central serotonergic neurons decreased REM sleep and attenuated arousal response. Front. Neurosci. 2018;12:535. DOI: 10.3389/fnins.2018.00535

[17] Venner A, Broadhurst RY, Sohn LT, Todd WD, Fuller PM. Selective activation of serotoninergic dorsal raphe neurons facilitates sleep through anxiolysis. Sleep. 2020;43(2):1-12. DOI: 10.1093/sleep/zsz231

[18] Blumberg MS, Lesku JA, Libourel P-A, Schmidt MH., Rattenborg NC. What is REM sleep? Current Biology. 2020; 30:R38–R49. DOI:10.1016/j.cub.2019.11.045

[19] Lyamin OI, Kibalnikov AS, Siegel JM. Sleep in ostrich chicks (*Struthio camelus*). Sleep. 2020; 1-14. DOI: 10.1093/sleep/zsaa259

[20] Berger M, van Calker D, Riemann D. Sleep and manipulations of the sleep–wake rhythm in depression. Acta Psychiatr. Scand. 2003:108(Suppl. 418):83-91.

[21] Campbell SS, Zulley J. Napping in time-free environments. In: Dinges DF, Broughton RJ, editors. Sleep and Alertness: Chronobiological, Behavioral, and Medical Aspects of Napping. N.Y.: Raven Press; 1989, p. 121-138.

[22] Yetish G, Kaplan H, Gurven M, Wood B, Pontzer H, Manger PR, Wilson C, McGregor R, Siegel JM. Natural sleep and its seasonal variations in three pre-industrial societies. Current Biology. 2015;25:2862-2868. DOI: 10.1016/j.cub.2015.09.046

[23] Shaffery J, Hoffmann R, Armitage R. The neurobiology of depression: Perspectives from animal and human sleep studies. Neuroscientist. 2003;9(1):82-98. DOI: 10.1177/1073858402239594

[24] D'Ambrosio S, Castelnovo A, Guglielmi O, Nobili L, Sarasso S, Garbarino S. Sleepiness as a local phenomenon. Front. Neurosci. 2019;13:1086. DOI: 10.3389/fnins.2019.01086

[25] Carskadon MA, Dement WC. Normal human sleep: an overview. In: Kryger M, Roth T, Dement WC, editors. Principles and Practice of Sleep Medicine. 6th edition. Philadelphia, PA: Elsevier; 2017. p.15-24.

[26] Banks S, Dorrian J, Basner M, Dinges DF. Sleep deprivation. In: Kryger M, Roth T, Dement WC, editors. Principles and Practice of Sleep Medicine. 6th edition. Philadelphia, PA: Elsevier; 2017.p. 49-54.

[27] Albert PR, Benkelfat C. The neurobiology of depression — revisiting the serotonin hypothesis. II. Genetic, epigenetic and clinical studies. Phil. Trans. R. Soc. B. 2013;368:20120535. DOI: 10.1098/rstb.2012.0535

[28] Albert PR, Benkelfat C, Descarries L. The neurobiology of depression — revisiting the serotonin hypothesis. I. Cellular and molecular mechanisms. Phil. Trans. R. Soc. B. 2012;367:2378-2381. DOI: 10.1098/rstb.2012.0190

[29] Lapin IP, Oxenkrug GF. Intensification of the central serotoninergic processes as a possible determinant of the thymoleptic effect. Lancet. 1969;293(7586):132-136. DOI: 10.1016/S0140-6736(69)91140-4

[30] Oxenkrug GF. This week's citation classic. Current Contents. 1987;2:16.

[31] Lapin IP. Neurokynurenines (NEKY) as common neurochemical links of stress and anxiety. Adv. Exp. Med. Biol. 2003;527:121-125.

[32] Oxenkrug GF. Serotonin – kynurenine hypothesis of

depression: historical overview and recent developments. Curr. Drug Targets. 2013;14(5):514-521. DOI: 10.2174/1389450111314050002

[33] Oxenkrug GF. Tryptophan–kynurenine metabolism as a common mediator of genetic and environmental impacts in major depressive disorder: The serotonin hypothesis revisited 40 years later. Isr. J. Psychiatry Relat. Sci. 2010;47(1):56-63.

[34] Maes M, Leonard BE, Myint AM, Kubera M, Verkerk R. The new '5-HT' hypothesis of depression: Cell-mediated immune activation induces indoleamine 2,3-dioxygenase, which leads to lower plasma tryptophan and an increased synthesis of detrimental tryptophan catabolites (TRYCATs), both of which contribute to the onset of depression. Progress in Neuro-Psychopharmacology & Biological Psychiatry. 2011;35:702-721. DOI: 10.1016/j.pnpbp.2010.12.017

[35] Savitz J. The kynurenine pathway: a finger in every pie. Molecular Psychiatry. 2019; DOI: 10.1038/s41380-019-0414-4

[36] Troubat R, Barone P, Leman S, Desmidt T, Cressant A, Atanasova B, Brizard B, El Hage W, Surget A, Belzung C, Camus V. Neuroinflammation and depression: a review. European Journal of Neuroscience. 2020; DOI: 10.1111/ejn.14720

[37] Palagini L, Baglioni C, Ciapparelli A, Gemignani A, Riemann D. REM sleep dysregulation in depression: State of the art. Sleep Med. Rev. 2013;17:377-390. DOI: 10.1016/j.smrv.2012.11.001

[38] Riemann D, Krone LB, Wulff K, Nissen C. Sleep, insomnia, and depression. Neuropsychopharmacology. 2020;45:74-89. DOI:10.1038/s41386-019-0411-y

[39] Fang H, Tu S, Sheng J, Shao A. Depression in sleep disturbance: A review on a bidirectional relationship, mechanisms and treatment. J. Cell. Mol. Med. 2019;23:2324-2332. DOI: 10.1111/jcmm.14170

[40] Ashcroft GW, Sharman DF. 5-Hydroxyindoles in human cerebrospinal fluids. Nature. 1960;186:1050-1051. DOI: 10.1038/1861050a0

[41] Baumeister AA, Hawkins MF, Uzelac SM. The myth of reserpine-induced depression: role in the historical development of the monoamine hypothesis. Journal of the History of the Neurosciences: Basic and Clinical Perspectives. 2003;12(2):207-220. DOI: 10.1076/jhin.12.2.207.15535

[42] Cowen PJ. Serotonin and depression: pathophysiological mechanism or marketing myth? Trends in Pharmacological Sciences. 2008;29(9):433-436. DOI: 10.1016/j.tips.2008.05.004

[43] Andrews PW, Bharwani A, Lee KR, Fox M, Thomson JA, Jr. Is serotonin an upper or a downer? The evolution of the serotonergic system and its role in depression and the antidepressant response. Neuroscience and Biobehavioral Reviews. 2015;51:164-188. DOI: 10.1016/j.neubiorev.2015.01.018

[44] Healy D. Serotonin and depression. The marketing of a myth. British Medical Journal. 2015;350:h1771 DOI: 10.1136/bmj.h1771

[45] van Dalfsen JH, Markus CR. The involvement of sleep in the relationship between the serotonin transporter gene-linked polymorphic region (5-HTTLPR) and depression: A systematic review. Journal of Affective Disorders. 2019;256:205-212. DOI: 10.1016/j.jad.2019.05.047

[46] Hasler G. Pathophysiology of depression: do we have any solid

evidence of interest to clinicians? World Psychiatry. 2010;9:155-161.

[47] Cline BH, Costa-Nunes JP, Cespuglio R, Markova N, Santos AI, Bukhman YV, Kubatiev A, Steinbusch HWM, Lesch K-P, Strekalova T. Dicholine succinate, the neuronal insulin sensitizer, normalizes behavior, REM sleep, hippocampal pGSK3 beta and mRNAs of NMDA receptor subunits in mouse models of depression. Frontiers in Behavioral Neuroscience. 2015; 9:37. DOI:10.3389/fnbeh.2015.00037

[48] Siegel JM. The REM sleep–memory consolidation hypothesis. Science. 2001;294:1058-1063.

[49] Siegel JM. The incredible shrinking sleep-learning connection. Behavioral and Brain Sciences. 2005;28:82-83.

[50] Vertes RP. Memory consolidation in sleep: dream or reality. Neuron. 2004;44:135-148.

[51] Vertes RP, Eastman K.E. The case against memory consolidation in REM sleep. Behavioral and Brain Sciences. 2000;23:793-1121.

[52] Strekalova T, Cespuglio R, Kovalzon V. Sleep structure during chronic stress and anhedonia in the mouse model of depression. In: Kalueff AV, LaPorte JL, editors. Experimental Animal Models in Neurobehavioral Research. Nova Science Publishers: N.Y.; 2009. p. 123-137.

Chapter 3

Roles of the Serotoninergic System in Coping with Traumatic Stress

Tania Vitalis and Catherine Verney

Abstract

Post-Traumatic Stress Disorder (PTSD) is characterized by substantial physiological and/or psychological distress following exposure to trauma. Intrusive fear memories often lead to persistent avoidance of stimuli associated with the trauma, detachment from others, irritability and sleep disturbances. Different key structures in the brain are involved with fear conditioning, fear extinction and coping. The limbic system, namely, the amygdala complex in close relationship with the hippocampal hub and the prefrontal cortex play central roles in the integration and in coping with fear memories. Serotonin acting both as a neurotransmitter and as a neurohormone participates in regulating the normal and pathological activity of these anatomic structures. We review the literature analyzing how the different actors of the serotoninergic system (5-HT receptors, transporters and anabolic and catabolic pathways) may be involved in regulating the sensitivity to highly stressful events and hopefully coping with them.

Keywords: 5-HT, 5-HT receptors, amygdala, hippocampus, limbic structures, PTSD, prefrontal cortex, SERT

1. Introduction

Following exposure to traumatic events as a succession of inescapable stressful stimuli or life-threatening accidents, most people adapt and cope with the stress and return to their normal life when the stressful event (s) has (ve) stopped. However a minority of them, 6-8% of people [1, 2] develop PTSD characterized by a variety of symptoms precisely defined by "the American Psychiatric Association's Diagnostic and Statistical manual of Mental Disorders" [3]. It includes intrusive memories of the traumatic event, nightmares, irritability, sleep impairment, attention deficit and/or emotional withdrawal. Post-traumatic stress disorder is often associated with several comorbidities such as inflammation [4], chronic pain and heightened risk of neurodegenerative disease. This disorder is more often than we believe difficult to treat as many patients suffer from it during several years after the traumatic event has stopped. For instance, 40 years after the Vietnam War, 11% of the veterans still experienced PTSD [5]. This disorder is primarily due to an overload of traumatic sensory stimuli inducing continuous overproduction of cortisol in the brain and body [6] generating secondary cascades of deregulations that prevent a return to the original homeostatic biological state by the parasympathetic brake, essential for the patient [6–8]. These biological impairments lead to the anchoring of fear memories in the limbic cerebral circuits which include primarily the amygdala complex (AMY) handling the emotional processing related to stress associated with memory processing of the hippocampal-cortical circuits [6, 9, 10].

The fact that a minority of people undergoing traumatic events don't recover and develop long-lasting PTSD suggests that among the population different genetic/epigenetic predispositions unique for each individual impact the way patients are able to cope or not with stressful events [6]. Impairments of the limbic circuitry and activity are among the key features explaining various PTSD symptoms. Numerous examples have shown that the serotoninergic system is well positioned to modulate the activity of the amygdalo-hippocampal-prefrontal hub. The serotoninergic system is widely known to play a critical role in mood regulation and it is not surprising that different pharmacological treatments initially proposed to relieve PTSD symptoms modulate serotoninergic systems [11–14]. Among them serotonin reuptake inhibitors (SSRIs; i.e. citalopram, escitalopram, fluoxetine, fluvoxamine, paroxetine, and sertraline) causing high extracellular 5-HT levels are classically used for their anxiolytic effects and treatment of depression and for their relative minor side effects [12–15].

We will review how the limbic system is modulated by changes in 5-HT homeostasis by acting through 5-HT transporter or receptors during development and in adults.

We analyze knowledge obtained from relevant adult rodent models and extend them to human data when possible. Indeed, rodent models, appear useful for understanding the etiology of PTSD, as the "fear circuitry" and the endocrine responses to stress are fairly conserved across species. However, they lack the complexity of the cognitive treatment mediated by highly developed cortical circuits observed in primates [6, 16–18]. We will also review literature clearly demonstrating that imbalance in the serotonergic system during development associated or not with genetic alterations may modify the way patients are able to cope with stressful events.

2. Anatomy and physiology of limbic circuits implicated in the stress response

Regardless of its intensity, stress induces primarily stimulation of the Hypothalamic-Pituitary-Adrenal (HPA) axis that coordinates the body-brain biological response through a highly regulated neurohormonal cascade. Corticotrophin releasing hormone (CRH) or factor (CRF) is released from hypothalamic neurons, letting adrenocorticotropic hormone (ACTH) out of pituitary cells, which in turn stimulates the secretion of cortisol (CORT) into the bloodstream by the adrenal cortex. Cortisol activates glucocorticoid receptors (GR) that are widely distributed in the brain, mainly along the HPA axis itself and in major limbic structures such as the amygdala complex (AMY), the hippocampal formation (HIP) and the prefrontal cortex (PFC). When the stress is qualified as « adaptive », activation of hypothalamic GR decreases HPA axis activity, creating a negative feedback loop leading to corticoid levels returning to normal with the stress responses turned off [6–8, 19]. In parallel the HPA axis interacts with the limbic structures afore mentioned which in turn participate to the feedback inhibition and feed-forward stimulation of the HPA axis that regulate stress responses [20–22]. When stressful events are perceived as particularly severe and/or persistent, the stressors can cause long-lasting changes in active stimulation of the HPA axis modifying the "body-brain" responses to CORT and CRH. In this context, corticoids flowing continuously in the brain and the body generate long lasting modifications/alterations of the limbic and cortical circuits contributing to induce a large array of PTSD symptoms [6–8] (**Figure 1**).

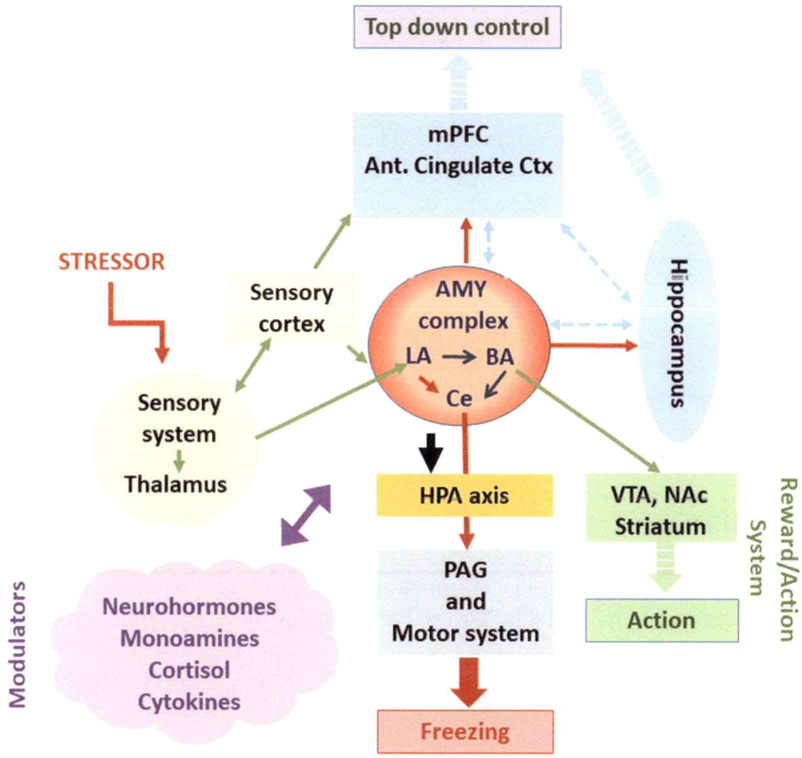

Figure 1.
The « reward/action » versus the « fear/inhibitory » circuits. Following a threat (stressor), sensory information arising from sensory stimuli is conveyed to the thalamus (light green) that relays information to the lateral amygdala (LA) of the amydgala complex (AMY; orange). The amygdala, in concert with the hippocampal and cortical memory circuits (blue), attributes an emotional valence to the stressor. When adaptive behaviour is possible, the basal nucleus (BA) of the amygdala complex is activated leading to stimulation of the « reward/action » systems (dark green) that includes the ventral tegmental area (VTA), the accumbens nucleus and the striatum. Action is also modulated by cognitive prefrontal circuits. If the threat is inescapable the central amygdala (CE) is activated, inducing an inhibition of the motor system (gray) and freezing behaviour (red). In parallel, the hypothalamus-pituitary-adrenal axis (HPA axis; yellow) induces a surge of neurohormones leading to the liberation of cortisol/corticosterone (violet) in the brain and body. When adaptive behaviour is possible and efficient, cortisol/corticosterone return to normal levels. If the stressor is too strong, HPA axis retrocontrol is blunted and cortisol production continues. In addition, inflammatory cytokines are released. Cortisol damages the prefrontal cortex and hippocampus that become hypotrophic. AMY is by contrast hypersollicitated and increased synaptic complexity of glutamatergic neurons induces its hypertrophy. Monoamines, including serotonin, that send axons in almost every brain regions mentioned are potent modulators (violet) of the reward/action and fear/freezing circuits.

The amygdala complex is considered as "a hub" of cerebral emotional processing, receiving inputs from sensory areas (including sensory thalamus), autonomic system, HIP and cortical regions such as the infra-limbic (IL) prefrontal cortex. By « computing » information stored in the HIP and cortical structures, AMY attributes an emotional valence to the event and plays a crucial role in fear learning and extinction [10, 23, 24]. In patients suffering PTSD, exaggerated responses to emotional stimuli induce hyperactivation of AMY, which become hypertrophic by the increased complexity of their glutamatergic neurons [6, 25]. Then in PTSD, the different subnuclei of AMY are modified in their connections and their complex regulation of inhibitory GABA neurons network. The basolateral nucleus (BLA) that receives sensory information stimulates abnormally the central nucleus (CE), which regulates the output of fear behavior [10, 26–28]. Different Pavlovian rodent models analyzed the neural basis for encoding association of two stimuli, a neutral stimulus (a sound, a light) and a painful stimulus (a footshock). They revealed that the lateral nucleus of the amygdala (LA) receives inputs of both stimuli, conveyed information to the basal nucleus (BA), then to the output CE which coordinates the expression of defensive behaviors such as freezing [29–31]. Recently, it was suggested that the BA may not be implicated in the defensive behavior but rather in avoidance [32]. The extended amygdala as the bed nucleus of the stria terminalis (BNST) is also largely implicated in anxiety [10, 26, 28] and its role will be developed later. The reciprocal connections of AMY with HIP and PFC, in particular IL cortex (in rodents) that participate in the inhibition of learned fears are defective in PTSD patients leading to the persistence of fearful memories and other emotional symptoms [24].

The HIP is known to play a critical role in learning and memory integrating contextual information to regulate behavior (Reviewed by [33]). In PTSD, it mediates memory-related problems including persistent re-experiencing of traumatic events and impaired context-dependent modulation of memory as well as increased salience of negative emotional memories deficits in working and verbal memory [6, 34]. Studies in rats have shown that the dorsal HIP (homologous to the human posterior HIP) is mostly associated with cognitive performance while the ventral HIP (homologous to the human anterior HIP) rather participates in the regulation of stress response and affect [35]. Hippocampal volume is reduced in individuals with PTSD compared to controls. The HIP morphology is highly plastic and size reduction could indicate predisposition for PTSD while increase in volume may underlie positive responses to treatment. The HIP reciprocal connections to other brain areas are critical in these regulations; importantly, the HIP interacts with the AMY to regulate emotional arousal and consolidation of fear memories (as previously mentioned [10, 27, 36] and with the PFC to regulate memory [37].

The prefrontal part (PFC) of the frontal lobe plays essential roles in attention, working memory, decision-making and regulation of emotion [38]. Its role is crucial for PTSD patients in the regulation of fear, learning, expression, and extinction [39]. Interestingly the anterior cingulate cortex (ACC) and the medial PFC (mPFC) display abnormal levels of activation in PTSD patients [40]. The human ventromedial PFC (vmPFC; analogous to the IL cortex in rodents) plays a key role in the extinction of fearful memories by processing "safety signals" and interacting with the AMY to inhibit fear expression [41]. In PTSD patients, impaired vmPFC activation leads to altered emotional processing and impaired retention of fear extinction learning. Other cortical structures such as the insular cortex (visceral regulation) intervene in the emotional processing and interoception that are altered in PTSD patients.

Going back to everyday life stress regulation, the response to an adaptive stress involves motivation and action giving rise to pleasure by activation of *reward circuit* or *strengthening/operant conditioning circuit* (as salivation in the Pavlovian conditioned dogs) present in most vertebrate species. Following a stress the dopaminergic neurons of ventral tegmental area (VTA) projecting towards limbic areas (the medial PFC, the AMY and the accumbens) "integrate" the emotional/pleasure valence linked to this event [42, 43]. When the stressor is adaptive, dopaminergic neurons of VTA and the accumbens are activated by different brain structures in particular AMY generating escape as adaptive behavior. When the stressor is too strong, the VTA-reward/action system becomes less efficient. When the stressor happens to be severe and/or permanent, the adaptive behavior VTA-reward/action system is decreased/abolished and the adaptive "way out" motor system is inhibited [44]. Interestingly, the activity of VTA neurons could be modulated by the noradrenergic and serotoninergic neurons. A small subset of the noradrenergic locus coeruleus (LC) neurons could activate VTA, playing therefore a role in resiliency to stress [45]. Similarly, several studies have shown that dorsal raphe serotoninergic neurons could modulate the activity of VTA neurons. Recently, it was shown using optogenic tools coupling to behavioral tests, that stimulation of dorsal raphe neurons induces reward seeking in mice. Moreover, this behavior was abolished by the specific inhibition of 5-HT-containing axons reaching the VTA and induces conditioned place aversion [46]. Depending on the targets reached by serotoninergic neurons their activation may lead to various and sometimes opposite roles in behavior [47]. We will discuss these recent findings in section 4.

3. Lay-out of the 5-HT system

3.1 Serotonin synthesis, storage and degradation

Serotonin is synthesized from the essential amino-acid L-tryptophan. In the blood stream, L-tryptophan is linked to serum-albumin but a free proportion that decreases with age and physiological status freely crosses the BBB (10% at postnatal day 12 when BBB is thought fully functional in rat [48]). In 5-HT-producing cells, tryptophan is then transported, accumulated and hydroxylated by the tryptophan hydroxylase (Tph) enzymes. Tryptophan hydroxylase type 2 (Tph2) is expressed in serotoninergic neurons of the raphe nuclei and myenteric neurons [49, 50] while Tph1 is expressed in the gut enterochromaffin cells, the pineal gland and various peripheral tissues [51, 52] and possibly in the placenta depending on the species [53]. 5-hydroxytryptophan is then further decarboxylated into 5-HT by the aromatic amino-acid decarboxylase (AADC). It has been shown that the availability of tryptophan to synthesize 5-HT depends on the inflammatory status of the organism. Interestingly, patients suffering PTSD develop a pro-inflammatory status with increased circulating pro-inflammatory cytokines [6]. Indoleamine 2,3-dioxygenase (IDO) is generated following inflammation and can lead to 5-HT depletion in the organism [54]. Such a state may impact the levels of 5-HT in PTSD patients and favor the emergence of depressive-like status.

5-HT producing cells express the SERT and vesicular monoamine transporter type 2 (VMAT2) allowing respectively 5-HT uptake and storage in those cells [55]. In the CNS these transporters regulate the level of 5-HT, not only at the synaptic cleft, but also when 5-HT is release along 5-HT-containing (5-HT+) axons in a « volume-transmission » manner [56]. The use of SSRIs have been used for treatment of PTSD symptoms [6]. In various rodent models, SSRIs were shown to relieve some of the PTSD-like symptoms (reviewed in [57]). Indeed, administration of SSRIs or ketamine ameliorate PTSD-like behavioral deficits in restraint paired forced swimming test (or other stressors) [58]. These models are attempting to reproduce unpredictable stress as those observed by soldiers experiencing war zones [59–61]. Similarly, exposure to a predator induces hyperarousal, avoidance and fear, [62–64] increases anxiety-like behavior and reduces fear extinction. In these models, animals also respond to sertraline reducing anxiety-like behavior and cue avoidance [65, 66]. Interestingly, SSRI treatment appears efficient only when administered chronically, at least for 3-6 month in patients. Initially depressive symptoms worsen by 5-HT increase activating the inhibitory 5-HT_1 autoreceptors in the raphe nuclei, before they get desensitized following chronic treatment. Alternatively, the delayed therapeutic effects of SSRIs may be due to neuroplastic changes that need time to develop in mature brain [62, 67].

5-HT is catabolized by monoamine oxidases A or B (MAOA or MAOB; located in the mitochondria and by catechol-O-methyltransferase (COMT) [68, 69]. MAOA has higher affinity for 5-HT than MAOB and is co-expressed with MAOB in rodent serotoninergic neurons [70]. MAOs are also expressed by many non-aminergic structures, in particular MAOB is expressed in glial cells throughout the brain [71] and our unpublished results). MAOA mRNA has been detected in the deep layers of the rodent prefrontal cortex [72]. MAOs may thus regulate the amount of 5-HT locally, throughout the brain and in the peripheral tissues where they are also expressed [70, 71]. Interestingly, MAOs expression and protein synthesis are tightly regulated and have been shown to be sensitive to environmental factors such as inflammation [73] and stress. Indeed, glucocorticoids increase MAOA in the brain through the stimulation of the Kruppel-like factor11 and cell-division associated 7-Like protein pathways [74]. Animals under chronic stress show increased MAOA and 5-HIAA/5-HT ratio suggesting a higher 5-HT turnover levels [75]. MAOA inhibitors have been shown to reverse the decreased neurogenesis and dendritic plasticity in the hippocampus of chronically stressed rats [76].

3.2 Transducing pathways

At least fourteen 5-HT receptor subtypes have been identified in the mammalian brain and periphery ([77–79]; see [80] for the latest classification). Isoform diversity, alternative splicing of some subtypes and RNA editing add to the complexity of serotoninergic receptor functions. With the exception of 5-HT_3 receptors, all 5-HT receptors are coupled to G-proteins. According to their second messenger coupling pathways, 5-HT receptors have been categorized into four groups. 5-HT_1 and 5-HT_5 receptors are coupled to Gi/Go proteins and exert their inhibitory effects on adenylate cyclase, inhibiting cAMP formation. Within the raphe nuclei, 5-HT_{1A} receptors are acting as autoreceptors inhibiting the release of 5-HT by serotoninergic neurons. After the start of SSRI treatment, they are proposed to be responsible for the initial worsening of depressive symptoms [13, 81]. 5-HT_2 receptors are coupled to Gq proteins and stimulate phospholipase C to increase the hydrolysis of inositol phosphates and elevate intracellular Ca^{2+}. 5-$HT_{4,6,7}$ receptors are coupled to Gs proteins and are positively linked to adenylate cyclase and increase cAMP formation. 5-HT_3 receptors are ligand-gated ion channel receptors and are a unique 5-HT receptor able to mediate fast response to neurotransmitter release [82]. It is generally admitted that, in the limbic structures 5-HT_{1A} receptors are mainly expressed by glutamatergic neurons. 5-HT_3 receptors are expressed by subtypes of interneurons expressing mainly the vasoactive intestinal peptide (VIP), cholecystokinin (CCK) or calretinin (CR) (but never expressing parvalbumin (PV) and rarely somatostatin (SOM)). 5-HT_2 receptors are expressed in both neuronal populations [83–85]. 5-HT_7 receptor expression has been shown in the deep layers of the rodent prefrontal cortex. For additional precision, see also [86].

4. Serotoninergic projections and modulation of limbic structures

4.1 Serotoninergic neurons and projections: focus on mature limbic systems

Different subsets of 5-HT+ neurons of brainstem raphe nuclei (average of 26 000 neurons in rodents) send diffuse axonal networks to specific brain areas throughout the brain. Pioneer studies using 5-HT or SERT Immunolabeling, coupled or not to retrograde tracing [87–89] provided a general description of these 5-HT projections towards numerous areas including the cerebral cortex. More recently, anterograde tracing (injection of adeno-associated viruses) in raphe nuclei of mice conditionally expressing the green fluorescent protein/channel rhodopsin under the control of the SERT or TPH2 promoter [47, 90, 91] have provided evidence that limbic structures receive 5-HT afferences from topographically organized subpopulations of dorsal DR (the largest 5-HT+ nuclei in rodent and primates) and median raphe nuclei (MnR). Using genetic activation of specific 5-HT+ projections, some studies allowed to correlate activation/inhibition of specific 5-HT+ subgroups/afferences to behaviour. Interestingly they revealed that DR and MnR 5-HT+ neurons should be apprehended as neuronal populations having the ability to release a large numbers of neurotransmitters and neuropeptides in addition to 5-HT [92, 93]. Such a diversity in subtypes, targeting and functions is already underlined by the complexity observed in 5-HT+ developmental programming (i.e. specification and axonal targeting; see [93, 94]).

As a whole, it is generally admitted that exposure to a severe/inescapable shock as in predator exposure, social defeat or other stress conditions [95] induces a surge of 5-HT in the vicinity of DR/MnR and in the corticolimbic structures such as the AMY, HIP and mPFC. Only a few studies have reported a decrease of serotoninergic activity following severe stressful situation. That may match with the genuine possibility of specific individual/strain to cope with stress [96]. Interestingly, around 80% of 5-HT+ neurons in the ventral portion of the DR (DRv) and MnR express the vesicular glutamate transporter type 3 (Vglut3) and send axons to AMY and HIP. These neurons can release 5-HT and/or glutamate and then modulate the activation of AMY and HIP [93, 94, 97]. Generally, low frequency stimulation (<10Hz) induces glutamate release resulting in fast excitation of the targeted neuron while higher frequency stimulations (10-20Hz) induce 5-HT release suggesting that these neurons could rapidly switch their neurotransmitter output depending on activation [97]. A subgroup of DR 5-HT+/Vglut3+ neurons projecting to the nucleus accumbens (NAc) and orbitofrontal cortex (OPFc) to specifically receive inputs and integrate information from "reward encoding regions" such as the ventral pallidum. Conversely, another group of DR 5-HT+/Vglut3+ neurons specifically receives inputs from the "fear encoding regions" (periacqueducal grey (PAG) and LC) and project to the BA. This last subpopulation appears to potentiate fear via the 5-HT_{1A} and 5-HT_{2A} receptor pathways and to impair fear extinction [98]. Interestingly, in rats some DRv 5-HT+/Vglut3+ neurons are sensitive to CRH released by the AMY that induces a decrease of TPH2 in them and ameliorates stress-induced anhedonia [99]. The level of TPH2 regulation by CRH could be the signature of a resilience status [99]. In the MnR 5-HT+/Vglut3+ neurons appear to integrate selectively negative events and may play a central role in depression-related mood disorders [100]. Subgroups of MnR 5-HT neurons express the type 2 CRH receptor. These examples illustrate the complexity of the 5-HT neuron-driven behaviors. Possible co-transmission based on gene expression suggests that DR and MnR 5-HT+ neurons could potentially also co-release GABA, dynorphin, galanin, cholecystokinin (CCK), nitric oxide (NO), CRH and other neuropeptides for which a role remains to be established (Reviewed in [93]).

4.2 The amygdala complex

Serotoninergic axonal projections to the AMY mainly arise from 5HT+ DR neurons while only rare axons arise from MnR. The 5-HT+ axonal density is strong in BA, moderate in LA, and moderate to low in CE, intercalated nuclei and BNST [87, 89, 91]. 5-HT axons target both glutamatergic principal neurons (PN, not interneurons) bearing 5-HT_{2C} receptors in LA and, 5-$HT_{2A}/_{1A}$ receptors in BA and a variety of GABAergic interneurons [101]. GABAergic interneurons expressing PV bear 5-HT_{2A}, receptors receive inputs from glutamatergic PN and project reciprocally on them and on somatostatin-expressing (SOM+) GABAergic neurons. 5-HT exerts most of its effects on PV+ GABAergic neurons that express the strongest levels of 5-HT_{2A} receptors and facilitate GABAergic inhibition. Following inescapable stress 5-HT_{2A}-receptor mediated facilitating actions are severely impaired. 5-HT_{2A} receptor-mRNA is downregulated following the surge of 5-HT in the AMY leading to hyperactivity of PN neurons [102]. Neuropeptide Y-containing (NPY+) (5-HT_{2C}+ and 5-HT_{1A}+ receptor) and CCK+ and VIP+ (5-HT_{3A}+receptor) also project on glutamatergic PN (**Figure 2** in [15]. Within the BA and LA the role of 5-HT_{3A} remains to be clarified. Glutamatergic principal neurons of LA and BA send numerous efferents to CE and to a lesser extent to BNST. These plastic efferent fields are sensitive to environmental conditions and in PTSD patients this could be

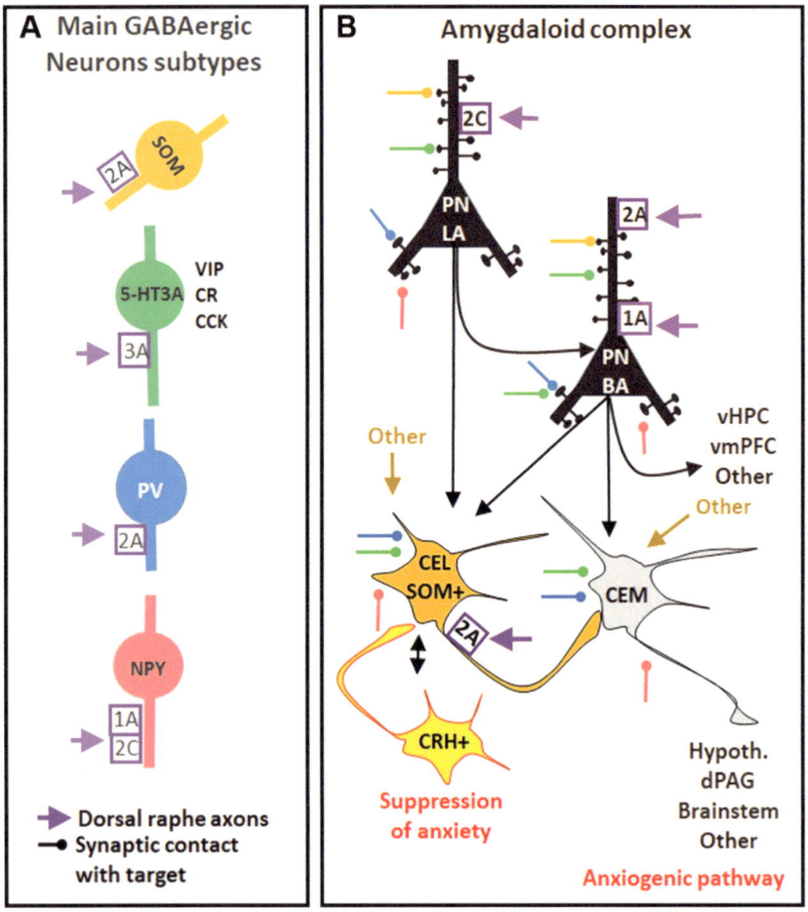

Figure 2.
The amygdala complex is modulated by serotonin via various 5-HT receptor expressions. A, The major GABAergic neuron subtypes modulating the function of the amygdala complex are represented in the left panel. They could be subdivided into four main classes: the somatostatin-containing (SOM; orange), the 5-HT_{3A}-expressing (5-HT_{3A}; green), the parvalbumin-containing (PV; bleu) and the neuropeptide Y-containing (NPY; pink). The 5-HT_{3A}-expressing GABAergic neurons could be further subdivided into three classes: the vasoactive intestinal peptide-containing (VIP), the cholecystokinin-containing (CCK) and the calretinin-containing (CR) GABAergic neurons. Their activities are modulated by serotoninergic axons arising from the dorsal raphe nucleus (violet arrows). B, In the amygdala complex, the lateral amygdala (LA) glutamatergic neurons (principal neurons, PN; black) that receive thalamic inputs stimulate glutamatergic neurons (principal neurons; PN) of the basal complex (BA; black). These neuronal populations are modulated by 5-HT_{2A}/$_{2C}$ receptors and 5-HT_{1A} autoreceptors. Glutamatergic BA neurons send outputs to the ventral hippocampus (vHPC) and to the ventromedial prefrontal cortex (vmPFC). LA and BA stimulate neurons of the central amygdala (CE). The central amygdala (CE) is mainly composed of GABAergic neurons. Lateral CE (CEL) contains GABAergic projection neurons that express somatostatin (SOM+) and are modulated by 5-HT_{2A} receptors. These neurons send outputs to the medial CE (CEM) that drives the anxiogenic pathway. CEM modulates the periaqueducal gray (PAG) and brainstem to induce freezing behaviour. By contrast, CEL receives corticotropin-releasing factor inputs (CRF+; yellow) that suppresses anxiety-like behaviour and anxiogenic pathway. Cross-talk between CRF+ and CEL neurons are continuous (double headed arrow).

responsible for the increased sensitivity of CE and BNST [103, 104]. The lateral part of the CE (CEL) receives major inputs from BA and LA but also from ventral HIP or sensory regions. CE is mainly populated by GABAergic interneurons. When avoidance of stressful stimulus is possible CRH+ GABAergic neurons are activated and SOM+ GABAergic projection neurons are inhibited [105]. Following fear conditioning, SOM+ GABAergic projection neurons disinhibiting the medial part of the CE (CEM) allowed a range of defensive behaviour as freezing [105–107] and fear recall [108]. Direct cross-talk between CRH+ and SOM+ neuronal populations allow the specific appropriate action [105].

Interestingly, 5-HT_{2A} receptors are expressed by SOM+ neurons of the CEL and the selective 5-HT_{2A} receptor inactivation in CEL increases innate freezing behaviour but decreases learned freezing induced by predator odor. Innate freezing behaviour and risk assessment are processed by the dorsal PAG while learned freezing is processed by the ventral PAG. These data suggest that 5-HT_{2A} receptor control innate freezing behaviour by the AMY-hypothalamus-dPAG pathway [109, 110]. As innate and acquired fears are controlled by antagonistic mechanisms, drugs that treat one type of fear could worsen the other one, leading to paradoxical results. Risperidon is largely used to treat various psychiatric disorders including PTSD. Although its main therapeutic target acts by antagonizing dopamine-D2 receptors, it is also targeting 5-HT_2 and therefore should be used carefully.

The activity of the bed nucleus of the stria terminalis (BNST) is correlated with fear mediated by uncertain threats [111]. It integrates fear, reward and stress-related circuits. BNST receives inputs from various limbic structures including BA and CE. The BNST displays a rich array of 5-HT receptors which define the three cell types I-III identified in this structure [112]. The 5-HT_{1A} receptor is the most abundant in BNST and the global effect of increased 5-HT in the BNST is a hyperpolarization of type I BNST neurons [113, 114]. Such hyperpolarization is associated with suppression of anxiety [115]. By contrast, type III cells express 5-HT_{2C} receptors and CRH and send outputs to the same hypothalamic and brainstem targets to which the CE projects and stimulate the anxiogenic pathway [116]. 5-HT_{2C} receptor-mRNA splicing/editing that leads to overexpression of 5-HT_{2C} receptors enhances anxiety and innate fear behaviour [117]. Specific 5-HT_{2C} receptor antagonists are now considered as possible compounds to treat anxiety disorders including PTSD as they relieve anxiety symptoms in patients and are well tolerated [118]. Interestingly, high-frequency BLA stimulations in rat models of anxiety or PTSD reduce anxiety-like behaviour following exposure to predator odor. These results can be compared to those observed after deep brain stimulation in humans [119].

4.3 The hippocampal formation

A dense serotoninergic innervation from the MnR is present in the hippocampus proper and has a powerful modulatory influence on hippocampal functions and memory formation [120]. In the CA1-CA3 hippocampal fields, stimulation of serotoninergic axons potentiates excitatory synapses and has positive effects on spatial memory processing in the dorsal hippocampus. Conversely, optogenetic silencing of CA1 5-HT terminals within the dorsal hippocampus inhibits spatial memory. Systemic modulation of 5-HT_4 receptor function can impact memory formation. PTSD patients display memory deficits in encoding and retrieval as well as in extinction learning such as fear extinction. In these patients, the hippocampal volume is smaller [121]. This is a consequence of the damage caused by the continuous release of cortisol associated with an increase of glutamate release (**Figure 3**).

MnR also sends axons to the ventral part of the hippocampus that is more specifically involved in anxiety-related disorders. Indeed, rats infused bilaterally

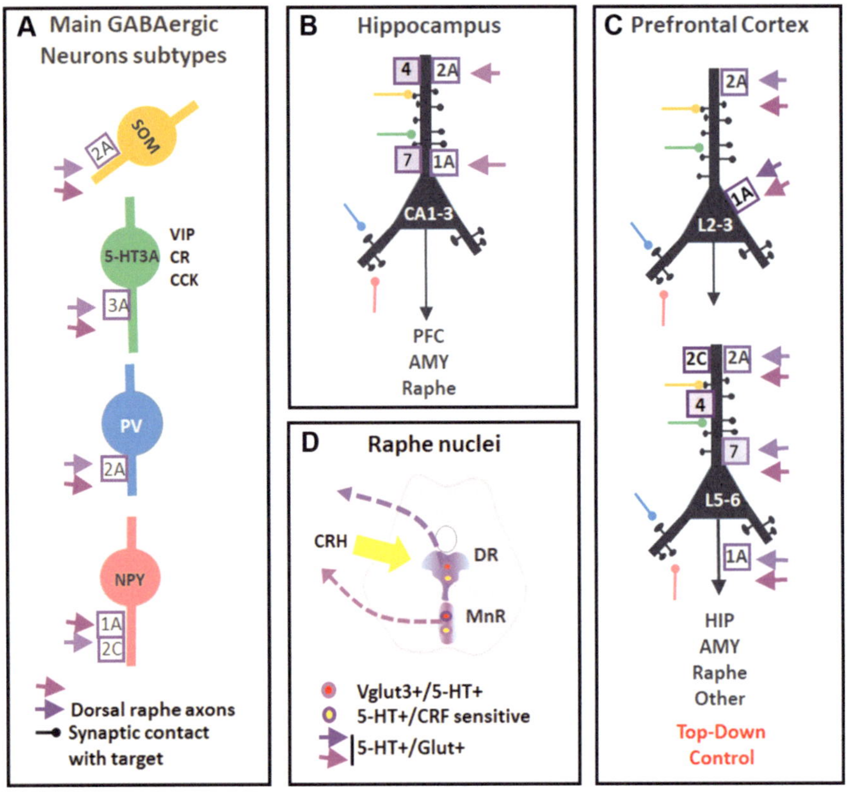

Figure 3.
The hippocampus and the medial prefrontal cortex are modulated by serotonin via various 5-HT receptors. A. The major GABAergic neuron subtypes modulating the function of the hippocampus and the medial prefrontal cortex are represented in the left panel. They could be subdivided into four main classes: the somatostatin-containing (SOM; orange), the 5-HT$_{3A}$-expressing (5-HT$_{3A}$; green), the parvalbumin-containing (PV; bleu) and the neuropeptide Y-containing (NPY; pink). The 5-HT$_{3A}$-expressing GABAergic neurons could be further subdivided into three classes: the vasoactive intestinal peptide-containing (VIP), the cholecystokinin-containing (CCK) and the calretinin-containing (CR) GABAergic neurons. Their activities are modulated by serotoninergic axons arising from the dorsal (violet arrows) and median (MnR) raphe nuclei (purple arrows). B, The CA1-CA3 hippocampal neurons express 5-HT$_{2A,4,7}$ receptors and 5-HT$_{1A}$ autoreceptors, they send axonal projections to the prefrontal cortex (mPFC), amygdala and the raphe. C, The prefrontal pyramidal glutamatergic neurons express 5-HT$_{2A,2C,4}$ receptors and 5-HT$_{1A}$ autoreceptors. In addition 5-HT$_7$ receptors are transiently expressed in layer 5-6 (L5-6) pyramidal neurons. The mPFC send axons to the hippocampus with which its activity is synchronized and to the amygdala and raphe nuclei. D, The dorsal (violet) and/or medial (purple) raphe nuclei send axons to the different structures mentioned above. A large number of raphe neurons located in the medial dorsal raphe (DR) and in the medial raphe (MnR) contain 5-HT and express the vesicular glutamate transporter type 3 (Vglut3; red dots in raphe). Some raphe neurons are sensitive to the corticotropin-releasing hormone (CRH; yellow).

with 5,7-dihydroxytryptamine (that induces a drastic reduction (80%) of 5-HT levels in the structure) in the ventral hippocampus spend less time in the open arm of an elevated plus maze. This suggests that reducing 5-HT level in the ventral hippocampus increases anxiety-like behavior [122]. In the same line of evidence, a rat strain selected for high levels of anxiety displayed reduced stress-induced 5-HT activation [123]. Increased anxiety-like behavior has been associated with decreased 5-HT$_{1A}$ receptor numbers in the ventral hippocampus [124] while reduced anxiety-like behavior has been reported to be associated with global overexpression of 5-HT$_{1A}$ receptors [125]. 5-HT$_2$ receptors are expressed in both glutamatergic and GABAergic neurons of the hippocampus. 5-HT$_2$ receptors modulate 5-HT-induced outward currents in hippocampal pyramidal neurons and facilitate GABAergic transmission [85]. The precise roles of hippocampal 5-HT$_2$ receptors in the control of anxiety-like phenotype remains to be investigated.

The modulation of 5-HT_7 receptors appears promising for the treatment of PTSD. 5-HT_7 receptors are expressed by CA3 neurons and activation of 5-HT_7 receptors hyperpolarizes these neurons and induces freezing. By contrast, infusion of 5-HT_7 antagonists in the ventral hippocampus decreases freezing behaviour induced by contextual fear conditioning [126, 127]. Since blockade of MnR 5-HT+/CRH2+ neurons reverse the effect mediated by 5-HT released in the ventral hippocampus, it has been speculated that 5-HT_7+ CA3 neurons would receive specific 5-HT+/CRH2+ inputs [127]. 5-HT_7 receptor antagonists are already used for the treatment of colonic intestinal symptoms and could be safely used for the treatment of fear-related disorders [128].

5-HT_4 receptor antagonists appear to modulate stress induced defecation but not freezing suggesting that this role may engage different sub-circuits [127]. 5-HT_4 receptor agonists may act rapidly and reduce immobility in forced swimming test, decrease sucrose intake following chronic mild stress and have been shown to display antidepressant potential. Drugs acting on 5-HT_4 receptors should be carefully considered and used depending on the level/type of stress induced by the trauma [129].

4.4 The prefrontal cortex

The serotoninergic system appears a potent regulator of the PFC circuitry acting through a variety of 5-HT receptors [85, 92, 130]. Throughout the rodent PFC, pyramidal neurons largely express 5-HT_{1A}, 5-HT_{2A} and 5-HT_{2c} receptors. Some pyramidal neurons co-express 5-HT_{1A}/5-HT_{2A} receptors [131] whereas 5-HT_{2A} and 5-HT_{2c} receptors are expressed by overlapping populations [132]. The 5-HT_{2A} receptor is more strongly expressed by layer 5 neurons [133–135]. 5-HT_4 receptors are expressed by PFC glutamatergic neurons [136] and pyramidal neurons of deep layers express transiently (P2-P14) 5-HT_7 receptors [137]. GABAergic interneurons express a large array of 5-HT receptors that mainly segregated in two subpopulations: 1/ the PV+ fast-spiking interneurons and the SOM+ interneurons both localized in deep cortical layers and expressing 5-HT_{1A} and 5-HT_{2A} receptors [130] and 2/the slow-spiking interneurons (VIP+, CR+) located in the superficial cortical layers and expressing 5-HT_{3A} receptors [83, 84, 138]. This variety of 5-HT receptor expression allows 5-HT to finely tune the excitability of pyramidal neurons, and therefore control the mPFC top-down exerted on other structures, such as the AMY, the HIP and raphe nuclei.

4.4.1 Prefrontal cortex and amygdala

The global effect of 5-HT application in vitro or the stimulation of endogenous 5-HT release in vivo in PFC is inhibitory and mediated by 5-HT_{1A} receptors. 5-HT_{1A} receptor stimulation (via LY341495) appears to play antidepressant role as shown by the reduction of the immobility time in 24h forced swim test which is partially reversed by infusion of the 5-HT_{1A} receptor antagonist WAY100635 in the mPFC [139]. Regulation of the GABAergic tone in the AMY (BLA) appears to be sensitive to mPFC top down-down control. 5-HT depletion in the mPFC increases expression of the immediate early gene c-fos in the BLA in the forced swimming test. It reduces GABA release induced by stress in the AMY [140, 141]. Moreover, unilateral 5-HT depletion in mPFC and infusion of an inhibitor of GABA synthesis into the contralateral BLA, selectively decrease immobility in the forced swimming test by inducing a “disconnection” between the PFC and the AMY [140].

The 5-HT_{2A} receptor is the major excitatory serotonin receptor in the brain. 5-HT_{2A} receptors have been implicated in mediating specific aspects of stress-induced responses. Indeed, stressful events as those induced by a six week isolation in rat, induces 5-HT_{2A} upregulation participating in anchoring the associative memory related to the stressful event [142, 143]. In humans, the density of 5-HT_{2A} receptors in the mPFC was negatively associated with reduced threat-related right AMY reactivity [144].

4.4.2 Medial prefrontal cortex and hippocampus

mPFC and HIP form a functional neural networks as their activities are highly synchronized. Specific oscillatory activities, detectable by EEG, correlate with specific behaviors [85] and may provide means for regulating neural communications. Synchronous firing between different neuronal populations should more efficiently in driving the firing of downstream neurons. Such process is important for complex cognitive tasks that require coordination of long-range networks across the brain. Interestingly, in humans transcranial stimulation or deep-brain stimulation in mPFC can assist major treatment-resistant depression probably by stimulating the afore-mentioned pathway [145].

4.4.3 Prefrontal cortex and raphe nuclei

PFC and raphe nuclei form a functional loop. PFC is reciprocally connected to both the DR and MnR [146] and exerts a top-down control on 5-HT neurons. Descending excitatory fibers from the PFC exert complex functional regulation of 5-HT neuronal activity with an overall inhibitory effect mediated by 5-HT_{1A} autoreceptors and feedforward inhibition [147, 148]. 5-HT_{2C} receptors, the targets of antidepressant (mirtazapine, agomelatine) and antipsychotic drugs are expressed by GABAergic interneurons of the PFC and may function in a negative feedback loop involving reciprocal interactions between GABAergic and serotonergic neurons [149]. 5-HT_4 and 5-HT_7 receptors also exert a top-down control on DR and MnR 5-HT+ neurons. 5-HT_4 receptor activation is associated with hypophagia induced by stress [150]. Selective activation of 5-HT_4 receptors in the PFC has been shown to induce modifications of SERT (dowregulation) and 5-HT_{1A} receptors and an increase in 5-HT release in the raphe [150]. 5-HT_7 receptors are transiently co-expressed with SERT in layers 5-6 neurons of mPFC during the P2-P14 period in mice, and modulate the development of mPFC neurons [137]. While SERT inhibition (SSRI treatment) during the P2-P14 period induces an increase in the number of mPFC synaptic contacts on DR neurons, ablation of 5-HT_7 (as observed in SERT-KO mice) induces a reduction of synaptic contacts in mPFC to DR [72, 137]. Therefore 5-HT_7 receptor inhibition counteracts the developmental effect mediated by SERT inhibition. SSRI treatment at P2-P14 or 5-HT_7 overexpression induces anxiety and depressive-like symptoms in adult mice. Such P2-P14 period is likely to correspond to the last trimester of pregnancy in humans [151]. During this period fetuses/babies (via the maternal milk) are highly impacted by maternal SSRI intake (see section 5). Since SERT-KO mice are not developing altered behavior, 5-HT_7 receptor antagonists appear as good candidate for the treatment of mood disorder during pregnancy or post-partum [152, 153].

Interestingly, the developmental maturation of the prefrontal cortex lasts far further into adolescence, up to the age of 20-24 years in humans [154]. Whether stress impacts the development apart the mature functions of mPFC is thus difficult to shape. Furthermore, the developmental expression of SERT in fetuses or infants is not known and much work has to be done to clarify the possible period of vulnerability to SSRI intake in humans (see [138] and section 5).

5. Sensitive periods for 5-HT in brain development: focus on limbic structures

When reviewing the role of 5-HT in the predisposition to develop PTSD or to cope with stress, it is necessary to untangle what is due to developmental modifications of the neuronal circuits apart from what is specifically due to modifications occurring at mature stages. During development, environmental stimuli sculpt neuronal circuits by an experience-dependent axon/synaptic refinement and pruning over the course of different critical periods, specific for each structure/function (i.e. the prefrontal system maturing all along development [154]). These processes have been shown to be highly sensitive to the imbalance in 5-HT levels depending on numerous genetic/epigenetic modifications of genes encoding the various actors of different 5-HT systems [93, 138, 151].

5.1 Subsets of 5-HT subgroups are differently implicated in response to stress

Although more complex, the development of 5-HT neurons largely depends on two transcription factors Lmx1b and Pet-1 [93, 94, 155, 156]. In Pet-1 knockout (KO) mice only few 5-HT+ neurons are preserved [155]. They correspond to 5-HT+ neurons located in the hypothalamic paraventricular nucleus (PVH), the ventral PAG and the ventral medulla, all projecting to the AMY while other brain targets are deprived of 5-HT+ axons. In conflict models, these mice show decreased levels of anxiety but enhanced freezing in fear conditioning tests. This suggests that 5-HT neurons could mediate anxiogenic effects in unconditioned anxiety tasks mainly through the innervation of forebrain areas such as the medial PFC and HIP, which receive no 5-HT innervation in Pet-1KO mice. Conversely data also suggests in Pet-1KO, that 5-HT might inhibit fear responses through the remaining 5-HT innervation toward specific AMY and PAG subnuclei [94, 156]. Further studies are needed for a better understanding of the contradictory effects of 5-HT on fear/anxiety responses in this model. Alternatively, compensatory mechanisms may occur in Pet1-KO mice that remain to go into in depth.

5.2 5-HT synthesis

In the mouse, a single-nucleotide polymorphism (SNP) has been identified in the *Tph2* gene that leads to a significant decrease in brain serotonin levels [157]. This polymorphism may account for the different susceptibility to anxiety and stress-related event across mouse strains (the C57BL/6J strain being more resistant). In humans, several polymorphisms inducing a loss of function of the *Tph2* gene have been detected and were associated with increased incidence of depression and anxiety or with exaggerated response of the AMY to, for instance, threatening faces. Such a loss of function appears relatively frequently in humans [158, 159]. TPH1 governs an average of 90% of 5-HT synthesis that occurs at the periphery. Peripheral 5-HT is then delivered in the blood (mainly stored in platelets) or during development by maternal/placental supply to the embryo prior BBB closure [160, 161]. Analysis of the impacts of maternal TPH1 deficiency on cortico-limbic development of the embryo is undergoing and suggests that TPH1 may durably alter vulnerability to stressful events (G. Vodjdani personal communication).

5.3 Vesicular storage of monoamines

In serotoninergic cell bodies and axons 5-HT is stored into vesicles preventing its degradation. Evidences that VMAT2 may play a role in regulating stress-related pathology was first discovered by reserpine treatment given to patients. Reserpine blocks VMATs function and induced depressive-like symptoms in humans. Reserpine's effect appears due to a defective storage of both catecholamine and 5-HT [162]. Mice displaying an altered copy of the VMAT2 allele display exaggerated corticosterone levels in response to forced swim test but respond normally to classic tests measuring anxiety-like behavior. Together this suggests that VMAT2 might play a role in regulating "depressive-like" behavior [163]. Magnitude to the antidepressant-like response appears to depend on the *VMAT2* gene that is differentially modified in the BALB/c versus A/J mouse strain [164]. However, the relative contribution of catecholamines and 5-HT remains to be clearly established.

5.4 5-HT transporter

As discussed above, SSRIs are largely used for their anti-depressant and anti-anxiogenic effects in adults. However, despite the fact that they are largely used in pregnant women (2-13% of women [165]) suffering mood disorders, it has been clearly shown that they have paradoxical long-term effects on fetuses and infant development. When administered during perinatal periods SSRIs increased the risk to develop anxiety and depression in infancy. SSRIs cross the placenta, are detectable in breast milk and reach the developing brain where they disturb the development of neuronal circuitry. During gestation SSRIs induced a reduction of blood flow in the middle cerebral artery and reduced fetal head growth [166, 167]. SSRIs impair motor movements, speech perception at 6-10 months of age, increased irritability and altered psychomotor development in children [168, 169]. When given during pregnancy, they induce a two-fold increased predisposition to develop autism-spectrum disorder [170]. Such alterations appeared correlated with higher dosage of SSRIs [171].

These various developmental roles are mainly related to the different developmental time windows in which SERT is expressed by a large array of glutamatergic neurons, increasing extracellular 5-HT levels and modulating the synaptic and axonal maturation of these neurons. Such a role has been first illustrated by pioneer studies analyzing the development of the somatosensory and visual system. In these systems, 5-HT excess acting via 5-HT_{1B} receptors, reduced glutamate release and induced the maintenance of immature features by SERT+ axons [172–177]. In the limbic system SERT expression has been described in the HIP, the AMY, the mPFC (for exhaustive list and time-window of expression see Table 1 in [173] and Figure 3 in [178]). However, in these regions, SERT+ neurons do not appear to express 5-HT_{1B} receptors during development and are modulated by excess 5-HT via other pathways that remained to be identified.

Similarly, genetic downregulation of the SERT causes depression-related behaviors of developmental origin. In humans, a lesser-expressing form of Slc6a4, the so-called short allele variant (Slc6a4s), has been associated with an increased risk of developing depression in response to early-life stress [179, 180]. This mutation also induces a decreased volume and activity of vmPFC, a structure actively implicated in the control of stress-coping response, which is hypoactive in depressive patients (review in [181]). Interestingly, in mice a subset of glutamatergic neurons located in the layer 5-6 of the IL cortex that transiently express SERT during early postnatal life (P2-P11) project to the DR. Conditional SERT ablation in those neurons leads to a 40% increase in the number of functional PFC synapses onto both 5-HT and GABA neurons of the DR, an effect that is reproduced by postnatal fluoxetine administration. Alteration of this neuronal population has been shown to mediate the depressive- and anxiety-like symptoms observed in adults previously subjected to early postnatal exposure to SSRIs. Thus, this neuronal population provides a top–down control of emotional deficits induced by exposure to SSRIs during early postnatal life, resulting in long-lasting effects on mood. Interestingly, 5-HT blockade during the P2-P11 period also impacts the development of prelimbic (PL) pyramidal neurons that neighbor IL neurons but in a reverse way. These neuronal populations which normally play a role in promoting fear extinction or inhibiting fear extinction respectively are permanently altered by SERT blockade leading to the emergence of affective and fear-related altered behaviours [72, 182].

Long life expression changes in SERT expression, such as those observed in mice knockout for SERT (SERT-KO) or overexpressing SERT (SERT-OE) result in altered development of limbic structures. SERT-KO mice display impaired recall of fear extinction compared to wild-type littermate controls. In these mice, BA and LA principal glutamatergic neurons display abnormal dendritic spine density [183]. Conversely, SERT-OE mice have lower extracellular 5-HT levels [184] and exhibit impaired fear learning [185]. Genetic manipulation of SERT during development induces compensatory mechanisms leading to modified levels of 5-HT_{1A} [11] and 5-HT_{2A} receptor expression [185, 186] in the AMY. Constitutive low levels of 5-HT_{2A} receptors in BA and LA may result in a reduced GABAergic tone in this structure that would be hyperresponsive to traumatic reminders or even innocuous stimuli [102].

It is to note that other risk alleles could interact within a context of SERT deficiency and further increase the risk for abnormal neural circuitry development. For instance, it has been observed in rodents that *PTEN* (a phosphatase and tensin homolog), a gene associated to autism spectrum disorders [187] interacts with SERT haploinsufficiency to modify brain size and social behaviors [188].

5.5 Monoamine oxidases

MAOA blockade was one of the first treatments used in humans to relieve symptoms of depression. However they showed side effects since they increased anxiety-like behavior and caused resistance to chronic mild stress habituation [189]. MAOA-KO mice display increase 5-HT levels in the brain that normalized with age (by 6 months). These mice show exaggerated unconditioned and conditioned fear behavior as well as increase aggressive-like behavior [190]. Such increased outbursts of aggressive behavior were also observed in a Dutch family by men lacking MAOA gene (MAOA is located on the X chromosome [191]). More common variants located on the MAOA promoter leading to a low MAOA activity induce, in humans, various social and emotional alterations. They were associated with increased responses of the HIP and AMY to threatening faces and with a reduction of grey matter volume in anterior cingulate cortex, insula and HIP and increased orbitofrontal volumes [192, 193]. Interestingly, human carrier of a hyperactive MAOA form tends to be more prone to depressive-like behavior [194]. By contrast, human carriers of the hypoactive form of MAOA show higher subjective stress, lesser glucocorticoid responses and blunted HPA axis response to chronic stress reflecting HPA axis exhaustion [195]. However, such alterations probably of developmental origin, could not be attributed specifically to 5-HT increase but could also be due to the norepinephrine increase characterized in early developmental and adulthood of MAOA-KO mice [190]. Various interindividual DNA methylations were detected on the promoter core of MAOA in peripheral circulating white cells and appear to predict efficiently the MAOA brain endophenotype and the susceptibility to stressful events [196]. Interestingly, the levels of MAOA methylation return to normal during the process of cognitive therapy of patients undergoing panic disorders. This study suggests that modification of MAOA methylation is part of a process that mediates fear extinction [197, 198].

6. Conclusion

5-HT appeared early on the scale of evolution and is highly conserved across species. 5-HT modulates nearly all the functions that are needed to sustain life and is also implicated in the formation of brain circuits. Despite the fact that 5-HT was one of the first neurotransmitters/neurohormones discovered, the large number of receptors that mediate its role make it difficult to apprehend how 5-HT regulate these functions. Indeed, some 5-HT receptor expressions and time of expressions (they may be transiently expressed) are still to be determined in rodents and in humans. Even regions and times of SERT expression remains to be established in humans. The treatment of PTSD is complex depending on the delay from the stressful event and although SSRIs associated with various psychotherapies were

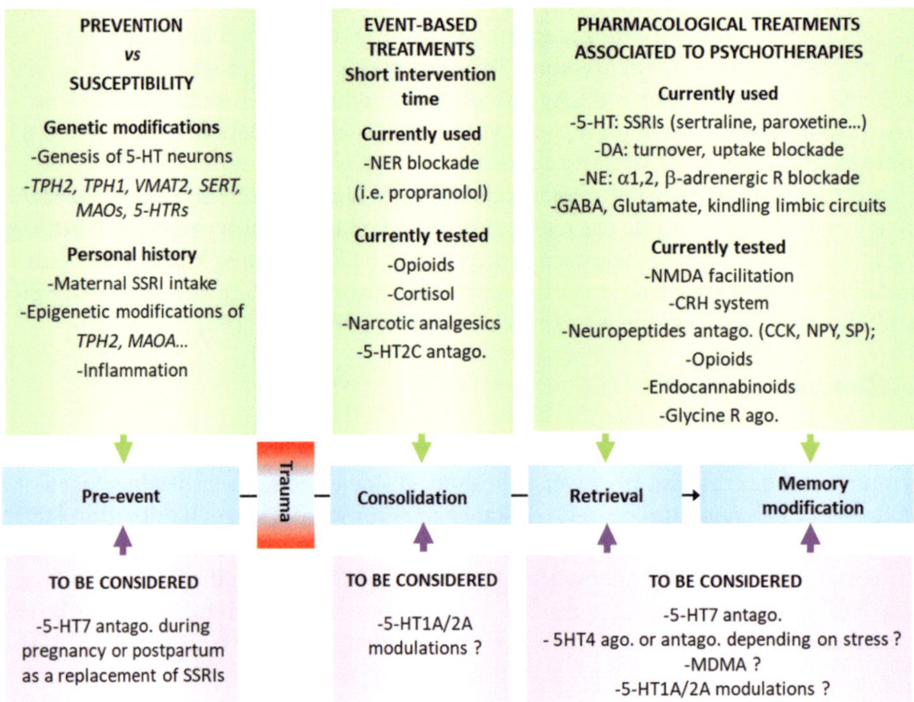

Figure 4.
Etiology of Post-traumatic Stress Disorder and possible treatments. Risk or protective factors may impact the way people cope with a stressor. This includes the genetic makeup specific to a patient and its personal history. We point here the role of epigenetic modifications impacting the serotoninergic system, the status of the mother during gestation and lactation. In particular, inflammatory status of the patient or of its mother while pregnant could lead to 5-HT depletion (central or peripheral). Maternal serotonin reuptake inhibitors (SSRIs) intake induces increase 5-HT levels in the embryo, the fetus and in the maternal milk. Recently 5-H7 antagonists were suggested to be used instead of classical SSRIs as they may induce fewer side effects. After the trauma, there is a short intervention time during which the weight of a traumatic memory could be decreased by pharmacological tools. In addition to the norepinephrine receptor (NER) blockade, alternative therapeutics are currently tested or considered. When Post-Traumatic Stress Disorder is clearly installed pharmacological treatment in combination with psychotherapy could be used to both alleviate the symptom and decrease the strength of traumatic memories. Alternative treatments are emerging some of them target the serotoninergic system. Blue Blocks depict the patient history and the emergence of PTSD induced by the resurgence of the traumatic event. Green blocks review what is already clearly established. Violet blocks review what should be considered and the interrogation point indicates that the cited compound should be tested with caution. 5-HT, 5-hydroxytryptamin; 5-HTRs, 5-hydroxytryptamin receptor; Ago., agonist; Antago., antagonist; CCK, cholecystokinin; CRH, corticotropin releasing hormone; DA, dopamine; GABA, gamma aminobutyric acid; MAOs, monoamine oxidase; MDMA, 3,4-Methylenedioxymethamphetamine; NE, norepinephrine; NER, norepinephrine receptor; NMDA, n-methyl-D-aspartate; NPY, neuropeptide Y; SERT, serotonin transporter; SSRIs, serotonin reuptake inhibitors; SP, substance P; TPH2, tryptophan hydroxylase 2; TPH1, tryptophan hydroxylase 1; VMAT2, vesicular.

initially largely prescribed, alternative pharmacological treatments are emerging. Some of them rely on 5-HT and modulate specific receptors, but a large array of pharmacological treatments currently used or clinically tested modulate other neurotransmitters, neurohormones or neuropeptides. They however all have a common goal: to decrease the strength of traumatic memories, to eliminate the pathological memories by reconsolidation blockade or even reducing the association between the traumatic event and the negative emotional valence. Anyway, the history of a patient and its genetic/epigenetic makeup he bears largely impact the way he will cope with a stressor. Regarding this last point it is clear that individual specificitics of the 5-HT system will influence how people are coping with stress (**Figure 4**).

Acknowledgment

TV was founded by the inserm and "The Fondation de France" grant No 00089602. TV and CV warmly thank Dr Pierre Gressens for constant support. TV wish to thank Drs Guilan Vodjdani and Sylvie Berard and, Oriane Bergiers and Renald Buzenet, two master students in the lab and H. Langzam for fruitful discussions.

Abbreviation list

5-HT	5-hydroxytryptamin
5-HIAA	5hydroxyindolacetic acid
AADC	aminoacid decarboxylase
ACTH	adrenocorticotropic hormone
AMY	amygdala complex
BA	basal nucleus of amygdala
BBB	brain blood barrier
BLA	basolateral nucleus of amygdala
BNST	bed nucleus of the stria terminalis
cAMP	cyclic adenosin monophosphate
CA1-CA3	hippocampal fields
CCK	cholecystokinin
CE	central nucleus of amygdala
CEL	lateral part of the CE
CEM	medial part of the CE
CNS	central nervous system
COMT	catéchol-O-méthyltransferase
CORT	cortisol/corticosterone
CR	calretinin
CRH or CRF	corticotrophin releasing hormone/factor
DR	dorsal raphe nuclei
vDR	ventral dorsal raphe
GABA	gamma aminobutyric acid
GR	glucocorticoid receptors
HIP	hippocampal formation
HPA	hypothalamic-pituitary-adrenal axis
IDO	indoleamine 2,3-dioxygenase
IL	infralimbic cortex
KO	knockout
LA	lateral nucleus of the amygdala

LC	locus coeruleus
MAOA	monoamine oxidase A
MAOB	monoamine oxidase B
MnR	median raphe nucleus
NAc	nucleus accumbens
NO	nitric oxide
NPY	neuropeptide Y
OPFc	orbitoprefrontal cortex
OE	over expression
PAG	periacqueductal grey
PFC	prefrontal cortex
PL	prelimbic cortex
PN	principal glutamatergic neurons
PTSD	post-traumatic stress disorder
PV	parvalbumin
PVH	paraventricular nucleus of the hypothalamus
SERT	serotonin transporter
SNP	single-nucleotide polymorphism
SOM	somatostatin
SSRI	serotonin reuptake inhibitor
TH	tyrosine Hydroxylase
Tph	tryptophan hydroxylase
Tph1	tryptophan hydroxylase type1
Tph2	tryptophan hydroxylase type 2
Vglut3	vesicular glutamate transporter 3
VIP	vasoactive intestinal polypeptide
VMAT 2	vesicular monoamine transporter 2
vmPFC	ventromedial prefrontal cortex
VTA	ventral tegmental area

Author details

Tania Vitalis* and Catherine Verney
Université de Paris, NeuroDiderot, Inserm U1141, Paris, France

*Address all correspondence to: tnvitalis@gmail.com and tania.vitalis@inserm.fr

References

[1] Kessler RC, et al. Posttraumatic stress disorder in the National Comorbidity Survey. Archives General Psychiatry. 1995;**52**(12):1048-1060

[2] Kessler RC, Wang PS. The descriptive epidemiology of commonly occurring mental disorders in the United States. Annual Review Public Health. 2008;**29**:115-129

[3] American Psychiatric Association. Diagnostic and Statistical Manual of Mental Disorders, Third Edition, Revised (American Psychiatric Association, 1987)

[4] Michopoulos V, et al. Association of CRP genetic variation and CRP level with elevated PTSD symptoms and physiological responses in a civilian population with high levels. American Journal Psychiatry. 2015;**172**(4):353-362

[5] Marmar CR, et al. Course of posttraumatic stress disorder 40 years after the Vietnam War: findings from the National Vietnam Veterans Longitudinal Study. JAMA Psychiatry. 2015;**72**:875-881

[6] Yehuda R. Status of glucocorticoid alterations in post-traumatic stress disorder. Annals New York Academy Sciences. 2009;**1179**:56-69

[7] Moisan MP, Le Moal M. Le stress dans tous ses états. Medecine/Science. 2012; **28**:612-617

[8] McEwen BS. Physiology and neurobiology of stress and adaptation: central role of the brain. Physiological Reviews. 2007;**87**(3):873-904

[9] Rodrigues SM, LeDoux JE, Sapolsky RM. The influence of stress hormones on fear circuitry. Annual Review Neuroscience. 2009;**32**: 289-313

[10] LeDoux JE, Pine DS. Using Neuroscience to Help Understand Fear and Anxiety: A Two-System Framework. American Journal Psychiatry. 2016;**173**(11):1083-1093

[11] Holmes A, Hariri AR. The serotonin transporter gene-linked polymorphism and negative emotionality: placing single gene effects in the context of genetic background and environment. Genes Brain & Behavior. 2003;**2**(6):332-335

[12] Celada P, et al. The therapeutic role of 5-HT1A and 5-HT2A receptors in depression. Journal Psychiatry & Neuroscience. 2004;**29**(4):252-265

[13] Homberg JR. Serotonergic modulation of conditioned fear. Scientifica (Cairo). 2012;**2012**:821549

[14] Burghardt NS, Bauer EP. Acute and chronic effects of selective serotonin reuptake inhibitor treatment on fear conditioning: implications for underlying fear circuits. Neuroscience. 2013;**247**:253-272

[15] Bocchio M, et al. Serotonin, Amygdala and Fear: Assembling the Puzzle. Frontiers Neural Circuits. 2016.**10**:24

[16] Adamec R, Shallow T. Lasting effects on rodent anxiety of a single exposure to a cat. Physiology & Behavior. 1993;**54:**101-109

[17] Adamec R. Transmitter systems involved in neural plasticity underlying increased anxiety and defense--implications for understanding anxiety following traumatic stress. Neuroscience & Biobehavioral Reviews. 1997;**21**(6):755-765

[18] Carlén M. What constitutes the prefrontal cortex? Science. 2017;**358**(6362):478-482

[19] Harris AP, et al. Mineralocorticoid and glucocorticoid receptor balance in control of HPA axis and behaviour. Psychoneuroendocrinology. 2013;**38**(5):648-658

[20] Gray TS, Carney ME, Magnuson DJ. Direct projections from the central amygdaloid nucleus to the hypothalamic paraventricular nucleus: possible role in stress-induced adrenocorticotropin release. Neuroendocrinology. 1989;**50**(4):433-446

[21] Tsigos C, Chrousos GP. Hypothalamic-pituitary-adrenal axis, neuroendocrine factors and stress. Journal Psychosomatic Research. 2002;**53**(4):865-871

[22] Penzo MA, et al. The paraventricular thalamus controls a central amygdala fear circuit. Nature. 2015;**519**(7544):455-459

[23] Duvarci S, Pare D. Amygdala microcircuits controlling learned fear. Neuron. 2014;**82**:966-980

[24] Asede D, et al. Sensory inputs to intercalated cells provide fear-learning modulated inhibition to the basolateral amygdala. Neuron. 2015;**86**:541-554

[25] Rauch SL, et al. Exaggerated amygdala response to masked facial stimuli in posttraumatic stress disorder: a functional MRI study. Biological Psychiatry. 2000; **47**:769-776

[26] LeDoux J. The amygdala. Current Biology. 2007;**17**(20):R868-874

[27] Johansen JP, et al. Molecular mechanisms of fear learning and memory. Cell. 2011;**147**(3):509-524

[28] LeDoux JE, Brown R. A higher-order theory of emotional consciousness. Proceedings National Academy Sciences USA. 2017;**114**(10):E2016-E2025

[29] Killcross S, Robbins TW, Everitt BJ. Different types of fear-conditioned behaviour mediated by separate nuclei within amygdala. Nature. 1997;**388**:377-380

[30] Amorapanth P, LeDoux JE, Nader, K. Different lateral amygdala outputs mediate reactions and actions elicited by a fear arousing stimulus. Nature Neuroscience. 2000;**3**:74-79

[31] Lázaro-Muñoz G, LeDoux JE, Cain CK. Sidman instrumental avoidance initially depends on lateral and basal amygdala and is constrained by central amygdala-mediated Pavlovian processes. Biological Psychiatry. 2010;**67**:1120-1127

[32] Manassero E, et al. Lateral and Basal Amygdal Account for Opposite Behavioral Responses during the Long-Term Expression of Fearful Memories. Scientific Reports. 2018;**8**:518

[33] Smith DM, Bulkin DA. The form and function of hippocampal context representations. Neuroscience & Biobehavioral Reviews. 2014;**40**:52-61

[34] Megías JL, et al. Comparisons of traumatic and positive memories in people with and without PTSD profile. Applied Cognitive Psychology. 2007;**21**:117-130

[35] Fanselow MS, Dong HW. Are the dorsal and ventral hippocampus functionally distinct structures? Neuron. 2010;**65**:7-19

[36] Fastenrath M, et al. Dynamic modulation of amygdala-hippocampal connectivity by emotional arousal. Journal Neuroscience. 2014; **34**:13935-13947

[37] Cohen MX. Hippocampal-prefrontal connectivity predicts midfrontal oscillations and long-term

memory performance. Current Biology. 2011;**21**:1900-1905

[38] Yuan P, Raz N. Prefrontal cortex and executive functions in healthy adults: a meta-analysis of structural neuroimaging studies. Neuroscience & Biobehavioral Reviews. 2014;**42**:180-192

[39] Gilmartin MR, Balderston NL, Helmstetter FJ. Prefrontal cortical regulation of fear learning. Trends Neuroscience. 2014;**37**(8):455-464

[40] Pitman RK, et al. Biological studies of post-traumatic stress disorder. Nature Review Neuroscience. 2012;**13**(11):769-787

[41] Giustino TF, Maren S. The role of the medial prefrontal cortex in the conditioning and extinction of fear. Frontiers in Behavioral Neuroscience. 2015;**9**:298

[42] Thierry AM, et al. Selective activation of the mesocortical dopaminergic system by stress. Nature.1976;**263**:242-244

[43] Douma EH, de Kloet ER. Stress-induced plasticity and functioning of ventral tegmental dopamine neurons. Neuroscience & Biobehavioral Reviews. 2020;**108**: 48-77

[44] Bouarab C, Thompson B, Polter AM. VTA GABA Neurons at the Interface of Stress and Reward. Frontiers Neural Circuits. 2019;**13**:78

[45] Isingrini E, et al. Resilience to chronic stress is mediated by noradrenergic regulation of dopamine neurons. Nature Neuroscience. 2016;**19**:560-563

[46] Nagai Y, et al. The Role of Dorsal Raphe Serotonin Neurons in the Balance between Reward and Aversion. Internal Journal Molecular Science. 2020;**21**(6):2160

[47] Ren J, et al. Anatomically Defined and Functionally Distinct Dorsal Raphe Serotonin Sub-systems. Cell. 2018;**175**(2):472-487

[48] Ribatti D, et al. Development of the blood-brain barrier: a historical point of view. Anatomical Record Part B New Anatomist. 2006;**289**(1):3-8

[49] Walther DJ, et al. Synthesis of serotonin by a second tryptophan hydroxylase isoform. Science. 2003;**299**(5603):76

[50] Patel PD, Pontrello C, Burke S. Robust and tissue-specific expression of TPH2 versus TPH1 in rat raphe and pineal gland. Biological Psychiatry. 2004;**55**(4):428-433

[51] Côte F, et al. Disruption of the nonneuronal tph1 gene demonstrates the importance of peripheral serotonin in cardiac function. Proceedings National Academy Sciences USA. 2003;**100**(23):13525-13530

[52] Côté F, et al. Maternal serotonin is crucial for murine embryonic development. Proceedings National Academy Sciences USA. 2007;**104**(1):329-334

[53] Wu HH, Choi S, Levitt P. Differential patterning of genes involved in serotonin metabolism and transport in extra-embryonic tissues of the mouse. Placenta. 2016;**42**:74-83

[54] Gupta V, et al. Molecular mechanism of monoamine oxidase A gene regulation under inflammation and ischemia-like conditions: key roles of the transcription factors GATA2, Sp1 and TBP. Journal Neurochemistry. 2015;**134**(1):21-38

[55] Hoffman BJ, et al. Localization and dynamic regulation of biogenic amine transporters in the mammalian central nervous system. Frontiers

Neuroendocrinology. 1998;**19**(3):187-231

[56] Torres GE, Amara SG. Glutamate and monoamine transporters: new visions of form and function. Current Opinion Neurobiology. 2007;**17**(3):304-312

[57] Siegmund A, Wotjak CT. A mouse model of posttraumatic stress disorder that distinguishes between conditioned and sensitised fear. Journal Psychiatric Research. 2007;**41**(10):848-860

[58] Sartori SB, Singewald N. Novel pharmacological targets in drug development for the treatment of anxiety and anxiety-related disorders. Pharmacology & Therapeutics. 2019;**204**:107402

[59] Wakizono T, et al. Stress vulnerabilities in an animal model of post-traumatic stress disorder. Physiology & Behavior. 2007;**90**(4):687-695

[60] Goswami S, et al. Animal models of post-traumatic stress disorder: face validity. Frontiers Neuroscience. 2013;**7**:89

[61] Shepard R, Page CE, Coutellier L. Sensitivity of the prefrontal GABAergic system to chronic stress in male and female mice: Relevance for sex differences in stress-related disorders. Neuroscience. 2016;**332**:1-12

[62] Adamec R, et al. Protein synthesis and the mechanisms of lasting change in anxiety induced by severe stress. Behavioral Brain Research. 2006;**167**(2):270-286

[63] Zoladz PR, et al. Psychosocial predator-based animal model of PTSD produces physiological and behavioral sequelae and a traumatic memory four months following stress onset. Physiology & Behavior. 2015;**147**:183-192

[64] Seetharaman S, et al. Influence of daily social stimulation on behavioral and physiological outcomes in an animal model of PTSD. Brain Behavior. 2016;**6**(5):e00458

[65] Zoladz PR, Diamond DM. Current status on behavioral and biological markers of PTSD: a search for clarity in a conflicting literature. Neuroscience & Biobehavioral Reviews. 2013;**37**(5):860-895

[66] Wilson CB, et al. Differential effects of sertraline in a predator exposure animal model of post-traumatic stress disorder. Frontiers Behavioral Neuroscience. 2014;**8**:256

[67] Pedraza LK, et al. Chronic fluoxetine prevents fear memory generalization and enhances subsequent extinction by remodeling hippocampal dendritic spines and slowing down systems consolidation. Translational Psychiatry. 2019;**9**(1):53

[68] Shih JC, Grimsby J. Chen K. The expression of human MAO-A and B genes. Journal Neural Transmission Supplementa. 1990;**32**:41-47

[69] Grimsby J, et al. Tissue distribution of human monoamine oxidase A and B mRNA. Journal Neurochemistry. 1990;**55**(4):1166-1169

[70] Vitalis T, et al. Developmental expression of monoamine oxidases A and B in the central and peripheral nervous systems of the mouse. Journal Comparative Neurology. 2002;**442**(4):331-347

[71] Vitalis T, et al. Developmental expression pattern of monoamine oxidases in sensory organs and neural crest derivatives. Journal Comparative Neurology. 2003;**464**(3):392-403

[72] Soiza-Reilly M, et al. SSRIs target prefrontal to raphe circuits during development modulating synaptic

connectivity and emotional behavior. Molecular Psychiatry. 2019;**24**(5):726-745

[73] Gupta V, et al. Molecular mechanism of monoamine oxidase A gene regulation under inflammation and ischemia-like conditions: key roles of the transcription factors GATA2, Sp1 and TBP. Journal Neurochemistry. 2015;**134**(1):21-38

[74] Higuchi Y, Soga T, Parhar IS. Regulatory Pathways of Monoamine Oxidase A during Social Stress. Frontiers Neuroscience. 2017;**11**:604

[75] Higuchi Y, Soga T, Parhar IS. Social Defeat Stress Decreases mRNA for Monoamine Oxidase A and Increases 5-HT Turnover in the Brain of Male Nile Tilapia (*Oreochromis niloticus*). Frontiers Pharmacology. 2019;**9**:1549

[76] Morais M, et al. The effects of chronic stress on hippocampal adult neurogenesis and dendritic plasticity are reversed by selective MAO-A inhibition. Journal Psychopharmacology. 2014;**28**(12):1178-1183

[77] Hoyer D, et al. International Union of Pharmacology classification of receptors for 5-hydroxytryptamine (Serotonin). Pharmacological Reviews. 1994;**46**(2):157-203

[78] Hoyer D, Hannon JP, Martin GR. Molecular, pharmacological and functional diversity of 5-HT receptors. Pharmacology Biochemistry & Behavior. 2002;**71**(4):533-554

[79] Millan MJ, et al. Signaling at G-protein-coupled serotonin receptors: recent advances and future research directions. Trends Pharmacological Science. 2008;**29**(9):454-464

[80] Barnes NM et al., International Union of Basic and Clinical Pharmacology. CX. Classification of Receptors for 5-hydroxytryptamine; Pharmacology and Function. Pharmacol Rev. 2021;**73**(1):310-520.

[81] Invernizzi R, Bramante M, Samanin R. Role of 5-HT1A receptors in the effects of acute chronic fluoxetine on extracellular serotonin in the frontal cortex. Pharmacology Biochemistry & Behavior.1996;**54**(1):143-147

[82] Chameau P, van Hooft JA. Serotonin 5-HT(3) receptors in the central nervous system. Cell Tissue Research. 2006;**326**(2):573-581

[83] Lee S, et al. The largest group of superficial neocortical GABAergic interneurons expresses ionotropic serotonin receptors. Journal Neuroscience. 2010;**30**(50):16796-16808

[84] Vucurovic K, et al. Serotonin 3A receptor subtype as an early and protracted marker of cortical interneuron subpopulations. Cerebral Cortex. 2010;**20**(10):2333-2347

[85] Puig MV, Gener T. Serotonin Modulation of Prefronto-Hippocampal Rhythms in Health and Disease. ACS Chemical Neuroscience. 2015;**6**(7):1017-1025.

[86] The Allen brain atlas (Brain Map - brain-map.org (brain-map.org)

[87] Steinbusch HW. Distribution of serotonin-immunoreactivity in the central nervous system of the rat-cell bodies and terminals Neuroscience.1981;**6**(4):557-618

[88] Vertes RP, Fortin WJ, Cranes AM. Projections of the Median Raphe Nucleus in the Rat. Journal Comparative Neurology.1999;**407**:555-582

[89] Linley SB, Olucha-Bordonau F, Vertes RP. Pattern of distribution of serotonergic fibers to the amygdala and extended amygdala in the rat. Journal Comparative Neurology. 2017;**525**(1):116-139

[90] Waselus M, Valentino RJ, Van Bockstaele EJ. Collateralized dorsal raphe nucleus projections: a mechanism for the integration of diverse functions during stress. Journal Chemical Neuroanatomy. 2011;**41**(4):266-280

[91] Muzerelle A, et al. Conditional anterograde tracing reveals distinct targeting of individual serotonin cell groups (B5–B9) to the forebrain and brainstem. Brain Structure - Function. 2016;**221**:535-561

[92] Celada P, Puig MV, Artigas F. Serotonin modulation of cortical neurons and networks. Frontiers Integrating Neuroscience. 2013;**19**;7-25

[93] Okaty BW, Commons KG, Dymecki SM. Embracing diversity in the 5-HT neuronal system. Nature Review Neuroscience. 2019;**20**(7):397-424

[94] Deneris E, Gaspar P. Serotonin neuron development: shaping molecular and structural identities. Wiley Interdisciplinary Reviews Developmental Biolology. 2018;**7(**1):10

[95] Amat J, et al. Medial prefrontal cortex determines how stressor controllability affects behavior and dorsal raphe nucleus. Nature Neuroscience. 2005:**8**(3):365-371

[96] Holmes A. Genetic variation in cortico-amygdala serotonin function and risk for stress-related disease. Neuroscience & Biobehavioral Reviews. 2008;**32**(7):1293-1314

[97] Sengupta A, et al. Control of Amygdala Circuits by 5-HT Neurons via 5-HT and Glutamate Cotransmission. Journal Neuroscience. 2017;**37**(7):1785-1796

[98] Sengupta A, Holmes A. A Discrete Dorsal Raphe to Basal Amygdala 5-HT Circuit Calibrates Aversive Memory. Neuron. 2019;**103**(3):489-505

[99] Prakash N, et al. Serotonergic Plasticity in the Dorsal Raphe Nucleus Characterizes Susceptibility and Resilience to Anhedonia. Journal Neuroscience. 2020;**40**(3):569-584

[100] Varga V, et al. Fast synaptic subcortical control of hippocampal circuits. Science. 2009;**326**:449-453

[101] Muller JF, Mascagni F, McDonald AJ. Serotonin-immunoreactive axon terminals innervate pyramidal cells and interneurons in the rat basolateral amygdala. Journal Comparative Neurology. 2007;**505**(3):314-335

[102] Jiang X, et al. Stress impairs 5-HT2A receptor-mediated serotonergic facilitation of GABA release in juvenile rat basolateral amygdala. Neuropsychopharmacology. 2009;**34**(2):410-423

[103] Adamec R, et al. Protein synthesis and the mechanisms of lasting change in anxiety induced by severe stress. Behavioral Brain Research. 2006;**167**(2):270-286

[104] Mitra R, Adamec R, Sapolsky R. Resilience against predator stress and dendritic morphology of amygdala neurons. Behavioral Brain Research. 2009;**205**(2):535-543

[105] Fadok JP, et al. A competitive inhibitory circuit for selection of active and passive fear responses. Nature. 2017;542(7639):96-100

[106] Ciocchi S, et al. Encoding of conditioned fear in central amygdala inhibitory circuits. Nature. 2010;**468**:277-282

[107] Yu K, et al. Central Amygdala Somatostatin Neurons Gate Passive and Active Defensive Behaviors. Journal Neuroscience. 2016;**36**(24):6488-6496

[108] Li H, et al. Experience-dependent modification of a central amygdala fear circuit. Nature Neuroscience. 2013;**16**:332-339

[109] Gross CT, Canteras NS. The many paths to fear. Nature Review Neuroscience. 2012;13(9):651-658

[110] Isosaka T, et al. Htr2a-Expressing Cells in the Central Amygdala Control the Hierarchy between Innate and Learned Fear. Cell. 2015;**163**(5):1153-1164

[111] Somerville LH, Jones RM, Casey BJ. A time of change: Behavioral and neural correlates of adolescent sensitivity to appetitive and aversive environmental cues. Brain cognition. 2010;**71**:12.

[112] Hammack SE, Mania I, Rainnie DG. Differential Expression of Intrinsic Membrane Currents in Defined Cell Types of the Anterolateral Bed Nucleus of the Stria Terminalis. Journal Neurophysiology. 2007;**98**: 638-656

[113] Guo JD, et al. Bi-directional modulation of bed nucleus of stria terminalis neurons by 5-HT: molecular expression and functional properties of excitatory 5-HT receptor subtypes. Neuroscience. 2009;**164**(4):1776-1793

[114] Hazra R, et al. Differential distribution of serotonin receptor subtypes in BNST(ALG) neurons: modulation by unpredictable shock stress. Neuroscience. 2012;**225**:9-21

[115] Daniel SE, Rainnie DG. Stress Modulation of Opposing Circuits in the Bed Nucleus of the Stria Terminalis. Neuropsychopharmacology. 2016;**41**(1):103-125

[116] Davis M, et al. Phasic vs sustained fear in rats and humans: role of the extended amygdala in fear vs anxiety. Neuropsychopharmacology. 2010;**35**(1):105-135

[117] Regue M, et al. Increased 5-HT2C receptor editing predisposes to PTSD-like behaviors and alters BDNF and cytokines signaling. Nature Translational Psychiatry. 2019;**9**:100

[118] De Berardis D, et al. The Melatonergic System in Mood and Anxiety Disorders and the Role of Agomelatine: Implications for Clinical Practice. *International Journal Molecular Sciences.* 2013;*14*(6):12458-12483

[119] Dengler BA, et al. Bilateral amygdala stimulation reduces avoidance behavior in a predator scent posttraumatic stress disorder model. Neurosurgical Focus. 2018; **45**(2):E16

[120] Teixeira CM, et al. Hippocampal 5-HT Input Regulates Memory Formation and Schaffer Collateral Excitation. Neuron. 2018;**98**(5):992-1004

[121] Logue MW, et al. Smaller Hippocampal Volume in Posttraumatic Stress Disorder: A Multisite ENIGMA-PGC Study: Subcortical Volumetry Results From Posttraumatic Stress Disorder Consortia. Biological Psychiatry. 2018;**83**:244-253

[122] Tu W, et al. Serotonin in the ventral hippocampus modulates anxiety-like behavior during amphetamine withdrawal. Neuroscience. 2014;**281**:35-43

[123] Keck ME, et al. Differences in serotonergic neurotransmission between rats displaying high or low anxiety/depression-like behaviour: effects of chronic paroxetine treatment. Journal Neurochemistry. 2005;**92**:1170-1179

[124] Fuss J, et al. Hippocampal serotonin-1A receptor function in a mouse model of anxiety induced by long-term voluntary wheel running. Synapse. 2013;**67**:648-655

[125] Kusserow H, et al. Reduced anxiety-related behaviour in transgenic mice overexpressing serotonin1A receptors. Brain Research. 2004;**129**:104-116

[126] Tanaka KF, Samuels BA, Hen R. Serotonin receptor expression along the dorsal-ventral axis of mouse hippocampus. Philosophical Transactions Royal Society B: Biological Sciences. 2012;**367**(1601):2395-2401

[127] Ohmura Y, et al. Serotonin 5-HT7 Receptor in the Ventral Hippocampus Modulates the Retrieval of Fear Memory and Stress-Induced Defecation. International Journal Neuropsychopharmacology. 2016;**19**(6):pyv131

[128] Dickson EJ, Heredia DJ, Smith TK. Critical role of 5-HT1A, 5-HT3, and 5-HT7 receptor subtypes in the initiation, generation, and propagation of the murine colonic migrating motor complex. American Journal Physiology-Gastrointestinal Liver Physiology. 2010;**299**(1):G144-157

[129] Lucas G, et al. Serotonin 5-HT4 receptor agonists are putative antidepressants with a rapid onset of action. Neuron. 2007;**55**(5):712-725

[130] Puig MV, Gulledge AT. Serotonin and prefrontal cortex function: neurons, networks, and circuits. Molecular Neurobiology. 2011;**44**(3):449-64

[131] Amargós-Bosch M, et al. Co-expression and in vivo interaction of serotonin1A and serotonin2A receptors in pyramidal neurons of prefrontal cortex. Cerebral Cortex. 2004;**14**(3):281-299

[132] Price AE, et al. Endogenous Serotonin 5-HT_{2A} and 5-HT_{2C} Receptors Associate in the Medial Prefrontal Cortex. ACS Chemical Neuroscience. 2019;**10**(7):3241-3248

[133] Cornea-Hebert V, et al. Cellular and subcellular distribution of the serotonin 5-HT2A receptor in the central nervous system of adult rat. Journal Comparative Neurology. 1999;**409**:187-209

[134] Jakab RL, Goldman-Rakic PS. Segregation of serotonin 5-HT2A and 5-HT3 receptors in inhibitory circuits of the primate cerebral cortex. Journal Comparative Neurology. 2000;**417**(3):337-348

[135] Miner LA, et al. Ultrastructural localization of serotonin2A receptors in the middle layers of the rat prelimbic prefrontal cortex. Neuroscience. 2003;**116**:107-117.

[136] Jean A, et al. Adaptive Control of Dorsal Raphe by 5-HT4 in the Prefrontal Cortex Prevents Persistent Hypophagia following Stress. Cell Reproduction. 2017;**21**(4):901-909

[137] Olusakin J, et al. Implication of 5-HT7 receptor in prefrontal circuit assembly and detrimental emotional effects of SSRIs during development. Neuropsychopharmacology. 2020;**45**(13):2267-2277

[138] Vitalis T, Ansorge MS, Dayer AG. Serotonin homeostasis and serotonin receptors as actors of cortical construction: special attention to the 5-HT3A and 5-HT6 receptor subtypes. Frontiers Cellular Neuroscience, 2013;**7**:93

[139] Fukumoto K, et al. 5-HT_{1A} receptor stimulation in the medial prefrontal cortex mediates the antidepressant effects of mGlu2/3 receptor antagonist in mice. Neuropharmacology. 2018;**137**:96-103

[140] Andolina D, et al. Prefrontal/amygdalar system determines stress coping behavior through 5-HT/GABA connection. Neuropsychopharmacology. 2013;**38**(10):2057-2067

[141] Puglisi-Allegra S, Andolina D. Serotonin and stress coping. Behavioral Brain Research. 2015;**277**:58-67

[142] Murnane KS. Serotonin 2A receptors are a stress response system: implications for post-traumatic stress disorder. Behavior Pharmacology. 2019(**2 and 3**-Spec Issue):151-162

[143] Gewirtz JC, Marek GJ. Behavioral evidence for interactions between a hallucinogenic drug and group II metabotropic glutamate receptors. Neuropsychopharmacology. 2000;**23**(5):569-576

[144] Fisher PM, et al. Medial prefrontal cortex 5-HT(2A) density is correlated with amygdala reactivity, response habituation, and functional coupling. Cerebral Cortex. 2009;**19**(11):2499-2507

[145] Boggio PS, et al. Noninvasive brain stimulation with high-frequency and low-intensity repetitive transcranial magnetic stimulation treatment for posttraumatic stress disorder. Journal Clinical Psychiatry. 2010;**71**(8):992-999

[146] Avesar, D, Gulledge AT. Selective serotonergic excitation of callosal projection neurons. Frontiers Neural Circuits. 2012;**6**:12

[147] Andolina D, et al. Strain-dependent variations in stress coping behavior are mediated by a 5-HT/GABA interaction within the prefrontal corticolimbic system. International Journal Neuropsychopharmacology. 2014;**18**(3):pyu074

[148] Pollak Dorocic I, et al. A whole-brain atlas of inputs to serotonergic neurons of the dorsal and median raphe nuclei. Neuron. 2014;**83**(3):663-664

[149] Liu S, et al. Serotonin2C receptor localization in GABA neurons of the rat medial prefrontal cortex: implications for understanding the neurobiology of addiction. Neuroscience. 2007;**146**(4):1677-1688

[150] Jean A, et al. Adaptive Control of Dorsal Raphe by 5-HT4 in the Prefrontal Cortex Prevents Persistent Hypophagia following Stress. Cell Reproduction. 2017;**21**(4):901-909

[151] *Vitalis T, Verney C. Sculpting cerebral cortex with serotonin in rodent and primate. 2017*. DOI: 10.5772/intechopen.69000. In serotonin a chemical messager between all types of living cells. Eds by Kaneez Fatima Shad.

[152] Nikiforuk A. Targeting the Serotonin 5-HT7 Receptor in the Search for Treatments for CNS Disorders: Rationale and Progress to Date. CNS Drugs. 2015;**29**(4):265-275

[153] Nikiforuk A, et al. Effects of the selective 5-HT7 receptor antagonist SB-269970 on premature responding in the five-choice serial reaction time test in rats. Behavior Brain Research. 2015;**289**:149-156

[154] Sowell ER, et al. Mapping continued brain growth and gray matter density reduction in dorsal frontal cortex: Inverse relationships during postadolescent brain maturation. Journal Neuroscience. 2001;**21**(22):8819-8829

[155] Liu C, et al. Pet-1 is required across different stages of life to regulate serotonergic function. Nature Neuroscience. 2010;**13**(10):1190-1198

[156] Kiyasova V, Gaspar P. Development of raphe serotonin neurons from specification to guidance. European Journal Neuroscience. 2011;**34**(10):1553-1562

[157] Zhang X, et al. Tryptophan hydroxylase-2 controls brain serotonin synthesis. Science. 2004;**305**(5681):217

[158] Delorme R, et al. No human tryptophan hydroxylase-2 gene R441H mutation in a large cohort of psychiatric patients and control subjects. Biological Psychiatry. 2006;**60**(2):202-203

[159] Christiansen L, et al. Candidate gene polymorphisms in the serotonergic pathway: influence on depression symptomatology in an elderly population. Biological Psychiatry. 2007;**61**(2):223-230

[160] Daneman R, et al. Pericytes are required for blood-brain barrier integrity during embryogenesis. Nature. 2010;**468**:562-566

[161] Ben-Zvi A, et al. Mfsd2a is critical for the formation and function of the blood-brain barrier. Nature. 2014;**509**: 507-511

[162] Bourin M. Is it possible to predict the activity of a new antidepressant in animals with simple psychopharmacological tests? Fundamental & Clinical Pharmacology. 1990;**4**(1):49-64

[163] Fukui M, et al. Vmat2 heterozygous mutant mice display a depressive-like phenotype. Journal Neuroscience. 2007;**27**(39):10520-10529

[164] Crowley JJ, et al. Pharmacogenomic evaluation of the antidepressant citalopram in the mouse tail suspension test. Neuropsychopharmacology. 2006;**31**(11):2433-2442

[165] Glover ME, Clinton SM. Of rodents and humans: A comparative review of the neurobehavioral effects of early life SSRI exposure in preclinical and clinical research. International Journal Developmental Neuroscience. 2016;**51**:50-72

[166] Rurak D, et al. Third trimester fetal heart rate and Doppler middle cerebral artery blood flow velocity characteristics during prenatal selective serotonin reuptake inhibitor exposure. Pediatric Research. 2011;**70**(1):96-101

[167] El Marroun H, et al., Maternal use of selective serotonin reuptake inhibitors, fetal growth, and risk of adverse birth outcomes. Archives General Psychiatry. 2012;**69**(7):706-714

[168] Oberlander TF, et al. Pain reactivity in 2-month-old infants after prenatal and postnatal serotonin reuptake inhibitor medication exposure. Pediatrics. 2005;**115**(2):411-425

[169] Casper RC, et al. Length of prenatal exposure to selective serotonin reuptake inhibitor (SSRI) antidepressants: effects on neonatal adaptation and psychomotor development. Psychopharmacology (Berl). 2011;**217**(2):211-219

[170] Croen LA, et al., Antidepressant use during pregnancy and childhood autism spectrum disorders. Archives General Psychiatry. 2011;**68**(11):1104-1112

[171] Oberlander TF, et al. Prenatal effects of selective serotonin reuptake inhibitor antidepressants, serotonin transporter promoter genotype (SLC6A4), and maternal mood on child behavior at 3 years of age. Archives Pediatrics & Adolescent Medecine. 2010;**164**(5):444-451

[172] Cases O, et al. Lack of barrels in the somatosensory cortex of monoamine oxidase A-deficient mice: role of a serotonin excess during the critical period. Neuron. 1996;**16**, 297-307

[173] Cases O, et al. Plasma membrane transporters of serotonin, dopamine, and norepinephrine mediate serotonin accumulation in atypical locations in the developing brain of monoamine oxidase A knock-outs. Journal Neuroscience. 1998;**18**(17):6914-6927

[174] Lebrand C, et al. Transient developmental expression of monoamine transporters in the rodent brain. Journal Comparative Neurology. 1998;**401**:506-524

[175] Lotto B, et al. Serotonin receptor activation enhances neurite outgrowth of thalamic neurones in rodents. Neuroscience Letters. 1999;**269**(2):87-90

[176] Laurent A, et al. Activity-dependent presynaptic effect of serotonin 1B receptors on the somatosensory thalamocortical transmission in neonatal mice. Journal Neuroscience. 2002;**22**(3):886-900

[177] Rebsam A, Seif I, Gaspar P. Refinement of thalamocortical arbors and emergence of barrel domains in the primary somatosensory cortex: a study of normal and monoamine oxidase a knock-out mice. Journal Neuroscience. 2002;**22**(19):8541-8552

[178] Narboux-Nême N, et al. Serotonin transporter transgenic (SERTcre) mouse line reveals developmental targets of serotonin specific reuptake inhibitors (SSRIs). Neuropharmacology. 2008;**55**(6):994-1005

[179] Murphy DL, Lesch KP. Targeting the murine serotonin transporter: insights into human neurobiology. Nature Review Neuroscience. 2008;**9**:85-96

[180] Pluess M, et al. 5-HTTLPR moderates effects of current life events on neuroticism: differential susceptibility to environmental influences. Progress Neuropsychopharmacology & Biological Psychiatry. 2010;**34**:1070-1074

[181] Gingrich JA, et al. New Insights into How Serotonin Selective Reuptake Inhibitors Shape the Developing Brain. Birth Defects Research. 2017;**109**(12):924-932

[182] Rebello TJ, et al. Postnatal day 2 to 11 constitutes a 5-HT-sensitive period impacting adult mPFC function. Journal Neuroscience. 2014;**34**(37):12379-12393

[183] Wellman CL, et al. Impaired stress-coping and fear extinction and abnormal corticolimbic morphology in serotonin transporter knock-out mice. Journal Neuroscience. 2007;**27**(3):684-691

[184] Jennings KA, et al. Increased expression of the 5-HT transporter confers a low-anxiety phenotype linked to decreased 5-HT transmission. Journal Neuroscience. 2006;**26**(35):8955-8964

[185] Bocchio M, et al. Increased Serotonin Transporter Expression Reduces Fear and Recruitment of Parvalbumin Interneurons of the Amygdala. Neuropsychopharmacology. 2015;**40**(13):3015-3026

[186] Li Q, et al. Brain region-specific alterations of 5-HT2A and 5-HT2C receptors in serotonin transporter knockout mice. Journal Neurochemistry. 2003;**84**(6):1256-1265

[187] Levitt P, Campbell DB. The genetic and neurobiologic compass points toward common signaling dysfunctions in autism spectrum disorders. Journal Clinical Investigation. 2009;**119**:747-754

[188] Page DT, et al. Haploinsufficiency for Pten and Serotonin transporter cooperatively influences brain size and social behavior. Proceedings National Academy Sciences USA. 2009;**106**:1989-1994

[189] Griebel G, et al. Differential modulation of antipredator defensive behavior in Swiss-Webster mice following acute or chronic administration of imipramine and

fluoxetine. Psychopharmacology (Berl). 1995;**120**(1):57-66

[190] Cases O, et al. Aggressive behavior and altered amounts of brain serotonin and norepinephrine in mice lacking MAOA. Science. 1995;**268**(5218):1763-1766

[191] Brunner HG, et al. Abnormal behavior associated with a point mutation in the structural gene for monoamine oxidase A. Science, 1993;**262**(5133):578-580

[192] Meyer-Lindenberg A. Neural connectivity as an intermediate phenotype: brain networks under genetic control. Human Brain Mapping. 2009;**30**(7):1938-1946

[193] Buckholtz JW, et al. Genetic variation in MAOA modulates ventromedial prefrontal circuitry mediating individual differences in human personality. Molecular Psychiatry. 2008;**13**(3):313-324

[194] Naoi M, Maruyama W, Shamoto-Nagai M. Type A monoamine oxidase and serotonin are coordinately involved in depressive disorders: from neurotransmitter imbalance to impaired neurogenesis. Journal Neural Transmission (Vienna). 2018;**125**(1):53-66

[195] Brummett BH, et al. Associations of a regulatory polymorphism of monoamine oxidase-A gene promoter (MAOA-uVNTR) with symptoms of depression and sleep quality. Psychosomatic Medecine. 2007;**69**(5):396-401

[196] Shumay E, et al.. Evidence that the methylation state of the monoamine oxidase A (MAOA) gene predicts brain activity of MAO A enzyme in healthy men. Epigenetics. 2012;**7**(10):1151-1160

[197] Ziegler C, et al. MAOA gene hypomethylation in panic disorder-reversibility of an epigenetic risk pattern by psychotherapy. Translational Psychiatry. 2016; **6**(4):e773

[198] Ziegler C, Domschke K. Epigenetic signature of MAOA and MAOB genes in mental disorders. Journal Neural Transmission (Vienna). 2018;**125**(11):1581-1588

Chapter 4

Small Molecule Drugs for Treatment of Alzheimer's Diseases Developed on the Basis of Mechanistic Understanding of the Serotonin Receptors 4 and 6

Charlotte Uldahl Jansen and Katrine M. Qvortrup

Abstract

Alzheimer's disease (AD) is the most common form of dementia affecting millions of people worldwide and currently, the only possible treatment is the use of symptomatic drugs. Therefore, there is a need for new and disease-modifying approaches. Among the numbers of biological targets which are today explored in order to prevent or limit the progression of AD, the modulation of serotonin receptors the subtype 4 and 6 receptors (5-HT4R and 5-HT6R) has received increasing attention and has become a promising target for improving cognition and limit the amyloid pathology through modulation of the neurotransmitter system. A large number of publications describing the development of ligands for these serotonin receptors have emerged, and their pharmaceutical potential is now quite evident. However, 5-HT4R and 5-HT6R functionality is much more complex than initially defined. This chapter describes recent advances in the understanding of this modulation as well as the medicinal chemistry efforts towards development of selective 5-HT4R or 5-HT6R ligands.

Keywords: serotonin pathways, Alzheimer's, 5-HT4R and 5-HT6R modulators, structure–activity relationship

1. Introduction

Alzheimer's disease (AD) is a devastating but poorly treated disease. Therefore, there is an urgent need for new and efficient treatment strategies, emphasized by recent statistics from WHO predicting that AD will become the second-most prevalent cause of death within 20 years.

Mounting evidence accumulated over the past years indicates that the neurotransmitter serotonin plays a significant role in cognition and memory. The intimate anatomical and neurochemical association of the serotonergic system and brain areas affected in AD have inspired researchers to focus on this system as a major therapeutic drug target.

Based on the current knowledge of mechanisms involved in serotonin regulation, we here provide structural insight into chemical compounds that have been developed for targeting of the serotonin receptors the subtype 4 and 6 receptors (5-HT4R and 5-HT6R) processes as potential treatments in AD.

2. The serotonergic system in Alzheimer's disease

Serotonin is a small molecule that functions both as a hormone in the periphery, and as neurotransmitter and neuromodulator in the central nervous system (CNS) [1]. In the CNS, it is produced by a small cluster of neurons located in the raphe nuclei of the midbrain. Through innervation of numerous brain regions, serotonin (5-hydroxytryptamine, 5-HT) modulates various physiological functions including circadian rhythms, mood, sleep, appetite, and learning and memory. The areas of the brain involved in learning and memory show high concentrations of 5-HT1AR, 5-HT4R, 5-HT6R and 5-HT7R, why modulation of these is of particular interest in for reversing the cognitive impairment associated with AD [2].

AD has been linked to a decrease of serotonergic neurons in the raphe nuclei, seemingly due to the accumulation of hyperphosphorylated Tau as well as deposits of amyloid beta in the projection sites of serotonergic neurons, causing retrograde degeneration of the neurons [3]. Furthermore, a significant decrease in the number of serotonin transporter (SERT) have also been reported [4]. Overall, this leads to a decrease in serotonin neurotransmission, suggesting that increasing serotonin level in the raphe nuclei can improve cognitive performance in AD patients. This is supported by studies showing that administration of selective serotonin reuptake inhibitors (SSRI) to mouse models of AD, reduced the production of toxic amyloid beta plaques [5, 6]. However, recent clinical trials concluded that treatment with amyloid beta lowering agents should be administered in the very early stages of the disease progression to have any impact on AD, limiting their use until better pre-symptomatic AD diagnostics have been developed.

Several 5-HT receptors (5-HTR) have been shown to influence processing of the amyloid protein precursor (APP), including 5-HT2AR, 5-HT2CR, and 5-HT4R [7, 8]. Among them, the 5-HT4R and 5-HT6R receptors have been of most interest. The 5-HT4R was identified as a most promising target, since activation of this receptor shift the equilibrium of APP cleavage towards formation of the soluble non-amyloidogenic form (sAPPα) fragment possessing neurotrophic and neuroprotective properties [7], while the 5-HT6R has caused much interest for potential roles in AD due to its modulatory effects on gamma-aminobytyric acid (GABA) and glutamate levels, [9] which facilitate the secondary release of other neurotransmitters including dopamine, noradrenaline and acetylcholine, all of which are compromised in AD. In addition, 5-HT6R are exclusively found in the CNS, indicating the possibility of selective CNS targeting to limit off-target toxic effects.

3. Serotonin subtype 4 receptor

Among the large family of 5-HTR, the 5-HT4R's are postsynaptic receptors. Although widely expressed throughout the body, the highest density is observed in the brain (olfactory tubercles, basal ganglia, substantia nigra, superior colliculi, hippocampus, and cortex). These are all CNS structures that are extensively involved in cognitive functions, suggesting that the 5-HT4R could be a therapeutic target for improving memory performance and hereby slowing memory deficits, such as those that occur in AD [10]. Moreover, it has been shown that 5-HT4R expression is reduced in AD patients. Furthermore, it has been shown that activation of these receptors enhances the release of acetylcholine in the frontal cortex and hippocampus [11], increases long term potentiation in the hippocampus [12] and induces a rapid and sustained increase in basal firing of 5-HT cells in the dorsal raphe nucleus [13, 14]. 5-HT4R activation also stimulates hippocampal expression of plasticity/learning-related proteins such as brain-derived-neurotrophic-factor, AKT, CREB, as well as neurogenesis in the dentate gyrus [15].

In addition, and a major advantage of using 5-HT4R agonists in treatment of AD, is their ability to shift the equilibrium of APP processing pathway from production of the neurotoxic amyloid-beta-peptide towards formation of the sAPPα [16]. In contrast to amyloid-beta-peptide, the soluble form has putative neurotropic and neuroprotective properties, see Maillet et al. [17] for a review. The ability of 5-HT4R agonists to stimulate the amyloidogenic pathway leading to release of soluble form of APP has been demonstrated in various cell-based animal models [18].

In early years, 5-HT4R agonists attracted much attention as potential gastrointestinal drugs used in the therapy of functional bowel illnesses such as constipation, irritable bowel syndrome, gastroparesis, and gastroesophageal reflux disease [19]. The first generations of 5-HT4R agonists used in clinical medicine were Tegaserod (**1**), Cisapride (**2**) and Procalupride (**3**) (**Figure 1A**), which showed clinically effective in treatment of gastrointestinal motility disorders; however, adverse cardiovascular events have resulted in the restricted availability of these drugs [20]. Therefore, in order to develop clinically relevant 5-HT4R agonists, the ligands must be potent and highly selective, which is hampered by high similarity of subtype receptors. In 1998, the molecular structure and functional characterization of four splice variants of the human 5-HT4R were described [21] that differ in the carboxy terminal cytoplasmic domain while extracellular and transmembrane domains are absolutely conserved [22].

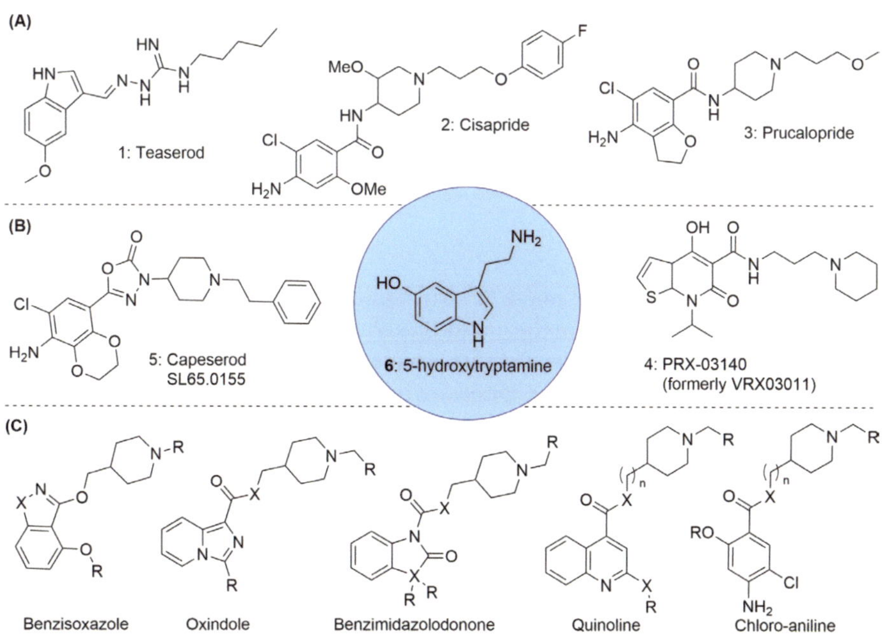

Figure 1.
5-HT4 receptor ligands (A) first generations of 5-HT4R agonists used in clinical medicine, (B) partial 5-HT4R for treatment of AD that reached Phase 2 studies, (C) Overview of structures studied for development of partial 5-HT4R for treatment of AD.

Another concern is the risk that prolonged or repeated exposure of the 5-HT4R to an agonist, may lead to receptor desensitization. The 5-HT4Rs are G-protein-coupled receptors (GPCRs), which can be desensitized following activation by agonists [23]. Agonist-induced desensitization of GPCRs is less common for partial agonists than strong agonists and therefore, most focus has been given to developing highly selective partial 5-HT4R agonists for treatment of AD. In order to being therapeutic useful in treatment of AD, the compound must therefore fulfill several requirements. In addition to being a selective partial 5-HT4R agonist, the target molecule must show good brain barrier penetration, which was also limited in the early generation agonists [24].

However, the potential for 5-HT4R partial agonists to offer clinical benefit for the treatment of AD has indeed been demonstrated. Data from a small Phase 2 study in patients with mild to moderate AD with the selective partial 5-HT4R agonist, PRX-03140 (**4**, EPIX Pharmaceuticals), [25] **Figure 1B**, showed a statistically significant improvement of cognitive processes after only two weeks of therapy [20]. Also, the partial agonist SL65.0155 (**5**, Sanofi-Aventis) reached phase II clinical trial for the treatment of AD [26]. However, these were both later discarded due to serious off-target effects.

This has stimulated much research aiming at designing and developing more selective 5-HT4R partial agonists.

3.1 Pharmacophore of the 5-HT4R ligand

In accordance with the natural ligand, 5-HT (**6**), the general pharmacophore of 5-HT4R agonists consists of an aromatic core connected via a chemical spacer to a basic amino moiety [27] to introduce affinity, while an extra hydrogen-bond donor-acceptor function (e.g., phenol in 5-HT) is required for high affinity ligands [28]. Furthermore, it is accepted that voluminous substituents of the basic nitrogen interact with a hydrophobic pocket in the 5-HT4R ligand recognition site [29]. Based on this pharmacophore framework, a broad range of substances has been investigated, aiming at introducing selectivity.

Suitable aromatic systems [30] include 4- amino-5-chloro-2-methoxy benzoic acid, indole, imidazopyridines and N-alkyl benzimidazolodonone among others (see **Figure 1C**). Several basic amines with voluminous substituents such as piperizines [31], and piperidines [30] have been used.

3.2 Agonists of 5-HT4R

Over the last years, a broad range of structural varied 5-HT4R agonists have been developed, which all share the common structural features presented by the pharmacophore described above. Below we have grouped them into 4 main groups and discuss the structural features for each of these groups.

3.2.1 Group 1: benzisoxazole, oxindole and benzimidazolodonone core

Much research aiming at developing new 5-HT4R agonists has focused on compounds possessing a benzyl ring linked to a 5 membered heterocycle, analogous to the indole ring in the natural 5-HTR ligand.

Inspired from early generations of 5-HT4R agonists (**1–3**, **Figure 1**), Brodney and coworkers [32] synthesized and studied a diverse set of structural varied chemical libraries aiming at identifying excellent CNS active 5-HT4R agonists. To improve chances of identifying compounds with brain barrier penetration, structures were selected based on a number of criteria: (1) reduced number of hydrogen

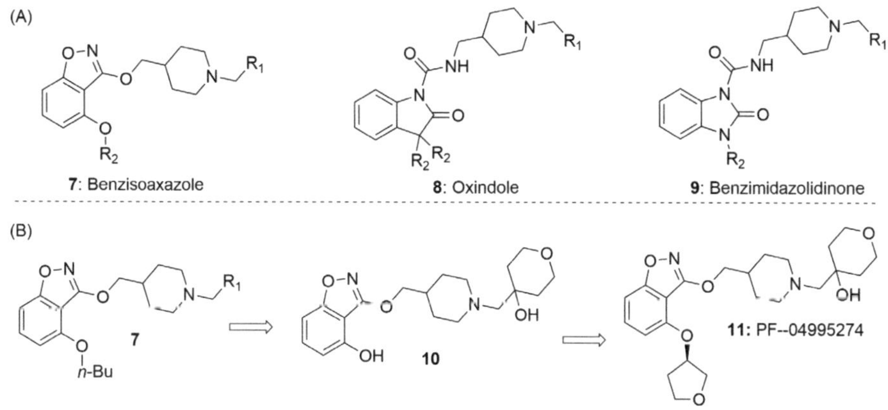

Figure 2.
*SAR studies of (A) benzisoxazole (7), oxindole (8) and benzimidazolodonone (9) core stuctures, (B) provided **11** as a potent partial 5-HT4R agonist [32].*

donors (≤ 1), (2) low molecular weight (<400) and (3) weakly basic amine centers (pKa < 8,5) [33]. Based on these criteria, the benzisoxazole (7), oxindole (**8**) and benzimidazolodonone (**9**) was chosen as core structural templates.

For benzisoaxazoles (7), the studies showed that manipulation of molecular size and shape of the R1 and R2 groups (structure 7, **Figure 2**) provided means to modulate intrinsic properties and ADME (adsorption-distribution-metabolism-excretion). Highly lipophilic compounds (R1 = n-butyl) resulted in high clearance from human liver and low passive permeability. Replacing the piperidine n-butyl group with hydroxyl-tetrahydropyran reduced the partition coefficient (ClogP), but analogue **10** still demonstrated high clearance. To further reduce ClogP, the isobytyl side chain was replaced with more polar groups. While the tertiary carbinol and tetrahydropyran analogues exhibited poor metabolic stability, the tetrahydrofyran **11** provided a potent partial agonist with low clearance.

Orjales and coworkers [33] provided a structure–activity-relationship (SAR) study of 2,3-dihydro-2-oxo-1H-benzimidazole-1-carboxamide derivatives bearing a piperazine moiety (**12a-h**, **Figure 3**). Both, the influence of the 3-substituent of the benzimidazole ring, the 4-substituent of the piperazine moiety, and the alkylene spacer was studied and especially the substituent in the 3-position was found to be critical for 5-HT4R affinity. While compounds with ethyl (**12a**), and cyclopropyl (**12b**) substituents showed moderate to high affinity for the receptor, derivatives having smaller alkyl substituents (H: **12c**, methyl: **12d**, propyl: **12e**) showed a significant drop in affinity. Also, introduction of large and bulky substituents (benzyl: **12f**, butyl: **12g** and phenylethyl: **12h**) severely reduced the affinity for the 5-HT4R. In addition to receptor affinity, also the 5-HT4R activity was dramatically influenced by substituents in the benzimidazolone 3-position. While ethyl- and cyclopropyl-functionalized derivatives (**12a**, **12b**) showed moderate antagonistic activity, the isopropyl derivatives (**12i** and **13c**) acted as partial agonists. The dramatic variation in the 5-HT4R pharmacological activity as a result of only small structural variations is in agreement with previous observations for benzoate derivatives [29].

A similar trend with benzimidazolone 5-HT4R ligands was reported by Langlois et al. [34] While the DAU-6215 ligand (**13a**) with no alkyl substituent on the nitrogen in the 3-position is in-active towards the 5-HT4R, the BIMU-1 (**13b**) and BIMU-8 (**13c**) compounds with ethyl and isopropyl substituents are potent 5-HT4R agonists [34, 35].

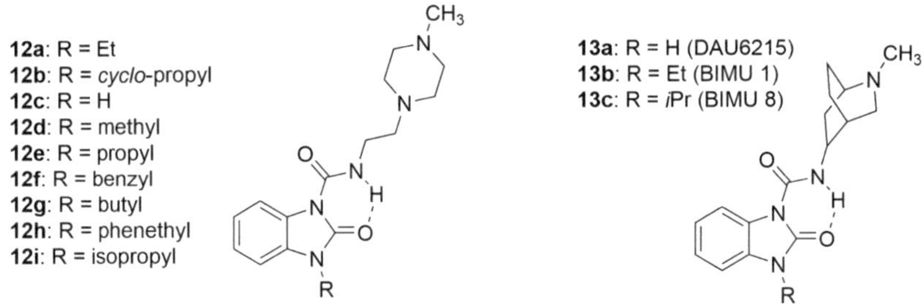

Figure 3.
Structures investigated in a SAR study of 2,3-dihydro-2-oxo-1H-benzimidazole-1-carboxamide derivatives bearing a piperazine moiety [33].

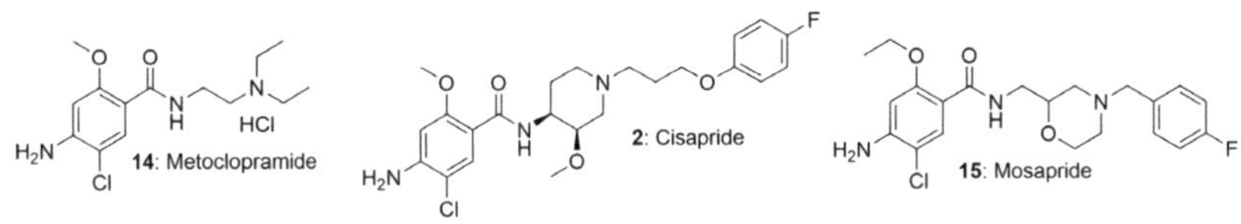

Figure 4.
Parent compounds of the chloro-aniline class of structures.

3.2.2 Group 2: chloro-aniline core

The parent compound of this class is metoclopramide [36, 37] (**14**, **Figure 4**), a drug well-known for its gastric prokinetic activity. Furthermore, compounds having the chloro-aniline core is already well known to confer 5-HT4R agonist activity, for example in Cisapride (**2**) [38] and Mosapride (**15**) [39]. Therefore, it is not surprising that several derivatives of 4-amino-5-chloro-2-methoxybenzoic acids have been investigates as 5-HT4R agonist in AD research.

Russo et al. [40] synthesized and studied a library of structures based on the 5-HT4R partial agonist, ML10302 (**16**, **Figure 5**) by introducing an amide group linked to the piperidine ring of ML10302 (**16**), **Figure 5**, hoping to introduce additional binding interactions. Displacements experiments with a 5-HT4R specific antagonist revealed that compounds in which the amide functionality was directly attached to the piperidine ring (**17**, n = 0) had weaker binding affinities compared to ML10302 (**16**). However, compounds where the amide moiety were attached to the piperidine ring through a methylene bridge, showed binding affinities that were globally better than ML10302 (**16**). Importantly, 4 compounds were identified that showed better functional properties than ML10302 (**16**) and induced up to 50% higher cyclic adenosinde monophosphate (cAMP) production. One compound (**18**) was further evaluated by in vivo biological tests, showing promising results for AD treatment.

RS67333 (**19**) [41] is a very affine 5-HT4R partial agonist, which also have high selectivity vs. other receptors. Its therapeutic relevance for treatment of AD is evident as it was shown to improve both object and place recognition in adult [42, 43] and aged animals [44, 45]. On this basis, Dallemagne and coworkers synthesized a series of analogues of RS6733 (**19**) [46], aiming at identifying a multitarget-directed ligand (MTDL) having both 5HT4R agonist and acetylcholinesterase (AChE) inhibitor activities. Among them, the compound donecopride (**20**) was designed: The cyclohexyl moiety was introduced to be a compromise between the N-butyl group of RS67333 (**19**) and the bulky benzyl group of the potent AChE inhibitor, donepezil (**21**). Donecopride (**20**) showed outstanding in vitro activity and was able to potentiate both the 5-HT4R partial agonist activities as well as the

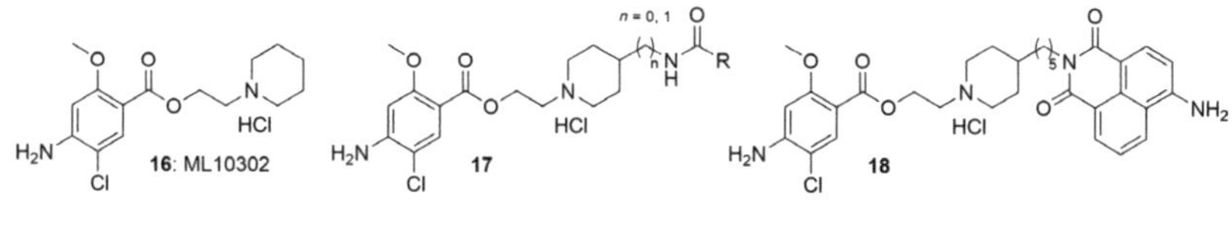

Figure 5.
Structures investigated in a SAR study of analogues of the 5-HT4R partial agonist, ML10302 [40].

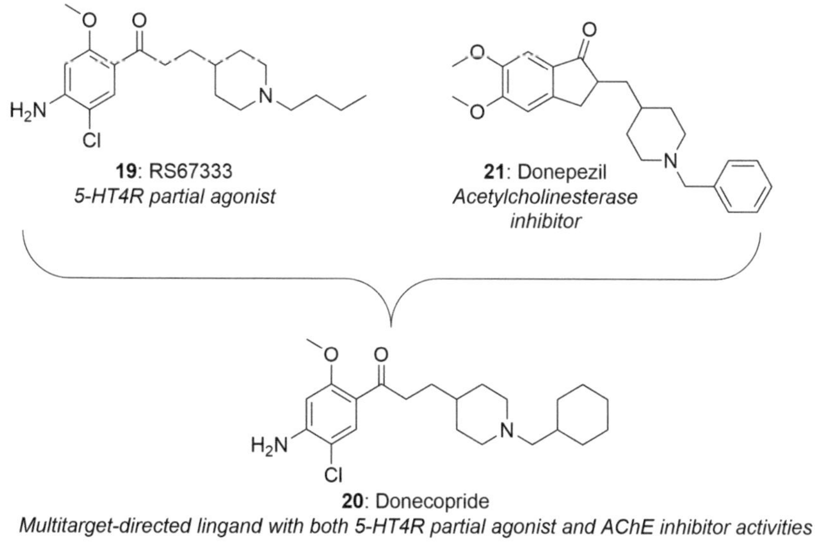

Figure 6.
A multitarget-directed ligand Donecopride (20) was developed to have both 5HT4R agonist and acetylcholinesterase inhibitor activities [46].

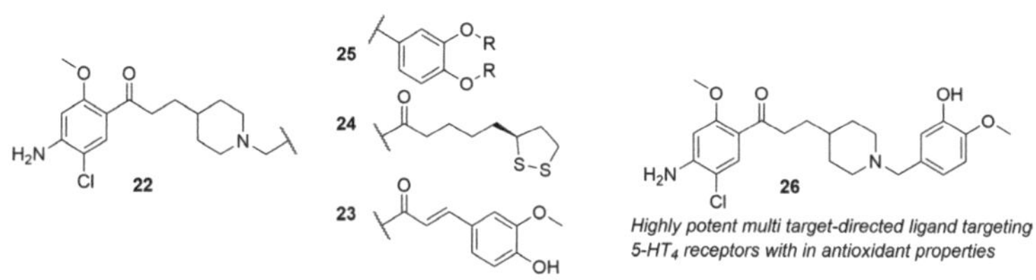

Figure 7.
Compound 26 was developed by combining the 5-HT4R chloro-aniline pharmacophore (22) and structures (23–25) having antioxidant properties [48].

inhibition of AChE, resulting in the alleviation of both amyloid aggregation and tau hyperphosphorylation, [47] which are known to be two major features in AD (**Figures 6** and 7).

In 2019, Lanthier et al. [48] generated a MTDL targeting both activation of the 5-HT4R while also bearing antioxidant activities; hereby being able to both control Ab protein accumulation and prevent toxicity of reactive oxygen species (ROS) in neuronal cells [48].

The chloro-aniline core connected via a chemical spacer to a basic piperidine ring (structure **22**) was introduced as the 5-HT4R binding moiety of the MDLT. As replacement of the butyl chain of RS67333 (**19**) by diverse alkyl moieties has been shown to have limited impact on both the affinity and the pharmacological profile towards the 5-HT4R [46], the chemical moiety having antioxidant activities was introduced as substituent on the central piperidine ring. A variety of structures was investigated, varying in spacer between the two pharmacophores. Also, various chemical structures known to exhibit antioxidant activities were investigated, including polyphenol [49], hydroxycinnamic acid (**23**) [50], lipoic acid (**24**) [51, 52], vanillin or isovanillin (**25**) [53, 54]. Hereby, Lanthier et al. were able to identify a potent 5-HT4R ligand (**26**) with promising antioxidant activity for future preclinical tests.

A similar approach was investigated by Yahiaoui et al., who reported the design of the dual compound **27** with 5-HT4R agonist and 5-HT6R antagonist effects (**Figure 8**) [55]. The dual 5-HT4R/5-HT6R ligand was designed through modulation of the 5-HT4R partial agonist, RS67333 (**19**) by introducing a 5-HT6R antagonist (**28,29**) pharmacophore (a positive ionizable atom, a hydrogen bond acceptor group, a hydrophobic site, and an aromatic-ring hydrophobic site) [56–60]. Yahiaoui et al. synthesized and tested a library of structures consisting of RS67333 (**19**) modulated with various arylsulfonyl groups (sulfonamides and sulfones) attached to the piperidine moiety through a variable number of methylene groups [61]. These studies resulted in identification of the compound **27** having nanomolar and submicromolar affinities towards 5-HT4R and 5-HT6R, acting as a partial agonist and antagonist, respectively.

To further elaborate on these studies, Hatat et al. [61] designing an anti-amnesic MTDL with balanced 5-HT4R agonist, 5-HT6R antagonist and AChE inhibitory activities. Starting from the dual MTDL **30** and the benzyl analog of Donecopride (**35**) [62], various analogues were designed and tested. However, counteracting requirements within the scaffold made the design difficult. While an unsubstituted benzyl group was the best substituent on the piperidine for affinity towards AChE and 5-HT4R, the 5-HT4R affinity appeared linked to substitution of the benzyl group. However, the analogue with a methyl group in the benzyl meta-position (**32**) showed balanced activities towards all three targets (**Figure 9**).

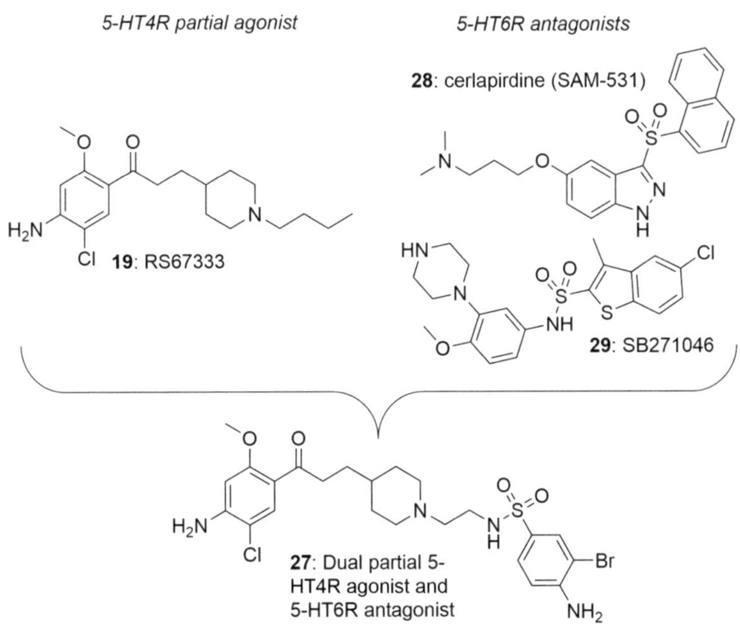

Figure 8.
The dual 5-HT4R/5-HT6R ligand was designed through modulation of the 5-HT4R partial agonist, RS67333 by introduction of a 5-HT6R antagonist pharmacophore [55].

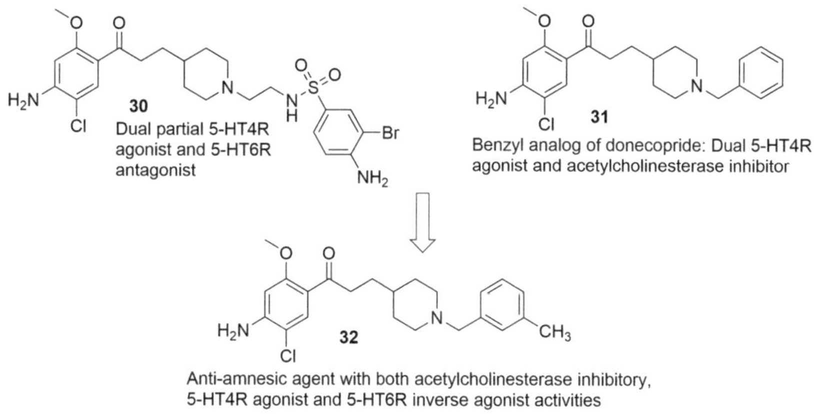

Figure 9.
Antiamnesic MTDL (32) with balanced 5-HT4R agonist, 5-HT6R antagonist and AChE inhibitory activities [61].

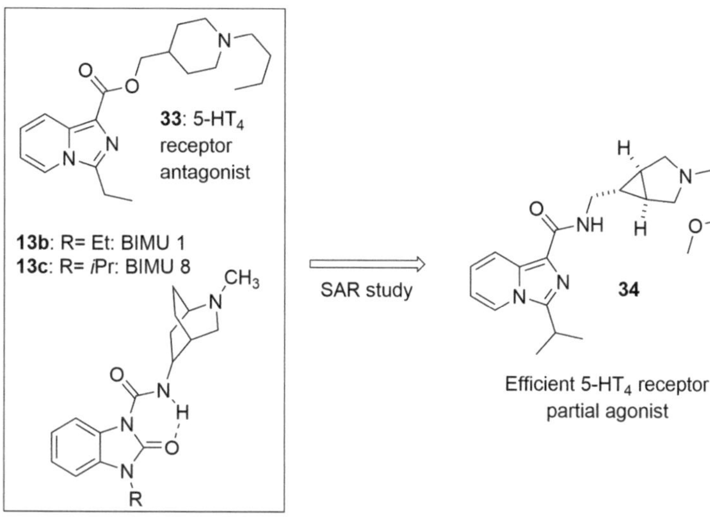

Figure 10.
SAR studies of imidazo[1,5-a]pyridine structures provided 34 as an efficient 5-HT4R partial agonist [66].

3.2.3 Group 3: imidazo[1,2-a]pyridine, imidazo[1,5-a]pyridine, imidazo[4,5-b] pyridine and imidazo[4,5-c]pyridine core

Compounds based on the imidazo[1,5-a]pyridine [63, 64] core were initially reported as dual mediators of 5-HT3R and 5-HT4R [65], see **Figure 10** (**33**). However, work from Nirogi et al. provided an understanding of the substitution patterns on both the imidazo[1,5-a]pyridine ring and piperidine ring, allowing for development of 5-HT4R partial agonists based on this core [66]. Derivatives were designed as bioisosteric analogues of the potent 5-HT4R agonists BIMU-1 and BIMU-8 (**Figure 10**, compounds **13b** and **13c**) [34] by replacing the benzimidazolone core with an imidazo[1,5-a] pyridine while preserving an alicyclic amine moiety, in accordance with the 5-HT4R pharmacophore (see section 3.1). Structural optimization was focused on modification of the alkyl substituent at the imidazopyridine ring, as well as the type of alicyclic amine. Also, a SAR iteration was carried out to understand the role of a methylene spacer between the amide group with the piperidine moiety, in addition to the effect of length and structure of the

N-alkyl/heteroalkyl chain. This process resulted in the discovery of a highly potent and selective partial 5-HT4R agonist **34** with pro-cognitive efficacy in rats and adequate ADME properties [66].

3.2.4 Group 4: quinoline core

Compounds containing the quinoline bicyclic aromatic core have attracted much attention in the design of 5-HT4R ligands [67–70]. To provide medicinal chemistry understanding of the quinoline 5-HT receptor ligands, Castriconi et al. [71] synthesized and studied binding affinity of potential 5-HT4R agonists with reference to the 5-HT4R ligands ML10302 (**16**) and PRX-03140 (**4**) by replacing the aromatic moieties with 2-methoxyquinoline. Interestingly, the flexible quinoline derivatives **35**, **36** showed remarkable differences in 5-HT4R affinity. In fact, while the ester derivative **35** showed a K_i value in the nanomolar range, the corresponding secondary amide **36** was at least two orders of magnitude less active. This was ascribed to the chemical nature of the amid bond linking the side chain with the quinoline moiety in **36** affecting the preferred conformation (**Figure 11**). To test this hypothesis, the flexible compounds **36** were transformed into the conformationally constrained derivatives **37**, **38** (**Figure 11**). This enhanced 5-HT4R affinity to the nanomolar range, suggesting that the conformationally constrained derivatives **37**, **38** represented the bioactive conformation of ester **35**, which cannot be populated by amide derivative **36** for steric reasons. The higher affinity of **38** compared to **37** suggests a secondary role of the second carbonyl group in the interaction with 5-HT4R binding site.

In later efforts, Cappelli and coworkers published a more comprehensive SAR study of receptor ligands with 2-methoxyquinoline as the aromatic system [72]. A series of piperidine containing functionalities were investigated, demonstrating N-butyl-4-piperidinylmethyl (also present in RS67333 (**19**), see **Figure 12**) to be a most promising basic moiety. Substituting the quinoline methoxy-substituent with a chloro- or cyclopropyl-substituent, did not have any significant effect on the activity (**39a-d**).

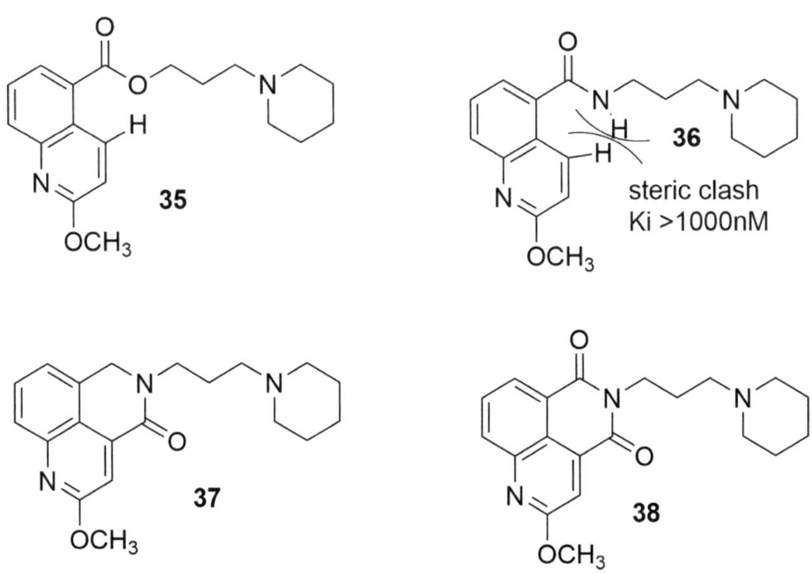

Figure 11.
Quinoline 5-HT$_4$ receptor ligands. Conformationally constrained derivatives 37, 38 showed improved affinity compared to the flexible compounds 35, 36 [71].

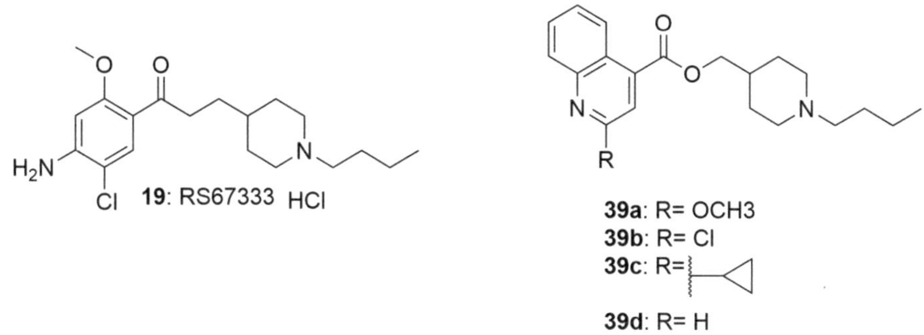

Figure 12.
A comprehensive SAR study of receptor ligands with 2-methoxyquinoline core structure provided 39a as an efficient 5-HT6R partial agonist [72].

4. Serotonin subtype 6 receptor

The 5-HT6R was discovered in 1993 by Monsma et al. [73–76]. These receptors are GPCRs, which are located postsynaptically to serotonergic neurons [77]. Since its identification, significant efforts have led to a better understanding of the biology of this receptor. The 5-HT_6 receptors are present in regions of the brain regions responsible for learning and memory, making them of high interest in AD research. Furthermore, blockade of 5-HT6R function was shown to increase acetylcholine- and glutamate-related neurotransmission, which enhances learning and memory [78, 79]. Evidence indicates that blockade of this receptor improve both cholinergic and glutamatergic system [79]. Furthermore, blockade of 5-HT6R alleviates memory deficits, such as age-related decline in cholinergic or glutamatergic neurons, [79, 80]. Studies conducted by Kotańska et al. [74] revealed that antagonism of the 5-HT6R enhanced neuroplasticity, helped maintain neurite growth and provided a neuroprotective effect against amyloid beta neurotoxicity [81, 82].

This has led to a high interest in this receptor in treatment of the cognitive decline associated with AD [75, 78, 79, 83]. In addition, the receptor is exclusively expressed in the CNS, primarily in the striatal, hippocampal and cortical areas of the brain [75] and therefore, could potentially provide therapeutics with limited peripheral side-effects [80].

Among the first reported selective antagonists are Ro-04-6790 (**40**) reported in 1998 [82, 84], SB-271046 (**29**) in 1999 [82, 85, 86] and SB-399885 (**41**) in 2002 [87] (see **Figure 13**) showed a 200-fold selectivity for the 5-HT6R. Although selective antagonists have been developed, no 5-HT6R antagonist has reached the pharmacological market to date. Thus, the search for new 5-HT6R agents is still of high focus in medicinal chemistry research. In this context, a better SAR understanding of the 5-HT6R pharmacophore is needed.

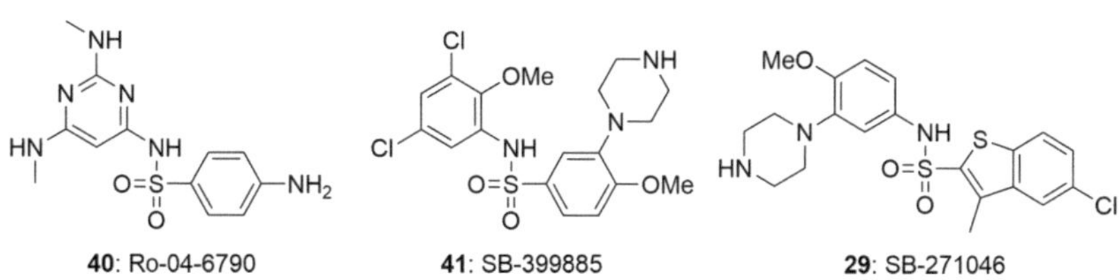

Figure 13.
*Illustrations of the some of the first selective 5-HT6R antagonists; Ro-04-6790 (**40**), SB-399885 (**41**) and SB-271046 (**29**).*

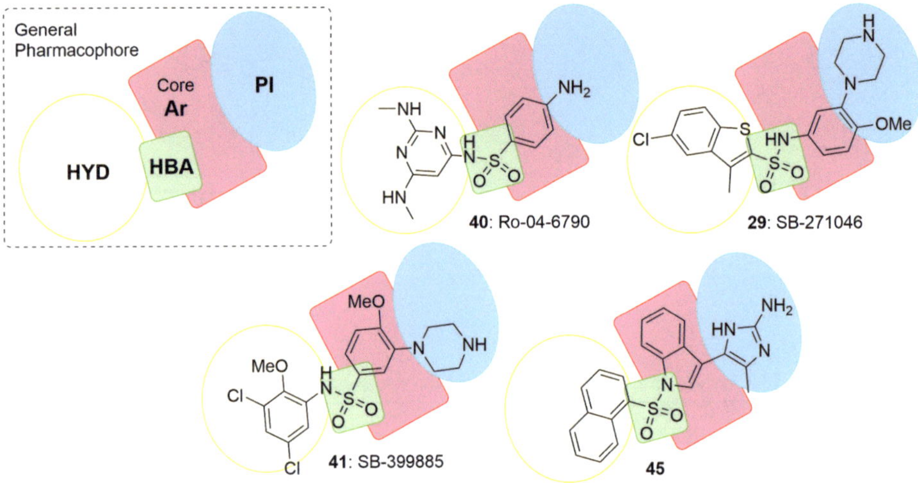

Figure 14.
*Schematic illustration of the pharmacophore (stripped box) along with overlays with using the first selective antagonist (**40, 29, 41**) and compound **45** from section 4.1. The figure is adapted from [88].*

4.1 Pharmacophore of the 5-HT6R ligand

From 1998 until today a fair number of studies have been conducted on 5-HT6R antagonists, which led to a good understanding of the pharmacophore. There are four main features responsible for interaction with the receptor: a polar positively ionizable (PI) group, a hydrogen bond acceptor (HBA), an aromatic area (AR) and a hydrophobic site (HYD) [75, 79] (see **Figure 14**).

In 2017, González-Vera and coworkers published [88] a SAR study regarding the hydrophobic moiety (HYD). In total 18 compounds were synthesized, all containing a sulfonamide as the HBA moiety. This study revealed that aromatic halogens in the HYD part of the structure increased affinity.

Based on this pharmacophore framework, a broad range of substances has been investigated as ligands for the 5-HT6R, aiming at introducing selectivity.

4.2 Antagonists for 5-HT6R

A comprehensive review was published by López-Rodríguez and colleagues in 2014 [79], which discussed the structural key features of 5-HT6R antagonists. In this review, they grouped them into 4 overall groups of structures that had been investigated for antagonism of 5-HT6R (see **Figure 15**). They made some general conclusions, which are summarized in **Figure 15**.

For more details about specific compounds, please refer to [79]. This chapter will focus on studies made since 2014, while the reader is referred to the following excellent reviews [75, 79] for investigations before 2014.

A SAR study published by Zajdel et al. in 2016 [89] studied analogues of the natural substrate 5-HT (**6**) for the receptor. Aiming to increase affinity by constraining the ligand into its preferred conformation, a substituent (R1) was introduced to the tryptamine core, hoping to obtain a more constrained basic amine (**Figure 16**). Furthermore, an aryl arylsulfonyl moiety was introduced in the N1 position of the indole moiety. A total of 28 compounds were tested, which provided two compounds, **42** and **43**, with both high affinity and selectivity for the 5-HT6R. The affinity data showed that R2 substituents were unfavored, while substituents in the indole C5 position improved properties

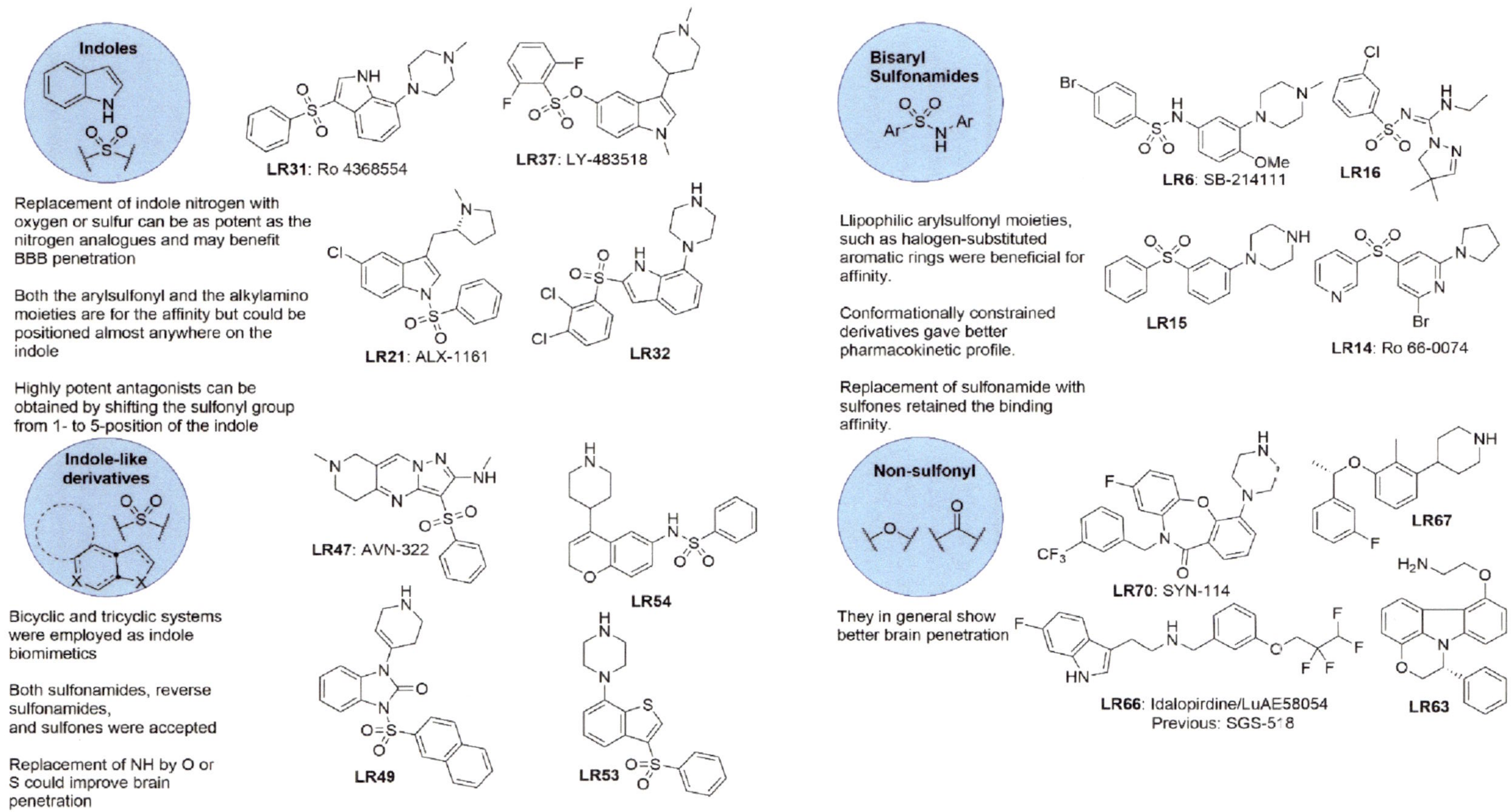

Figure 15.
Representative examples from review by López-Rodríguez and colleagues [79]. The compound notation/numbering correlates with that of the review.

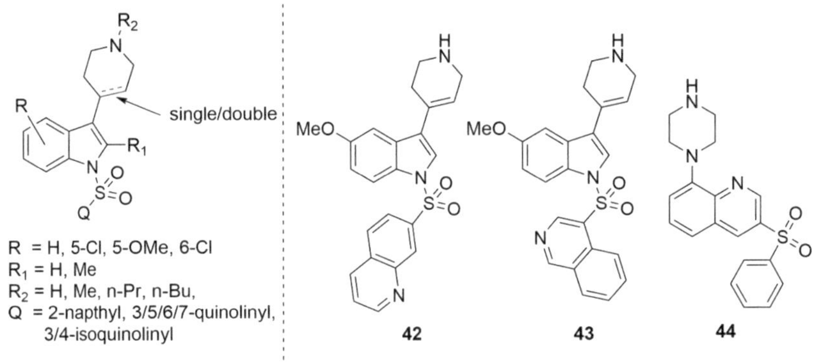

Figure 16.
*Summarizing the structures from the SAR, followed by two potential antagonists (**42** and **43**), along with reference compound SB-742457 (**44**). [89].*

(**Figure 16**). When reducing the double bond in compound **42** and **43**, a slight decrease in affinity was observed, probably due to higher flexibility.

The two compounds were further tested for their functional activity *in vitro* and compared with reference compound SB-742457 (**44**). The compounds behaved as potent antagonist in a cAMP assay, while only displaying weak affinity for off-target receptors. Preliminary pharmacokinetic profiling of **43** showed good blood–brain-barrier (BBB) penetration, improved recognition of novel objects in mice, in addition to a putative antidepressant activity in lower doses compared to the reference compound. Furthermore, **43** did not show any anxiolytic activity.

In 2019 Hogendorf et al. [90] published a comprehensive SAR study involving more than 50 compounds, all containing an aminoimidazole moiety as a new bioisoster of the classical PI amino-group. These were found to form strong hydrogen bonds with electronegative acceptors, such as carbonyls, in the enzyme active site. In total six different series were investigated, but only the two series that were found to be most important for activity are included in **Figure 17**.

Based on affinity, physiochemical properties (ClogP, pKa, topological polar surface area, water solubility, etc.), metabolic stability, mutagenic/toxicity and BBB permeation, compound **45**, **Figure 17**, was chosen as the lead structure. The compound showed high selectivity and displayed ability to reverse scopolamine-induced cognitive impairment. Crystallographic studies of the 2-aminoimidazole-based antagonists revealed that the high receptor affinity was reached due to a resonance driven conformational change [90] upon protonation of the imidazole fragment.

AD is more than just an imbalance in the cholinergic or glutamatergic systems and therefore, it was speculated whether better therapeutics could be achieved by using MTDLs affecting several neurotransmitter pathways [77]. In recent years, various MTDLs have been studied [81].

Marcinkowska et al. [81] designed MTDLs combining 5-HT6R antagonism, inhibitory effect against butyrylcholinesterase (BuChE) [91] and antioxidant properties [81], aiming at achieving both cognition-enhancing properties and neuroprotective activity. Both series were based on typical the 5-HT6R antagonist scaffold with a N-substituted 4-(piperazin-1-yl)-1H-indole core [79]. The indole 1-position was occupied with a benzyl group for series 1 and a 2-chloro benzene moiety for series 2 (marked with blue in **Figure 18**). The piperazine was N-substituted with an alkyl-phthalimide moiety with variation of the length of the alkyl chain (see **Figure 18**). The phthalimide group (marked with yellow in **Figure 18**) is known for interacting with the hydrophobic pocket in BuChE [92]. The indole moiety (marked with red in **Figure 18**), in addition to being important for 5-HT6R antagonism, had antioxidant properties: Indoles are known for their ability to capture free radicals and protect biological systems against peroxidation [93]. From their screen they found that longer alkyl chains, connecting the phthalimide to the piperazine ring, decreased affinity for the 5-HT6R, while substituents on the benzyl group did not alter affinity significantly.

However, counteracting requirements within the scaffold complicated the design. From the BuChE inhibitor (BuChEI) screen they concluded that generally the unsubstituted benzyl analogues showed highest activity, with compound **46** (R = H, n = 1) being the best inhibitor, while best 5-HT6R affinity was obtained with substrates having chloride in meta position on the benzyl moiety (**47**). Taking both targets into account, compound **48** (R = Cl, n = 1) showed the best overall properties, with good affinity for 5-HT6R, promising BuChE inhibitory effect and satisfying antioxidant properties. This SAR study demonstrated promise for MTDLs as AD therapeutics and inspired further research in the field.

Zajdel et al. recently [94] investigated MTDLs combining 5-HT6R inverse agonist activities and a monoamine oxidase B (MAO-B) inhibitory effect. The

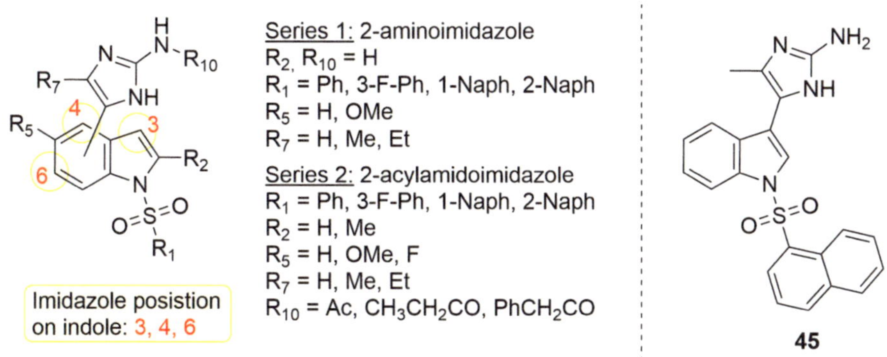

Figure 17.
*SAR illustration covering two out of six series along with lead compound **45**. [90].*

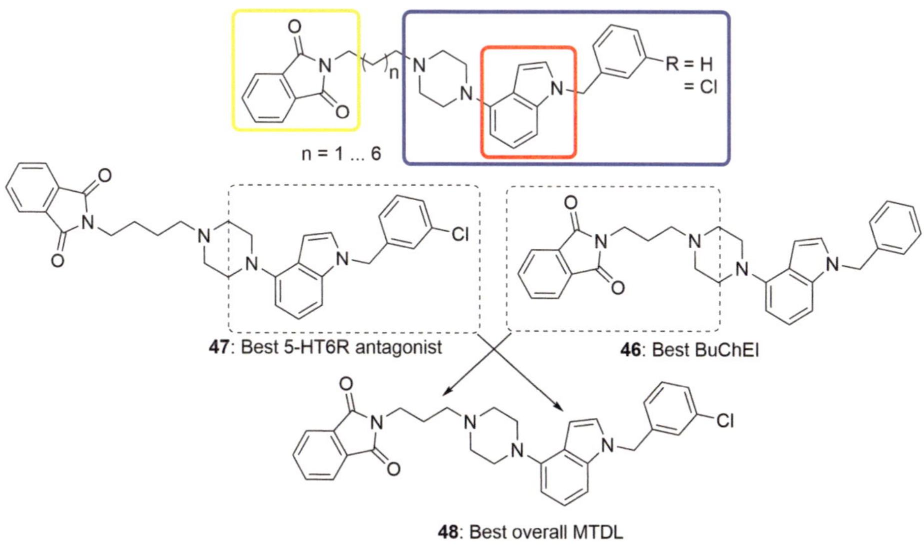

Figure 18.
*Schematic illustration of the model compound highlighting important feature for the MTDL. Compound **47** was the best 5-HT6R antagonist from the study, compound **46** the best BuChE inhibitor and lead compound **48** with the best overall results. [81].*

design included a 5-HT6R antagonist scaffold and fragments of either a reversible or an irreversible MAO-B inhibitor (see **Figure 19**) attached through an alkyl spacer of different lengths.

Their results indicate that the sulfone group was crucial for affinity to the 5-HT6R, while non-substituted phenyl groups (R = H) seemed to result in the best 5-HT6R binding. However, it is relevant to mention that no compounds containing the sulfone group together with the chloride-substituent were tested, making it difficult to make an overall conclusion. Among the 18 synthesized compounds, the very promising lead compound **49** was discovered. This compound displayed moderate metabolic stability, good artificial membrane permeability as well as good distribution in the brain. Furthermore, the compound showed glioprotective properties and fully reversed scopolamine-induced memory deficits.

In 2016 Grychowska et al. [83] published a study for a new core design based on a scaffold-hopping approach, with swapping of carbon and nitrogen atom in the indole ring [95], starting from the SSRI 6-nitroquipazine (**50**) to achieve the 1H-pyrrolo [3,2-c] quinoline core (**51**). They afterwards studied alternating substitution patterns on the arylsulfonyl fragment, which resulted in identification of **52**, see **Figure 20**, as their lead structure for further studies. The SAR revealed that substituents in the meta-position of the phenyl were beneficial. However, it is difficult to make any general conclusions of this effect, as both electron-withdrawing and -donating substituents resulted in compounds with good affinity for the receptor. Of all the compounds tested, compounds containing a chloro-substituent were found to induce strong antagonistic properties. In general, the S enantiomers of the aminopyrrolidine were more favored than the R enantiomers and compound **52** showed to be the best candidate with high selectivity for the 5-HT6R over the 5-HT1AR, 5-HT2AR, 5-HT2CR, 5-HT2BR, 5-HT7R as well as dopamine (D2), adrenergic (alpha1A), histamine (H1), muscarinic acetylcholine (M1) receptors and SERT.

From a GPCR signaling assay it was determined that compound **52** behaved as neutral antagonist, whereas the reference SB-742457 (**44**) behaved as an inverse agonist. *In vivo* studies demonstrated that both **52** and SB-742457 (**44**) have pro-cognitive properties, as they were able to reverse pharmacological-induced memory deficits in rats and improve recognition of novel objects. Additionally, **52** showed antidepressant properties. Compound **52** was later used as scaffold for development of a MTDL with both neuroprotective and precognitive activities (5-HT6R and dopamine subtype 3 receptor (D3R) antagonism).

In an attempt to obtain the desired MTDL, Grychowska et al. [96] designed a series of 11 compounds combining structural elements of the 5-HT6R antagonist **52**, (blue box in **Figure 21**) with structural elements of a D3R antagonist (Eticlopride [97] and Nafadotride [98]), red box in **Figure 21**. All compounds synthesized in the study showed moderate-to-high affinity for 5-HT6R; however, only four compounds showed acceptable affinity for D3R. An elongation in the length of the alkyl chain (R, **Figure 21**) provided a better binding to D3R, however, decreased the affinity for the 5-HT6R. A chloride-substituted phenyl (X = Cl) showed significantly higher affinity for the 5-HT6R compared to the unsubstituted phenyl (X = H), in accordance with the previous mentioned importance of a halogen substituent (see section 4.1). Rewardingly, the S enantiomers were favored over the R enantiomers for both receptors. Based on all results, **53** showed overall good properties and its selectivity for the 5-HT6R compared to other receptors was studied. Fortunately, it did not bind to 5-HT1AR, 5-HT2AR or 5-HT7R and also showed a 10-fold selectivity over D2Rs. Furthermore, compound **53** proved to be a neutral antagonist, as it did not significantly affect the cAMP level. Its therapeutic potential was nicely demonstrated from animal studies, where both a neuroprotective effect and reversal of pharmacological-induced memory decline was observed.

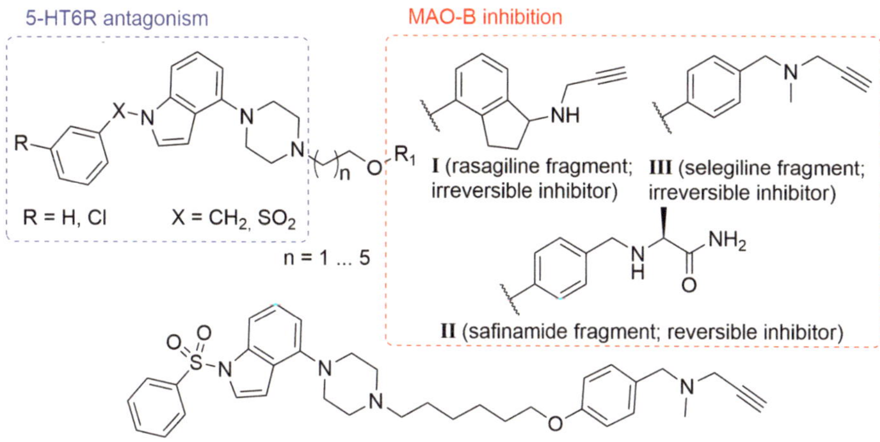

49

Figure 19.
*Schematic illstration outlining the scope of the SAR study and potential MTDL compound **49**. [94].*

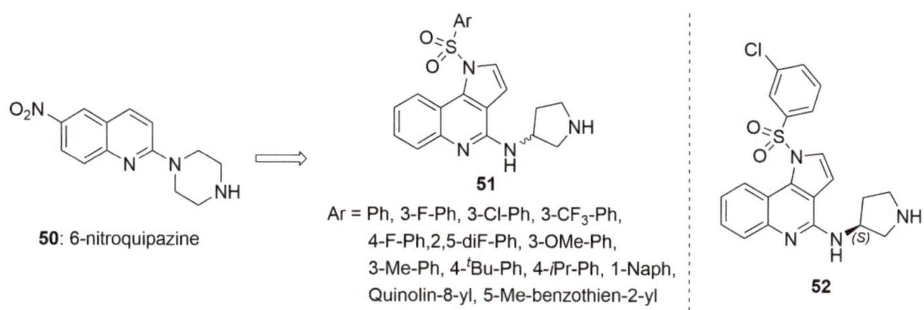

Figure 20.
*SAR scaffold-hopping approach from SSRI (**50**) to 1H-pyrrolo[3,2-c] quinoline core (**51**) to lead compound **52**. [83].*

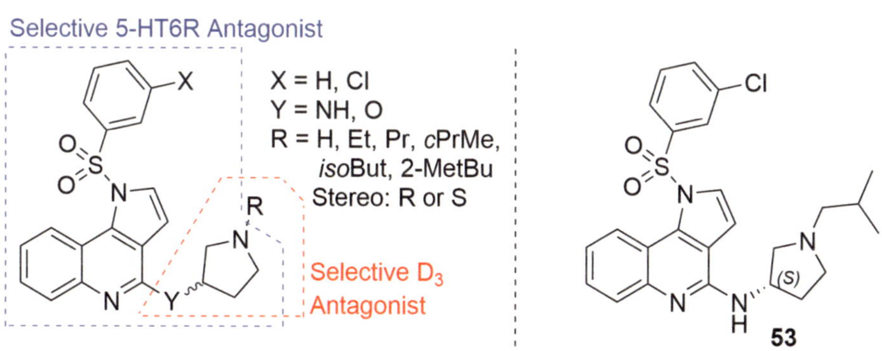

Figure 21.
*Schematic illustration from MTDL SAR combining 5-HT6R antagonist core with selective D3R antagonist fragment, to give lead compound **53**. [96].*

Structure **54** (see **Figure 22**) was identified through a drug discovery strategy based on a virtual screening platform [75, 99]. In total 45 compounds, all possessing the aryl-sulfonamide, was held up against the knowledge of the binding pocket and 5-HT6R ligand pharmacophore, while also adding knowledge from the GPCR ligand database.

For several of the antagonists developed over the years, clinical trials seemed promising until the late studies. One example is the well-known non-sulfonyl

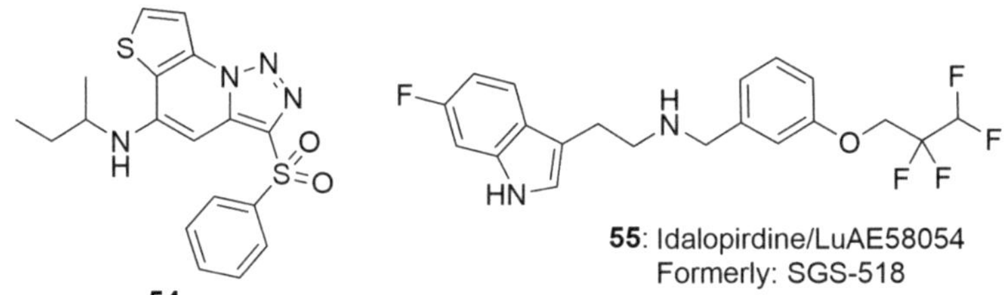

54

55: Idalopirdine/LuAE58054
Formerly: SGS-518

Figure 22.
*(left) Compound **54** obtained from a virtual screening platform [75, 99]. (right) Idalopirdine/LuAE58054 (55) [100].*

compound Idalopirdine or Lu AE58054 (**55**, **Figure 22**), discovered by Lilly. Idalopirdine was found to have high affinity for the 5-HT6R (>50-fold) compared to more than 70 targets studied [79] and reversed pharmacological-induced cognitive impairment. Lilly licensed the compound to Saegis for clinical development. Phase I was started in 2005 by Saegis and phase II in 2009 by Lundbeck (Lundbeck acquired Saegis in 2006) [100]. In phase II, Idalopirdine (**55**) was given to AD patients already receiving donepezil (**21**, an AChE inhibitor). It was found that Idalopirdine (55) provided an inhibitory effect on CYP206, which is involved in the metabolism of donepezil (21), therefore, it cannot be ruled out that the initial positive results originated from an increase in donepezil bioavailability [85]. Three Phase III studies with idalopirdine were initiated in 2013 involving patients with mild to moderate AD. Patients were treated with idalopirdine in combination with either donepezil (two of the studies; NCT02006641 and NCT01955161) or an unspecified AChE inhibitor (the third study; NCT02006654). Idalopirdine seemed to be highly tolerated with very few side effects. However, all three studies did not meet the necessary efficacy and Idalopirdine was therefore removed from the pipeline in 2017. (for more detail on the clinical trials the reader is referred to [101, 102]).

4.3 Neutral antagonists and inverse agonists for the 5-HT6R

An important feature of the 5-HT6R is its ability to exist in different conformational states depending on the ligand bound, which can lead to initiation of different signal transduction pathways. The engagement of the 5-HT6R in several pathways has now been demonstrated. In addition to the canonical Gs adenylyl cyclase signaling pathway implicated in the control of neuronal migration [103], the 5-HT6R is also involved in pathways engaged in brain development of synaptic plasticity, more specifically the rapamycin [104] and cyclin-dependent kinase 5 (Cdk5) signaling pathways [105]. Another relevant feature is the high level of constitutive activity of the 5-HT6R. The 5-HT6R has different pathways that can be activated upon different antagonistic and agonistic approaches, and the above-mentioned problems during clinical trials, stimulated interest for investigating other mechanistic approaches against the receptor.

It is worth having in mind that Cdk5-dependent neurite growth has been found to involve the 5-HT6Rs [105] and being agonist dependent. An inverse agonist of this signaling system, like SB-258585 (**56**, **Figure 23**) prevents neurite growth, neuronal migration and dendritic spine morphogenesis [96, 105]. For this purpose, both neutral antagonists and inverse agonists have been investigated.

Utilizing a scaffold-hopping approach based on swapping one carbon with a nitrogen atom in the indole ring, Vanda et al. [95] synthesized 33 compounds varying in both the position of the nitrogen, alkyl-substituents on the C2 position (R-group, **Figure 23**) and substituents on the benzyl group and based on biological testing, they made some general conclusions. Localization of the nitrogen was crucial for 5-HT6R affinity and compounds with the imidazole[4,5-b]pyridine fragment were in general the best binders. Elongation of the benzyl to a phenethyl group decreased affinity. Furthermore, while bulky and aromatic substituents were not tolerated in the C2 position, small alkyl substituents was in general accepted, with the ethyl-group being the most favored. Furthermore, substituents in the benzyl 3-position were generally preferred, while substituents in the 2- and 4-position lowered affinity compared to the non-substituted analogue. The studies resulted in identification of compound **57** as a new and potent 5-HT6R partial inverse agonist at the Gs signaling pathway, while being a neutral antagonist in the Cdk5 pathway.

4.4 Agonists for the 5-HT6R

Interestingly, it has been suggested that not only 5-HT6R antagonists but also 5-HT6R agonists may have pro-cognitive activities [107]. The 5-HT6R agonist WAY-181187 (**58**) was shown to enhance GABA concentrations, which may potentially

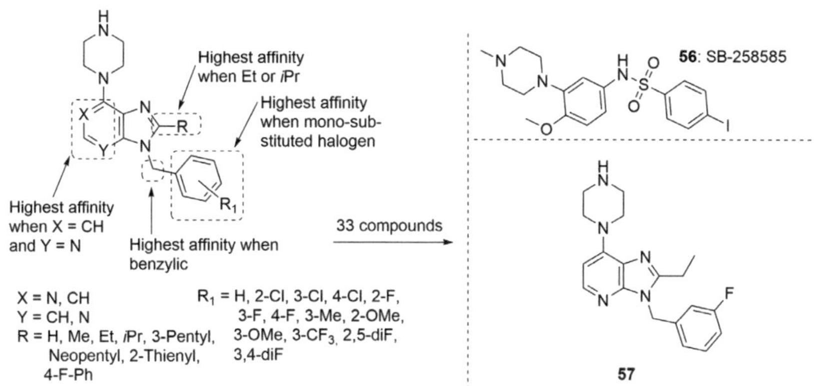

Figure 23.
Illustration of conducted SAR study adapted from [106] and the obtained lead compound (57), along with compound 56.

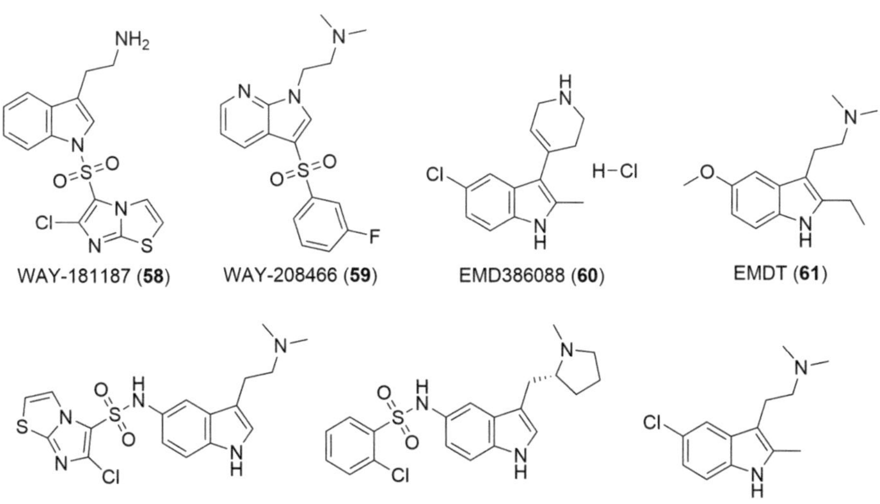

Figure 24.
5-HT6R agonists; WAY-181187 (58) [108, 109], WAY-208466 (59) [109], EMDT (60) [110], EMD386088 (61) [111], E-6801 (62) [112], R-13c (63) [113], ST1936 (64) [114].

have a positive effect on the neuronal plasticity [76], likewise enhancing cholinergic and glutamatergic mechanisms [80], indicating that both activation and inhibition of this receptor evoke similar responses. Although, the mechanism behind these paradoxical similar effects of 5-HT6R agonists and antagonists is not fully understood, it has been suggested that they could be acting on receptors located on distinct neuronal populations. Further discussing of these paradoxical effects can be found in [80], where also other possible explanations are presented.

Several 5-HT6R agonists have been identified, some of them are summarized in **Figure 24** [80].

The effectiveness of the antagonist vs. the agonist approach is further discussed in reviews by Meneses et al. [115] and Fone [80].

5. Conclusion

Alzheimer's disease is increasingly being recognized as one of the most challenging medical and social challenging health concerns in older people. To date, only treatments offering symptomatic relief to patients exist for this disease, limiting benefit to patients. As there is no curable medical treatment available, much effort has been focusing on identifying novel potential targets for drug development. The rich involvement of serotonin (5-HT) in both cognition and memory; some of the most symptomatic areas being affected in AD, has directed current drug discovery programs to focus on this system as a major therapeutic drug target.

Thus, serotonin receptor modulators offer an attractive option for a future treatment of AD patients and modulation of 5-HT4R has indeed demonstrated to improve neurotransmission and enhance the release of acetylcholine resulting in the memory formation. Furthermore, in various cell based and animal models, partial 5-HT4R agonists were demonstrated to promote the release of sAPPα and block the release of amyloid beta peptide. Remarkably, 5-HT4R agonists were also reported to induce neurogenesis in hippocampus as well as enteric system through the activation of cyclic AMP response element binding protein in rodents.

During the past 20 years, also the 5-HT6R has received increasing attention and is now a promising target for improving cognition. However, 5-HT6R functionality is much more complex. Several studies with structurally different compounds have shown that not only antagonists but also 5-HT6R agonists improve learning and memory in animal models. This paradoxical effect may explain why several compounds that reached phase III clinical trials failed to replicate the positive impact on cognition [76, 94]. Therefore, even though preclinical and clinical trials show that the 5-HT6R is a promising target for treatment of neurodegenerative diseases such as AD, there is an urgent need for a better understanding of the pathways involved in modulation of the receptor. However, there is hope that with the recent advances in molecular biological techniques, including improved cloning and sequencing methods, strategies for the development of in silico GPCR models, will advance our understanding of the molecular mechanisms underlying the impact of serotoninergic signaling in AD to provide beneficial treatments for AD.

Taken together, 5-HT4R and 5-HT6R modulators address all major facets of AD. However, although important progress has been made with developing relevant modulators to improve both cognition and memory, crucial challenges still need to be overcome before a promising cure to AD has been found. Most importantly, an in depth understanding of the pathways involved in modulation of the serotonin receptors is urgently needed. Also, to limit side-effects the identification of CNS specific molecules is crucial.

Abbreviations

AChE	acetylcholinesterase
AD	Alzheimer's disease
ADME	absorption, distribution, metabolism, and excretion
alpha1A	adrenergic
APP	amyloid protein precursor
AR	aromatic area
BBB	blood–brain barrier
BuChE	butyrylcholinesterase
cAMP	cyclic adenosinde monophosphate
Cdk5	cyclin dependent kinase 5
ClogP	calculated logarithm of octanol/water partition coefficient
CNS	central nervous system
D2	dopamine
D3R	dopamine subtype 3 receptor
GABA	gamma-aminobytyric acid
GPCR	G protein-coupled receptor
H1	histamine
HBA	hydrogen bond acceptor
HYD	hydrophobic site
M1	muscarinic acetylcholine
MAO-B	monoamine oxidase B
MTDL	multitarget-directed ligands
PI	positively ionizable
ROS	reactive oxygen species
sAPPα	soluble non-amyloidogenic form
SAR	structure–activity relationship
SERT	serotonin transporter
SSRI	selective serotonin reuptake inhibitors
5-HT	5-hydroxytryptamine
5-HT4R	5-hydroxytryptamine receptor 4
5-HT6R	5-hydroxytryptamine receptor 6
5-HTR	5-hydroxytryptamine receptor

Author details

Charlotte Uldahl Jansen and Katrine M. Qvortrup*
Technical University of Denmark, Kongens Lyngby, Denmark

*Address all correspondence to: kaqvo@kemi.dtu.dk

References

[1] S. N. Young, "How to increase serotonin in the human brain without drugs," *J Psychiatry Neurosci*, vol. 32, no. 6, pp. 394-399, Nov. 2007.

[2] M. King, C. Marsden, and K. Fone, "A role for the 5-HT1A, 5-HT4 and 5-HT6 receptors in learning and memory," *Trends in Pharmacological Sciences*, vol. 29, no. 9, pp. 482-492, Sep. 2008, doi: 10.1016/j.tips.2008.07.001.

[3] G. Simic, G. Stanic, M. Mladinov, N. Jovanov-Milosevic, I. Kostovic, and P. R. Hof, "Does Alzheimer's disease begin in the brainstem?," *Neuropathology and Applied Neurobiology*, vol. 35, no. 6, pp. 532-554, Nov. 2009, doi: 10.1111/j.1365-2990.2009.01038.x.

[4] S. M. Tejani-Butt, J. Yang, and A. C. Pawlyk, "Altered serotonin transporter sites in Alzheimer' s disease raphe and hippocampus:," *NeuroReport*, vol. 6, no. 8, pp. 1207-1210, May 1995, doi: 10.1097/00001756-199505300-00033.

[5] J. R. Cirrito *et al.*, "Serotonin signaling is associated with lower amyloid- levels and plaques in transgenic mice and humans," *Proceedings of the National Academy of Sciences*, vol. 108, no. 36, pp. 14968-14973, Sep. 2011, doi: 10.1073/pnas.1107411108.

[6] Y. I. Sheline *et al.*, "An Antidepressant Decreases CSF A Production in Healthy Individuals and in Transgenic AD Mice," *Science Translational Medicine*, vol. 6, no. 236, pp. 236re4-236re4, May 2014, doi: 10.1126/scitranslmed.3008169.

[7] M. Cochet *et al.*, "5-HT $_4$ Receptors Constitutively Promote the Non-Amyloidogenic Pathway of APP Cleavage and Interact with ADAM10," *ACS Chem. Neurosci.*, vol. 4, no. 1, pp. 130-140, Jan. 2013, doi: 10.1021/cn300095t.

[8] A. Thathiah and B. De Strooper, "The role of G protein-coupled receptors in the pathology of Alzheimer's disease," *Nat Rev Neurosci*, vol. 12, no. 2, pp. 73-87, Feb. 2011, doi: 10.1038/nrn2977.

[9] L. Ciranna, "Serotonin as a Modulator of Glutamate- and GABA-Mediated Neurotransmission: Implications in Physiological Functions and in Pathology," *CN*, vol. 4, no. 2, pp. 101-114, Apr. 2006, doi: 10.2174/157015906776359540.

[10] S. E. Murphy, L. C. Wright, M. Browning, P. J. Cowen, and C. J. Harmer, "A role for 5-HT $_4$ receptors in human learning and memory," *Psychol. Med.*, vol. 50, no. 16, pp. 2722-2730, Dec. 2020, doi: 10.1017/S0033291719002836.

[11] S. Consolo, S. Arnaboldi, S. Giorgi, G. Russi, and H. Ladinsky, "5-HT4 receptor stimulation facilitates acetylcholine release in rat frontal cortex:," *NeuroReport*, vol. 5, no. 10, pp. 1230-1232, Jun. 1994, doi: 10.1097/00001756-199406020-00018.

[12] E. Marchetti, F. A. Chaillan, A. Dumuis, J. Bockaert, B. Soumireu-Mourat, and F. S. Roman, "Modulation of memory processes and cellular excitability in the dentate gyrus of freely moving rats by a 5-HT4 receptors partial agonist, and an antagonist," *Neuropharmacology*, vol. 47, no. 7, pp. 1021-1035, Dec. 2004, doi: 10.1016/j.neuropharm.2004.06.033.

[13] G. Lucas and G. Debonnel, "5-HT $_4$ receptors exert a frequency-related facilitatory control on dorsal raphé nucleus 5-HT neuronal activity: 5-HT $_4$ receptors and 5-HT neuronal activity," *European Journal of Neuroscience*, vol. 16, no. 5, pp. 817-822, Sep. 2002, doi: 10.1046/j.1460-9568.2002.02150.x.

[14] G. Lucas *et al.*, "Frontocortical 5-HT4 receptors exert positive

feedback on serotonergic activity: Viral transfections, subacute and chronic treatments with 5-HT4 agonists," *Biological Psychiatry*, vol. 57, no. 8, pp. 918-925, Apr. 2005, doi: 10.1016/j.biopsych.2004.12.023.

[15] H. Hagena and D. Manahan-Vaughan, "The serotonergic 5-HT4 receptor: A unique modulator of hippocampal synaptic information processing and cognition," *Neurobiology of Learning and Memory*, vol. 138, pp. 145-153, Feb. 2017, doi: 10.1016/j.nlm.2016.06.014.

[16] I. Ahmad and R. Nirogi, "5-HT₄ Receptor Agonists for the Treatment of Alzheimer's Dsease," *NM*, vol. 02, no. 02, pp. 87-92, 2011, doi: 10.4236/nm.2011.22013.

[17] M. Maillet, S. Robert, and F. Lezoualc'h, "New Insights into Serotonin 5-HT4 Receptors : A Novel Therapeutic Target for Alzheimers Disease?," *CAR*, vol. 1, no. 2, pp. 79-85, May 2004, doi: 10.2174/1567205043332252.

[18] S. Cho and Y. Hu, "Activation of 5-HT4 receptors inhibits secretion of β-amyloid peptides and increases neuronal survival," *Experimental Neurology*, vol. 203, no. 1, pp. 274-278, Jan. 2007, doi: 10.1016/j.expneurol.2006.07.021.

[19] N. Manabe, B. S. Wong, and M. Camilleri, "New-generation 5-HT $_4$ receptor agonists: potential for treatment of gastrointestinal motility disorders," *Expert Opinion on Investigational Drugs*, vol. 19, no. 6, pp. 765-775, Jun. 2010, doi: 10.1517/13543784.2010.482927.

[20] J. H. De Maeyer, R. A. Lefebvre, and J. A. J. Schuurkes, "5-HT4 receptor agonists: similar but not the same: 5-HT4 receptor agonists: similar but not the same," *Neurogastroenterology & Motility*, vol. 20, no. 2, pp. 99-112, Jan. 2008, doi: 10.1111/j.1365-2982.2007.01059.x.

[21] O. Blondel, M. Gastineau, Y. Dahmoune, M. Langlois, and R. Fischmeister, "Cloning, Expression, and Pharmacology of Four Human 5-Hydroxytryptamine4 Receptor Isoforms Produced by Alternative Splicing in the Carboxyl Terminus," *Journal of Neurochemistry*, vol. 70, no. 6, pp. 2252-2261, Nov. 2002, doi: 10.1046/j.1471-4159.1998.70062252.x.

[22] J. Bockaert, S. Claeysen, V. Compan, and A. Dumuis, "5-HT4 receptors: History, molecular pharmacology and brain functions," *Neuropharmacology*, vol. 55, no. 6, pp. 922-931, Nov. 2008, doi: 10.1016/j.neuropharm.2008.05.013.

[23] R. R. Gainetdinov, R. T. Premont, L. M. Bohn, R. J. Lefkowitz, and M. G. Caron, "DESENSITIZATION OF G PROTEIN–COUPLED RECEPTORS AND NEURONAL FUNCTIONS," *Annu. Rev. Neurosci.*, vol. 27, no. 1, pp. 107-144, Jul. 2004, doi: 10.1146/annurev.neuro.27.070203.144206.

[24] D. E. Johnson *et al.*, "The 5-Hydroxytryptamine $_4$ Receptor Agonists Prucalopride and PRX-03140 Increase Acetylcholine and Histamine Levels in the Rat Prefrontal Cortex and the Power of Stimulated Hippocampal θ Oscillations," *J Pharmacol Exp Ther*, vol. 341, no. 3, pp. 681-691, Jun. 2012, doi: 10.1124/jpet.112.192351.

[25] J. T. Megerian, "Results of a Phase 2A study of a novel 5HT4 agonist for the treatment of Alzheimer's Disease," presented at the American Society for Experimental Neuro Therapeutics Annual Meeting, Arlington, Mar. 2009.

[26] P. C. Moser *et al.*, "SL65.0155, A Novel 5-Hydroxytryptamine $_4$ Receptor Partial Agonist with Potent Cognition-Enhancing Properties," *J Pharmacol Exp Ther*, vol. 302, no. 2, pp. 731-741, Aug. 2002, doi: 10.1124/jpet.102.034249.

[27] J. M. Schaus, D. C. Thompson, W. E. Bloomquist, A. D. Susemichel, D. O. Calligaro, and M. L. Cohen, "Synthesis and Structure−Activity Relationships of Potent and Orally Active 5-HT $_4$ Receptor Antagonists: Indazole and Benzimidazolone Derivatives," *J. Med. Chem.*, vol. 41, no. 11, pp. 1943-1955, May 1998, doi: 10.1021/jm970857f.

[28] K.-H. Buchheit *et al.*, "The Serotonin 5-HT4 Receptor. 1. Design of a New Class of Agonists and Receptor Map of the Agonist Recognition Site," *J. Med. Chem.*, vol. 38, no. 13, pp. 2326-2330, Jun. 1995, doi: 10.1021/jm00013a009.

[29] D. Yang *et al.*, "New Esters of 4-Amino-5-chloro-2-methoxybenzoic Acid as Potent Agonists and Antagonists for 5-HT $_4$ Receptors," *J. Med. Chem.*, vol. 40, no. 4, pp. 608-621, Feb. 1997, doi: 10.1021/jm960320m.

[30] R. M. McKinnell *et al.*, "A Multivalent Approach to the Design and Discovery of Orally Efficacious 5-HT $_4$ Receptor Agonists," *J. Med. Chem.*, vol. 52, no. 17, pp. 5330-5343, Sep. 2009, doi: 10.1021/jm900881j.

[31] I. Tapia *et al.*, "2,3-Dihydro-2-oxo-1 *H* -benzimidazole-1-carboxamides with Selective Affinity for the 5-HT $_4$ Receptor: Synthesis and Structure−Affinity and Structure−Activity Relationships of a New Series of Partial Agonist and Antagonist Derivatives," *J. Med. Chem.*, vol. 42, no. 15, pp. 2870-2880, Jul. 1999, doi: 10.1021/jm981098j.

[32] M. A. Brodney *et al.*, "Identification of Multiple 5-HT $_4$ Partial Agonist Clinical Candidates for the Treatment of Alzheimer's Disease," *J. Med. Chem.*, vol. 55, no. 21, pp. 9240-9254, Nov. 2012, doi: 10.1021/jm300953p.

[33] T. T. Wager *et al.*, "Defining Desirable Central Nervous System Drug Space through the Alignment of Molecular Properties, in Vitro ADME, and Safety Attributes," *ACS Chem. Neurosci.*, vol. 1, no. 6, pp. 420-434, Jun. 2010, doi: 10.1021/cn100007x.

[34] M. Langlois and R. Fischmeister, "5-HT $_4$ Receptor Ligands: Applications and New Prospects," *J. Med. Chem.*, vol. 46, no. 3, pp. 319-344, Jan. 2003, doi: 10.1021/jm020099f.

[35] R. Bureau, M. Boulouard, F. Dauphin, F. Lezoualc'h, and S. Rault, "Review of 5-HT4R Ligands: State of Art and Clinical Applications," *CTMC*, vol. 10, no. 5, pp. 527-553, Apr. 2010, doi: 10.2174/156802610791111551.

[36] R. M. Pinder, R. N. Brogden, P. R. Sawyer, T. M. Speight, and G. S. Avery, "Metoclopramide: A Review of its Pharmacological Properties and Clinical Use," *Drugs*, vol. 12, no. 2, pp. 81-131, 1976, doi: 10.2165/00003495-197612020-00001.

[37] R. M. Eglen, Ed., *5-HT4 Receptors in the Brain and Periphery*. Berlin, Heidelberg: Springer Berlin Heidelberg, 1998.

[38] N. M. Gray and J. W. Young, "Methods for treating gastrointestinal motility dysfunction using optically pure (+) cisapride," US5955478A, Sep. 21, 1999.

[39] T. Odaka, T. Suzuki, A. Seza, T. Yamaguchi, and H. Saisho, "[Serotonin 5- HT4 receptor agonist (mosapride citrate)]," *Nihon Rinsho*, vol. 64, no. 8, pp. 1491-1494, Aug. 2006.

[40] O. Russo *et al.*, "Design, Synthesis, and Biological Evaluation of New 5-HT $_4$ Receptor Agonists: Application as Amyloid Cascade Modulators and Potential Therapeutic Utility in Alzheimer's Disease," *J. Med. Chem.*, vol. 52, no. 8, pp. 2214-2225, Apr. 2009, doi: 10.1021/jm801327q.

[41] R. M. Eglen, D. W. Bonhaus, L. G. Johnson, E. Leung, and R. D. Clark,

"Pharmacological characterization of two novel and potent 5-HT4 receptor agonists, RS 67333 and RS 67506, in vitro and in vivo," *British Journal of Pharmacology*, vol. 115, no. 8, pp. 1387-1392, Aug. 1995, doi: 10.1111/j.1476-5381.1995.tb16628.x.

[42] M. Hotte, F. Dauphin, T. Freret, M. Boulouard, and G. Levallet, "A Biphasic and Brain-Region Selective Down-Regulation of Cyclic Adenosine Monophosphate Concentrations Supports Object Recognition in the Rat," *PLoS ONE*, vol. 7, no. 2, p. e32244, Feb. 2012, doi: 10.1371/journal.pone.0032244.

[43] G. Levallet, M. Hotte, M. Boulouard, and F. Dauphin, "Increased particulate phosphodiesterase 4 in the prefrontal cortex supports 5-HT4 receptor-induced improvement of object recognition memory in the rat," *Psychopharmacology*, vol. 202, no. 1-3, pp. 125-139, Jan. 2009, doi: 10.1007/s00213-008-1283-8.

[44] L. Lamirault and H. Simon, "Enhancement of place and object recognition memory in young adult and old rats by RS 67333, a partial agonist of 5-HT4 receptors," *Neuropharmacology*, vol. 41, no. 7, pp. 844-853, Dec. 2001, doi: 10.1016/S0028-3908(01)00123-X.

[45] L. Lamirault, C. Guillou, C. Thal, and H. Simon, "Combined treatment with galanthaminium bromide, a new cholinesterase inhibitor, and RS 67333, a partial agonist of 5-HT4 receptors, enhances place and object recognition in young adult and old rats," *Progress in Neuro-Psychopharmacology and Biological Psychiatry*, vol. 27, no. 1, pp. 185-195, Feb. 2003, doi: 10.1016/S0278-5846(02)00351-2.

[46] C. Lecoutey *et al.*, "Design of donecopride, a dual serotonin subtype 4 receptor agonist/acetylcholinesterase inhibitor with potential interest for Alzheimer's disease treatment," *Proceedings of the National Academy of Sciences*, vol. 111, no. 36, pp. E3825–E3830, Sep. 2014, doi: 10.1073/pnas.1410315111.

[47] C. Rochais *et al.*, "Donecopride, a Swiss army knife with potential against Alzheimer's disease," *Br J Pharmacol*, vol. 177, no. 9, pp. 1988-2005, May 2020, doi: 10.1111/bph.14964.

[48] C. Lanthier *et al.*, "Novel multi target-directed ligands targeting 5-HT4 receptors with in cellulo antioxidant properties as promising leads in Alzheimer's disease," *European Journal of Medicinal Chemistry*, vol. 182, p. 111596, Nov. 2019, doi: 10.1016/j.ejmech.2019.111596.

[49] C. Spagnuolo, M. Napolitano, I. Tedesco, S. Moccia, A. Milito, and G. Luigi Russo, "Neuroprotective Role of Natural Polyphenols," *CTMC*, vol. 16, no. 17, pp. 1943-1950, Apr. 2016, doi: 10.2174/1568026616666160204122449.

[50] X. Zhang, X. He, Q. Chen, J. Lu, S. Rapposelli, and R. Pi, "A review on the hybrids of hydroxycinnamic acid as multi-target-directed ligands against Alzheimer's disease," *Bioorganic & Medicinal Chemistry*, vol. 26, no. 3, pp. 543-550, Feb. 2018, doi: 10.1016/j.bmc.2017.12.042.

[51] M. Bolognesi, A. Minarini, V. Tumiatti, and C. Melchiorre, "Lipoic Acid, a Lead Structure for Multi-Target-Directed Drugs for Neurodegeneration," *MRMC*, vol. 6, no. 11, pp. 1269-1274, Nov. 2006, doi: 10.2174/138955706778742731.

[52] M. L. Bolognesi *et al.*, "Toward a Rational Design of Multitarget-Directed Antioxidants: Merging Memoquin and Lipoic Acid Molecular Frameworks," *J. Med. Chem.*, vol. 52, no. 23, pp. 7883-7886, Dec. 2009, doi: 10.1021/jm901123n.

[53] C. Rice-Evans, N. Miller, and G. Paganga, "Antioxidant properties

of phenolic compounds," *Trends in Plant Science*, vol. 2, no. 4, pp. 152-159, Apr. 1997, doi: 10.1016/S1360-1385(97)01018-2.

[54] A. Tai, T. Sawano, F. Yazama, and H. Ito, "Evaluation of antioxidant activity of vanillin by using multiple antioxidant assays," *Biochimica et Biophysica Acta (BBA) - General Subjects*, vol. 1810, no. 2, pp. 170-177, Feb. 2011, doi: 10.1016/j.bbagen.2010.11.004.

[55] S. Yahiaoui *et al.*, "Design, synthesis, and pharmacological evaluation of multitarget-directed ligands with both serotonergic subtype 4 receptor (5-HT4R) partial agonist and 5-HT6R antagonist activities, as potential treatment of Alzheimer's disease," *European Journal of Medicinal Chemistry*, vol. 121, pp. 283-293, Oct. 2016, doi: 10.1016/j.ejmech.2016.05.048.

[56] M. Hao, Y. Li, H. Li, and S. Zhang, "Investigation of the Structure Requirement for 5-HT6 Binding Affinity of Arylsulfonyl Derivatives: A Computational Study," *IJMS*, vol. 12, no. 8, pp. 5011-5030, Aug. 2011, doi: 10.3390/ijms12085011.

[57] K. G. Liu *et al.*, "Identification of 3-sulfonylindazole derivatives as potent and selective 5-HT6 antagonists," *Bioorganic & Medicinal Chemistry*, vol. 19, no. 1, pp. 650-662, Jan. 2011, doi: 10.1016/j.bmc.2010.10.033.

[58] R. V. S. Nirogi *et al.*, "Indole-3-piperazinyl derivatives: Novel chemical class of 5-HT6 receptor antagonists," *Bioorganic & Medicinal Chemistry Letters*, vol. 21, no. 1, pp. 346-349, Jan. 2011, doi: 10.1016/j.bmcl.2010.11.001.

[59] K. G. Liu and A. J. Robichaud, "5-HT6 Medicinal Chemistry," in *International Review of Neurobiology*, vol. 94, Elsevier, 2010, pp. 1-34.

[60] A. Bali and S. Singh, "Serotonergic 5-HT_6 Receptor Antagonists: Heterocyclic Chemistry and Potential Therapeutic Significance," *CTMC*, vol. 15, no. 17, pp. 1643-1662, Jun. 2015, doi: 10.2174/1568026615666150427110420.

[61] B. Hatat *et al.*, "A Novel in vivo Anti-amnesic Agent, Specially Designed to Express Both Acetylcholinesterase (AChE) Inhibitory, Serotonergic Subtype 4 Receptor (5-HT4R) Agonist and Serotonergic Subtype 6 Receptor (5-HT6R) Inverse Agonist Activities, With a Potential Interest Against Alzheimer's Disease," *Front. Aging Neurosci.*, vol. 11, p. 148, Jun. 2019, doi: 10.3389/fnagi.2019.00148.

[62] C. Rochais *et al.*, "Novel Multitarget-Directed Ligands (MTDLs) with Acetylcholinesterase (AChE) Inhibitory and Serotonergic Subtype 4 Receptor (5-HT_4 R) Agonist Activities As Potential Agents against Alzheimer's Disease: The Design of Donecopride," *J. Med. Chem.*, vol. 58, no. 7, pp. 3172-3187, Apr. 2015, doi: 10.1021/acs.jmedchem.5b00115.

[63] D. P. Becker, D. L. Flynn, A. E. Moormann, and C. I. Villamil, "New meso-azacyclic amides of imidazopyridine carboxylic acids and analogs thereof," US5430040A, Jul. 04, 1995.

[64] F. D. King, L. M. Gaster, and G. F. Joiner, "Imidazopyridines and indolizines as 5-ht4 antagonists," WO1993008187A1, Apr. 29, 1993.

[65] H. Noguchi and C. Uchida, "Imidazopyridine compounds having 5-ht4 receptor agonistic activity and 5-ht3 receptor antagonistic activity," CA2523077A1, Nov. 04, 2004.

[66] R. Nirogi *et al.*, "Synthesis and SAR of Imidazo[1,5-a]pyridine derivatives as 5-HT4 receptor partial agonists for the treatment of cognitive disorders associated with Alzheimer's disease," *European Journal of Medicinal Chemistry*,

vol. 103, pp. 289-301, Oct. 2015, doi: 10.1016/j.ejmech.2015.08.051.

[67] J. Hannon and D. Hoyer, "Molecular biology of 5-HT receptors," *Behavioural Brain Research*, vol. 195, no. 1, pp. 198-213, Dec. 2008, doi: 10.1016/j.bbr.2008.03.020.

[68] G. Furlotti *et al.*, "Discovery and Pharmacological Profile of New 1 *H* -Indazole-3-carboxamide and 2 *H* -Pyrrolo[3,4- *c*]quinoline Derivatives as Selective Serotonin 4 Receptor Ligands," *J. Med. Chem.*, vol. 55, no. 22, pp. 9446-9466, Nov. 2012, doi: 10.1021/jm300573d.

[69] A. Hinschberger *et al.*, "New Benzo[*h*][1,6]naphthyridine and Azepino[3,2- *c*]quinoline Derivatives as Selective Antagonists of 5-HT $_4$ Receptors: Binding Profile and Pharmacological Characterization," *J. Med. Chem.*, vol. 46, no. 1, pp. 138-147, Jan. 2003, doi: 10.1021/jm020954v.

[70] E. Dubost *et al.*, "Synthesis and Structure–Affinity Relationships of Selective High-Affinity 5-HT $_4$ Receptor Antagonists: Application to the Design of New Potential Single Photon Emission Computed Tomography Tracers," *J. Med. Chem.*, vol. 55, no. 22, pp. 9693-9707, Nov. 2012, doi: 10.1021/jm300943r.

[71] F. Castriconi *et al.*, "Synthesis and structure–activity relationship studies in serotonin 5-HT4 receptor ligands based on a benzo[de][2,6]naphthridine scaffold," *European Journal of Medicinal Chemistry*, vol. 82, pp. 36-46, Jul. 2014, doi: 10.1016/j.ejmech.2014.05.015.

[72] F. Castriconi *et al.*, "Development of subnanomolar-affinity serotonin 5-HT $_4$ receptor ligands based on quinoline structures," *Med. Chem. Commun.*, vol. 9, no. 9, pp. 1466-1471, 2018, doi: 10.1039/C8MD00233A.

[73] F. J. Monsma, Y. Shen, R. P. Ward, M. W. Hamblin, and D. R. Sibley, "Cloning and expression of a novel serotonin receptor with high affinity for tricyclic psychotropic drugs," *Mol Pharmacol*, vol. 43, no. 3, pp. 320-327, Mar. 1993.

[74] M. Kotańska, K. Lustyk, A. Bucki, M. Marcinkowska, J. Śniecikowska, and M. Kołaczkowski, "Idalopirdine, a selective 5-HT6 receptor antagonist, reduces food intake and body weight in a model of excessive eating," *Metab Brain Dis*, vol. 33, no. 3, pp. 733-740, Jun. 2018, doi: 10.1007/s11011-017-0175-1.

[75] W. J. Geldenhuys and C. J. Van der Schyf, "The serotonin 5-HT $_6$ receptor: a viable drug target for treating cognitive deficits in Alzheimer's disease," *Expert Review of Neurotherapeutics*, vol. 9, no. 7, pp. 1073-1085, Jul. 2009, doi: 10.1586/ern.09.51.

[76] R. Khoury, N. Grysman, J. Gold, K. Patel, and G. T. Grossberg, "The role of 5 HT6-receptor antagonists in Alzheimer's disease: an update," *Expert Opinion on Investigational Drugs*, vol. 27, no. 6, pp. 523-533, Jun. 2018, doi: 10.1080/13543784.2018.1483334.

[77] N. Upton, T. T. Chuang, A. J. Hunter, and D. J. Virley, "5-HT6 receptor antagonists as novel cognitive enhancing agents for Alzheimer's disease," *Neurotherapeutics*, vol. 5, no. 3, pp. 458-469, Jul. 2008, doi: 10.1016/j.nurt.2008.05.008.

[78] W. J. Geldenhuys and C. J. Van der Schyf, "Triquinane-based compounds as possible serotonin 5-HT6 receptor antagonists for the treatment of Alzheimer's disease," *Medical Hypotheses*, vol. 68, no. 1, pp. 81-86, Jan. 2007, doi: 10.1016/j.mehy.2006.06.032.

[79] B. Benhamú, M. Martín-Fontecha, H. Vázquez-Villa, L. Pardo, and M. L. López-Rodríguez, "Serotonin 5-HT $_6$ Receptor Antagonists for the Treatment of Cognitive Deficiency in Alzheimer's Disease," *J. Med. Chem.*, vol. 57, no. 17,

pp. 7160-7181, Sep. 2014, doi: 10.1021/jm5003952.

[80] K. C. F. Fone, "An update on the role of the 5-hydroxytryptamine6 receptor in cognitive function," *Neuropharmacology*, vol. 55, no. 6, pp. 1015-1022, Nov. 2008, doi: 10.1016/j.neuropharm.2008.06.061.

[81] M. Marcinkowska *et al.*, "Anti-Alzheimer's multitarget-directed ligands with serotonin 5-HT $_6$ antagonist, butyrylcholinesterase inhibitory, and antioxidant activity," *Arch. Pharm. Chem. Life Sci*, vol. 352, no. 7, p. 1900041, Jul. 2019, doi: 10.1002/ardp.201900041.

[82] A. Foley *et al.*, "The selective 5-HT6 receptor antagonists SB-271046 and SB-399885 potentiate NCAM PSA immunolabeling of dentate granule cells, but not neurogenesis, in the hippocampal formation of mature Wistar rats," *Neuropharmacology*, vol. 54, no. 8, pp. 1166-1174, Jun. 2008, doi: 10.1016/j.neuropharm.2008.03.012.

[83] K. Grychowska *et al.*, "Novel 1H-Pyrrolo[3,2-c]quinoline Based 5-HT6 Receptor Antagonists with Potential Application for the Treatment of Cognitive Disorders Associated with Alzheimer's Disease," *ACS Chem. Neurosci.*, vol. 7, no. 7, pp. 972-983, Jul. 2016, doi: 10.1021/acschemneuro.6b00090.

[84] A. J. Sleight, F. G. Boess, M. Bös, B. Levet-Trafit, C. Riemer, and A. Bourson, "Characterization of Ro 04-6790 and Ro 63-0563: potent and selective antagonists at human and rat 5-HT $_6$ receptors: Selective 5-HT $_6$ receptor antagonists," *British Journal of Pharmacology*, vol. 124, no. 3, pp. 556-562, Jun. 1998, doi: 10.1038/sj.bjp.0701851.

[85] S. M. Bromidge *et al.*, "5-Chloro- *N* -(4-methoxy-3-piperazin-1-yl- phenyl)-3-methyl-2-benzothiophenesulfon-amide (SB-271046): A Potent, Selective, and Orally Bioavailable 5-HT $_6$ Receptor Antagonist," *J. Med. Chem.*, vol. 42, no. 2, pp. 202-205, Jan. 1999, doi: 10.1021/jm980532e.

[86] C. Routledge *et al.*, "Characterization of SB-271046: A potent, selective and orally active 5-HT $_6$ receptor antagonist: SB-271046: a 5-HT $_6$ receptor agonist," *British Journal of Pharmacology*, vol. 130, no. 7, pp. 1606-1612, Aug. 2000, doi: 10.1038/sj.bjp.0703457.

[87] W. D. Hirst *et al.*, "SB-399885 is a potent, selective 5-HT6 receptor antagonist with cognitive enhancing properties in aged rat water maze and novel object recognition models," *European Journal of Pharmacology*, vol. 553, no. 1-3, pp. 109-119, Dec. 2006, doi: 10.1016/j.ejphar.2006.09.049.

[88] J. A. González-Vera *et al.*, "A new serotonin 5-HT6 receptor antagonist with procognitive activity – Importance of a halogen bond interaction to stabilize the binding," *Sci Rep*, vol. 7, no. 1, p. 41293, Feb. 2017, doi: 10.1038/srep41293.

[89] P. Zajdel *et al.*, "N1-Azinylsulfonyl-1H-indoles: 5-HT6 Receptor Antagonists with Procognitive and Antidepressant-Like Properties," *ACS Med. Chem. Lett.*, vol. 7, no. 6, pp. 618-622, Jun. 2016, doi: 10.1021/acsmedchemlett.6b00056.

[90] A. S. Hogendorf *et al.*, "2-Aminoimidazole-based antagonists of the 5-HT6 receptor – A new concept in aminergic GPCR ligand design," *European Journal of Medicinal Chemistry*, vol. 179, pp. 1-15, Oct. 2019, doi: 10.1016/j.ejmech.2019.06.001.

[91] N. H. Greig, D. K. Lahiri, and K. Sambamurti, "Butyrylcholinesterase: An Important New Target in Alzheimer's Disease Therapy," *Int. Psychogeriatr.*, vol. 14, no. S1, pp. 77-91, Feb. 2002, doi: 10.1017/S1041610203008676.

[92] A. Więckowska *et al.*, "Synthesis of new N-benzylpiperidine derivatives as cholinesterase inhibitors with β-amyloid anti-aggregation properties and beneficial effects on memory in vivo," *Bioorganic & Medicinal Chemistry*, vol. 23, no. 10, pp. 2445-2457, May 2015, doi: 10.1016/j.bmc.2015.03.051.

[93] S. Suzen, S. S. Cihaner, and T. Coban, "Synthesis and Comparison of Antioxidant Properties of Indole-Based Melatonin Analogue Indole Amino Acid Derivatives: Antioxidant Properties of Indole Amino Acids," *Chemical Biology & Drug Design*, vol. 79, no. 1, pp. 76-83, Jan. 2012, doi: 10.1111/j.1747-0285.2011.01216.x.

[94] V. Canale *et al.*, "A dual-acting 5-HT6 receptor inverse agonist/MAO-B inhibitor displays glioprotective and pro-cognitive properties," *European Journal of Medicinal Chemistry*, vol. 208, p. 112765, Dec. 2020, doi: 10.1016/j.ejmech.2020.112765.

[95] D. Vanda *et al.*, "Novel non-sulfonamide 5-HT 6 receptor partial inverse agonist in a group of imidazo[4,5- b]pyridines with cognition enhancing properties," *European Journal of Medicinal Chemistry*, vol. 144, pp. 716-729, Jan. 2018, doi: 10.1016/j.ejmech.2017.12.053.

[96] K. Grychowska *et al.*, "Dual 5-HT6 and D3 Receptor Antagonists in a Group of 1H-Pyrrolo[3,2-c]quinolines with Neuroprotective and Procognitive Activity," *ACS Chem. Neurosci.*, vol. 10, no. 7, pp. 3183-3196, Jul. 2019, doi: 10.1021/acschemneuro.8b00618.

[97] H. Hall, C. Köhler, and L. Gawell, "Some in vitro receptor binding properties of [3H]eticlopride, a novel substituted benzamide, selective for dopamine-D2 receptors in the rat brain," *European Journal of Pharmacology*, vol. 111, no. 2, pp. 191-199, May 1985, doi: 10.1016/0014-2999(85)90756-3.

[98] F. Sautel *et al.*, "Nafadotride, a potent preferential dopamine D3 receptor antagonist, activates locomotion in rodents," *J Pharmacol Exp Ther*, vol. 275, no. 3, pp. 1239-1246, Dec. 1995.

[99] H.-J. Kim *et al.*, "New Serotonin 5-HT $_6$ Ligands from Common Feature Pharmacophore Hypotheses," *J. Chem. Inf. Model.*, vol. 48, no. 1, pp. 197-206, Jan. 2008, doi: 10.1021/ci700160t.

[100] D. Galimberti and E. Scarpini, "Idalopirdine as a treatment for Alzheimer's disease," *Expert Opinion on Investigational Drugs*, vol. 24, no. 7, pp. 981-987, Jul. 2015, doi: 10.1517/13543784.2015.1052402.

[101] A. Atri *et al.*, "Effect of Idalopirdine as Adjunct to Cholinesterase Inhibitors on Change in Cognition in Patients With Alzheimer Disease: Three Randomized Clinical Trials," *JAMA*, vol. 319, no. 2, p. 130, Jan. 2018, doi: 10.1001/jama.2017.20373.

[102] D. A. Bennett, "Lack of Benefit With Idalopirdine for Alzheimer Disease: Another Therapeutic Failure in a Complex Disease Process," *JAMA*, vol. 319, no. 2, p. 123, Jan. 2018, doi: 10.1001/jama.2017.19700.

[103] O. Riccio *et al.*, "Excess of serotonin affects embryonic interneuron migration through activation of the serotonin receptor 6," *Mol Psychiatry*, vol. 14, no. 3, pp. 280-290, Mar. 2009, doi: 10.1038/mp.2008.89.

[104] J. Meffre *et al.*, "5-HT $_6$ receptor recruitment of mTOR as a mechanism for perturbed cognition in schizophrenia," *EMBO Mol Med*, vol. 4, no. 10, pp. 1043-1056, Oct. 2012, doi: 10.1002/emmm.201201410.

[105] F. Duhr *et al.*, "Cdk5 induces constitutive activation of 5-HT6 receptors to promote neurite growth," *Nat Chem Biol*, vol. 10, no.

7, pp. 590-597, Jul. 2014, doi: 10.1038/nchembio.1547.

[106] D. Vanda, P. Zajdel, and M. Soural, "Imidazopyridine-based selective and multifunctional ligands of biological targets associated with psychiatric and neurodegenerative diseases," *European Journal of Medicinal Chemistry*, vol. 181, p. 111569, Nov. 2019, doi: 10.1016/j.ejmech.2019.111569.

[107] M. J. Ramírez, "5-HT6 receptors and Alzheimer's disease," *Alz Res Therapy*, vol. 5, no. 2, p. 15, Apr. 2013, doi: 10.1186/alzrt169.

[108] D. C. Cole *et al.*, "Discovery of N $_1$ -(6-Chloroimidazo[2,1- *b*][1,3]thiazole-5-sulfonyl)tryptamine as a Potent, Selective, and Orally Active 5-HT $_6$ Receptor Agonist," *J. Med. Chem.*, vol. 50, no. 23, pp. 5535-5538, Nov. 2007, doi: 10.1021/jm070521y.

[109] L. E. Schechter *et al.*, "Neuropharmacological Profile of Novel and Selective 5-HT6 Receptor Agonists: WAY-181187 and WAY-208466," *Neuropsychopharmacol*, vol. 33, no. 6, pp. 1323-1335, May 2008, doi: 10.1038/sj.npp.1301503.

[110] P. Svenningsson *et al.*, "Biochemical and Behavioral Evidence for Antidepressant-Like Effects of 5-HT6 Receptor Stimulation," *Journal of Neuroscience*, vol. 27, no. 15, pp. 4201-4209, Apr. 2007, doi: 10.1523/JNEUROSCI.3110-06.2007.

[111] M. Jastrzębska-Więsek *et al.*, "Partial agonist efficacy of EMD386088, a 5-HT6receptor ligand, in functionalin vitroassays.pdf," *Pharmacological Reports*, vol. 65, pp. 998-1005, 2013.

[112] G. Romero *et al.*, "Efficacy of selective 5-HT6 receptor ligands determined by monitoring 5-HT6 receptor-mediated cAMP signaling pathways: 5-HT6 receptor ligand efficacy properties," *British Journal of Pharmacology*, vol. 148, no. 8, pp. 1133-1143, Aug. 2006, doi: 10.1038/sj.bjp.0706827.

[113] D. C. Cole *et al.*, "Discovery of 5-Arylsulfonamido-3- (pyrrolidin-2-ylmethyl)-1 *H* -indole Derivatives as Potent, Selective 5-HT $_6$ Receptor Agonists and Antagonists," *J. Med. Chem.*, vol. 48, no. 2, pp. 353-356, Jan. 2005, doi: 10.1021/jm049243i.

[114] H.-M. Yun and H. Rhim, "The Serotonin-6 Receptor as a Novel Therapeutic Target," *Exp Neurobiol*, vol. 20, no. 4, pp. 159-168, Dec. 2011, doi: 10.5607/en.2011.20.4.159.

[115] A. Meneses, G. Pérez-García, T. Ponce-Lopez, and C. Castillo, "5-HT6 Receptor Memory and Amnesia: Behavioral Pharmacology – Learning and Memory Processes," in *International Review of Neurobiology*, vol. 96, Elsevier, 2011, pp. 27-47.

Chapter 5

Aggression and Sexual Behavior: Overlapping or Distinct Roles of 5-HT_{1A} and 5-HT_{1B} Receptors

Berend Olivier and Jocelien D.A. Olivier

Abstract

Distinct brain mechanisms for male aggressive and sexual behavior are present in mammalian species, including man. However, recent evidence suggests a strong connection and even overlap in the central nervous system (CNS) circuitry involved in aggressive and sexual behavior. The serotonergic system in the CNS is strongly involved in male aggressive and sexual behavior. In particular, 5-HT_{1A} and 5-HT_{1B} receptors seem to play a critical role in the modulation of these behaviors. The present chapter focuses on the effects of 5-HT_{1A}- and 5-HT_{1B}-receptor ligands in male rodent aggression and sexual behavior. Results indicate that 5-HT_{1B}-heteroreceptors play a critical role in the modulation of male offensive behavior, although a definite role of 5-HT_{1A}-auto- or heteroreceptors cannot be ruled out. 5-HT_{1A} receptors are clearly involved in male sexual behavior, although it has to be yet unraveled whether 5-HT_{1A}-auto- or heteroreceptors are important. Although several key nodes in the complex circuitry of aggression and sexual behavior are known, in particular in the medial hypothalamus, a clear link or connection to these critical structures and the serotonergic key receptors is yet to be determined. This information is urgently needed to detect and develop new selective anti-aggressive (serenic) and pro-sexual drugs for human applications.

Keywords: aggression, sexual behavior, serotonin, 5-HT_{1A} receptor, 5-HT_{1B} receptor, serenics, neural circuit

1. Introduction

Early studies into the role of various brain structures in aggression focused merely on the hypothalamus already starting in the 1920s by Hess [1]. Electrical stimulation in the hypothalamus induced stimulation-evoked (or –bound) attack behavior, where rat studies [2–5] created an important framework underlying the functional organization of attack circuitry [6]. Lesion experiments in mice [7] and rats [8, 9] also implicate parts of the hypothalamus in offensive and defensive aggression [9, 10].

Anterior hypothalamic lesions, damaging large parts of the anterior hypothalamus (AH), rostral parts of the ventromedial hypothalamus (VMH), and smaller parts of the caudal preoptic area (PA), indeed, strongly increase defensive behavior toward a male intruder. Mammillary body lesions, damaging large parts of the ventral (vPMV) and dorsal premammillary nucleus (dPMV), caudal parts of the

IntechOpen

arcuate nucleus, medial mammillary nucleus (mMM), posterior mammillary nucleus (pMM), supramammillary peduncle induced strong increases in offensive aggression [9]. These findings suggested the existence of at least two distinct neural substrates in the hypothalamus normally modulating defensive (anterior medial hypothalamus) and offensive (posterior medial hypothalamus) aspects of intermale aggression. Concomitant studies strongly support the ventral premammillary nucleus as a possible central hub of aggression [11]. Because electrolytical lesions are rather nonspecific, i.e., it is virtually impossible to wipe out, on both sides of the brain, one structure without damaging other structures including neurons and fibers of passage. Alternatively, electrical (micro) stimulation can be used to study the role of the underlying substrate (again neurons and fibers of passage) in certain behaviors, including aggression (and sexual behavior).

Already early in the twentieth century [1], hypothalamic stimulation in cats induced attacks. In the seventies [2, 3], this research extended to rats where electrical stimulation in the (ventrolateral) hypothalamus induced attack behavior, although rather nonspecific in that different subjects (mice (live or dead), rat pups, guinea pigs, and adult rats) were attacked. At the end of the seventies, the groups of Koolhaas in Groningen and Kruk in Leiden extensively investigated that upon electrical stimulation in hypothalamic structures, specific behavioral responses were elicited [4, 5]. The Kruk group [12] described, after extensive and meticulous studies, an "aggressive area," later named the "Hypothalamic Aggression Area (HAA)," lateral from the ventrolateral lobe of the ventromedial hypothalamus (VMH) into the frontal pole of the VMH and the anterior hypothalamic nucleus (AHN). This area extends medially to the arcuate nucleus through the ventrolateral and medial parts of the VMH (see for a 3D-picture, Fig. 1 in [13]. The HAA largely (or completely) coincides with the area in the hypothalamus that upon lesioning leads to reduced aggression [9]. In female rats, aggression can be evoked in the same (HAA) area as in males [14].

Recent studies applying genetically defined functional manipulations showed that the VMH and in particular the ventrolateral part (vlVMH) and the medial amygdala are critical sites to evoke aggression [15]. The VMH receives direct and indirect input from the medial amygdala and from the bed nucleus of the stria terminalis (principal nucleus:BNSTpr), but also from various other structures [16], such as the ventral premammillary nucleus (vPMN), the lateral septum (LS), and subparaventricular zone (SPZ) [17].

Newman [18] argued already that the neurobiology of aggressive behavior is embedded in a larger and integrated network of various social behaviors, including sexual and parental behavior. This implies that the neural circuitry involved in these behaviors must consist of a number of commonly activated brain areas (sensitive to a variety of shared cues) and separately by brain areas specifically involved in a specific function or a selective role in each behavior, as, e.g., occurs in the vomeronasal circuitry [19].

The putative "dual" or "multiple" involvement of a specific neural area (node) in, e.g., aggression and sexual behavior necessitates testing the effects of manipulations of this node in other behaviors, e.g., exploratory or other behaviors. Veening and coworkers [20] approached this question by studying whether the patterns of brain activation during male rat aggression and sexual behavior are specific for either behavior or show (partly) overlapping patterns. By using Fos-immunoreactivity, it was shown that some brain areas (caudal medial preoptic area and medial amygdala) were commonly activated, whereas other areas (posterodorsal parts of the medial amygdala, rostral preoptic and premammillary hypothalamus) show differences in neural activation. This is in line with the idea that aggressive and sexual behaviors share partly integrated neural pathways, next to more specific "aggressive" and "sexual" brain areas. In general, the medial preoptic nucleus (MPN) and the VMHvl are essential regions for male sexual and aggressive behavior, respectively. Estrogen receptor alpha (ESR1)-expressing cells in the posterior amygdala (PA) are a main source of excitatory input to the hypothalamus and are main mediators for mating and fighting in male mice [21]. PA^{Esr1+} neurons to the MPN are activated during sexual behavior and also induce sexual behavior. PA^{Esr1+} neurons that project to the VMHvl promote attacks. The PA can be considered a key node in male aggressive and sexual behavior circuitry. Optogenetic activation of VMHvl cells expressing estrogen receptor alpha-progesterone receptors induced attack, whereas pharmacogenetic optogenetic inactivation of the VMHvl inhibited naturally occurring aggression [17], Moreover, the VMHvl is also involved in generating preparatory (learned) behaviors associated with the attacks [22]. Available evidence gives an essential role to the medial hypothalamus in the generation of aggression, the hypothalamic aggression area or circuit. This hypothalamic aggression circuit is embedded, upstream and downstream, in other circuits that modulate the aggression outcome, e.g., the dopaminergic mesolimbic dopamine pathway. Its connection from the ventral tegmental area (VTA) to the nucleus accumbens (NAc) is a key circuit in the rewarding control of aggression [17, 23].

Optogenetic stimulation of the network in the HAA that evokes aggression [15] was also able to evoke mounting. The neurons involved (estrogen-1 (Esr1)-expressing) in the VMHvl evoke mounting upon stimulation with lower frequencies [24]. The VMHvl neurons are sensitive to varying levels of optogenetic stimulation and the (behavioral) outcome ranges from highly prosocial (sexual) to antisocial (aggression). Apparently, one could assume that the VMHvl, and specifically one type of neuron ($Esr1^{+}$), is an overlapping node in male aggression and sexual behavior circuits [25].

For a long time, it was a common belief that male aggressive and sexual behavior shares many of the underlying neurobiological, neurological, pharmacological, physiological, and neuroendocrine mechanisms. This seems, at least partly, true for aggression and sexual behavior. Apparently, such a shared structure (e.g., the VMHvl) mediates multiple social behaviors and processes [26]). Factors such as social experience, behavioral context, hormonal state, spatial and sensory cues probably (co)-influence which behavior is generated at a specific moment and time [27].

2. Serotonin and sexual behavior

Sexual behavior systems operate under rather constant inhibitory control to ascertain that sexual behavior is performed only under appropriate circumstances. Serotonergic neurotransmission is involved in inhibitory and disinhibitory processes regulating proper sexual behavior. 5-HT release, facilitating transmission, is regulated via negative feedback mechanisms, through different presynaptic (5-HT_{1A}, 5-$HT_{1B/1D}$) autoreceptors. Moreover, postsynaptic serotonergic heteroreceptors are also involved in negative feedback on serotonergic cell firing [28]. The 5-HT transporter (5-HTT or SERT) plays an important role in homeostatic modulation of the magnitude, duration, and spatial distribution of signals reaching serotonin receptors [29, 30]. Although 5-HT is not considered a central modulator of sexual behavior, but rather modulatory or facilitating, 5-HT activity plays an important role during sexual behavior, via its machinery of pre- and postsynaptic interactions, thereby critically interfering with GABA-ergic and glutamatergic neurons in various brain areas (prefrontal cortex, hypothalamus, lateral habenula, and dorsal raphe nucleus). Serotonergic fibers are abundant in many areas of the spinal cord implicated in ejaculatory processes [31]. Postsynaptic 5-HT receptors are located at lumbar spinothalamic cells [32], indicative of a role of 5-HT in ejaculation at the level of the spinal cord, descending from supraspinal areas such as the nPGI. These descending 5-HTergic neurons from supraspinal areas innervate spinal cord mechanisms that control bulbospongiosus muscles, which have inhibitory effects on ejaculation [32]. At hypothalamic level, the medial preoptic area (mPOA) is involved in lowering an ejaculatory threshold via inhibition of an inhibitory serotonergic tone exerted by the nPGI [33, 34], removing a brake on ejaculatory processes. The lateral hypothalamic area (LHA) is also involved in ejaculation: lesions affect ejaculation, but not preceding mounts and intromission [35]. Because 5-HT is released in the LHA at the occurrence of ejaculation and infusion of selective serotonin reuptake inhibitors (SSRIs) into this area influences sexual behavior [36], a role of serotonin is clearly implicated. The main sources of 5-HTergic innervation of the forebrain emerge from the dorsal (DRN) and medial (MRN) raphe nuclei. Ascending 5-HTergic fibers are divided into a meso-limbic pathway from the MRN and a meso-striatal pathway derived from the DRN [31, 37, 38]. Although DRN and MRN have (partly) overlapping projections, they do not overlap in the projected structure but go to different subareas [38]. MRN and DRN have reciprocal connections, and both structures express high densities of 5-HT_{1A} receptors. An unanswered question is whether and how these extremely complex interactions (including those with non-serotonergic structures) interact during sexual behavior [39, 40]. Most research in these areas is performed in males (mostly rodents).

Notwithstanding an extensive role of serotonin in aggression and sexual behavior [29, 41] in the present chapter, we focus on the role of two receptors, 5-HT_{1A} and 5-HT_{1B} receptors because they appear as most relevant in interactions between aggressive and sexual behaviors (**Figure 1** shows a cartoon of a serotonergic neuron

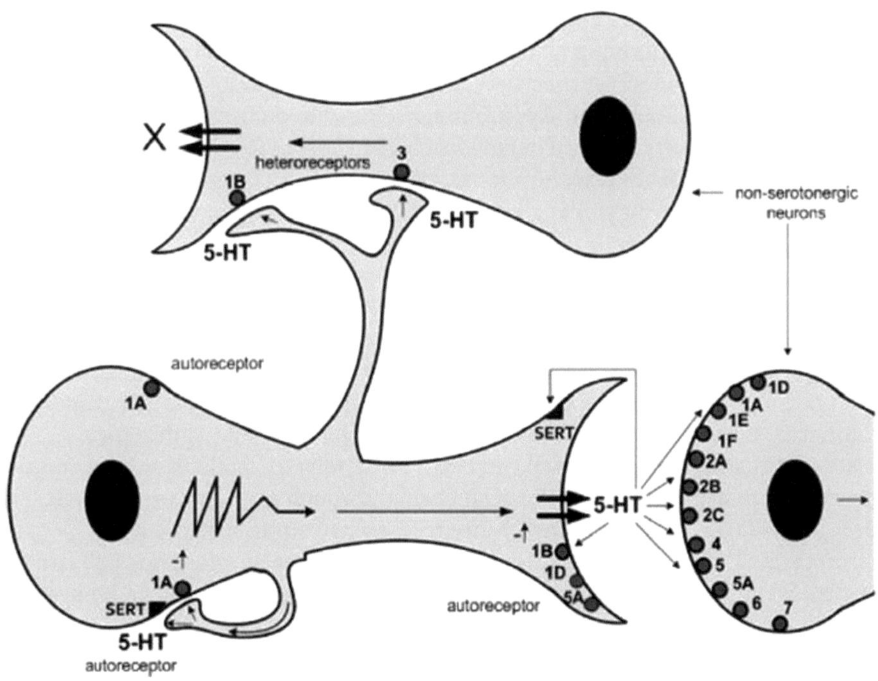

Figure 1.
Cartoon of a serotonergic neuron projecting to two non-serotonergic neurons. Fourteen different serotonergic receptors are located either as presynaptic autoreceptors (5-HT_{1A}, 5-HT_{1B}) or as postsynaptic heteroreceptors (all 14 receptors). The 5-HT transporter (SERT) is located at the somadendritic and synaptic part of the serotonergic neuron. See text for further details.

with all 14 different 5-HT receptors). 5-HT$_{1A}$ receptors are present as somatodendritic autoreceptors on serotonergic neurons that present upon activation as negative feedback on cell firing, thus inhibiting 5-HT release and thereby exerting a broad influence on 5-HTergic tone. 5-HT$_{1A}$ receptors are also widely distributed in terminal areas of the brain expressed as postsynaptic heteroreceptors in a variety of different brain structures and influence a wide scale of neuropsychopharmacological events [42]. 5-HT$_{1B}$ receptors and its counterpart 5-HT$_{1D}$ receptor have a long, complex, and debated history (see Figure 3 in [42]), because of species differences in function and structure. It was finally confirmed that 5-HT$_{1B}$ and 5-HT$_{1D}$ receptors represent two different receptor classes, and the 5-HT$_{1B}$-receptor (including the rat 5-HT$_{1B}$-receptor) plays the most prominent functional role, although the pharmacology of ligands for the human and rodent 5-HT$_{1B}$ receptors can be quite deviating. Most of animal behavioral data on 5-HT$_{1B}$ receptor ligands have been gathered in rodents, which makes prediction for human applications sometimes unreliable [42]. 5-HT$_{1B}$ receptors are present as inhibitory autoreceptor on the presynaptic part of 5-HT neurons (see **Figure 1**) and as inhibitory heteroreceptor on non-serotonergic neurons [42]. Although it is unclear whether every single 5-HT neuron is equipped with similar autoreceptors, at least for the MRN and DRN it is known that they possess somatodendritically localized autoreceptors and presynaptically localized 5-HT$_{1B}$ autoreceptors and 5-HT transporters. 5-HT activity has to be terminated, which is effectuated via reuptake of 5-HT by the serotonin transporter (SERT), a complex molecule with 13 transmembrane loops. After this uptake over the cell membrane via the SERT from the synapse, 5-HT is subsequently taken up by the vesicular-monoamine transporter (VMAT2) and stored in the synaptic vesicles for reuse. Another major route to end serotonergic activity is a process whereby 5-HT is taken up by the surrounding glia cells and degraded by the enzyme monoamine-oxidase-A (MAO-A) [43] to its metabolite 5-hydroxyindole acetic acid (5-HIAA). Simultaneously, the released 5-HT activates 5-HT$_{1B}$ autoreceptors leading to inhibition of further 5-HT release from the vesicles and activates also the somatodendritical 5-HT$_{1A}$ autoreceptors, leading to inhibition of cell firing [44, 45]. The interplay between these three mechanisms (5-HT reuptake, inhibition of release via activation of 5-HT$_{1B}$ autoreceptors, and inhibition of cell firing via activation of somatodendritic 5-HT$_{1A}$ autoreceptors) reduces the activity of the serotonergic neurons after activity, preparing the neuron for a new discharge [44, 45]. Of course, many non-serotonergic inputs are acting on serotonergic cells in the raphé nuclei (a nice schematic overview is shown in Fig. 2 in [46]).

3. 5-HT$_{1A}$ and 5-HT$_{1B}$ receptors in aggressive and sexual behavior

The prototypic 5-HT$_{1A}$-receptor agonist (±)-8-OH-DPAT was developed in the early eighties and when tested on male rats, showed a remarkable stimulation of male sexual behavior [47]. The effects of the racemic (±)-8-OH-DPAT and its active enantiomer (+)-8-OH-DPAT have been confirmed in many subsequent studies [31]. Veening and Coolen [48] presented a so-called "funnel-model" of sexual behavior in the rat, based on experiments on feeding, sexual and aggressive behavior combined with electrical stimulation in the ventromedial hypothalamus [49]. The "funnel-model" also applies to other behavioral systems, including aggressive behavior. In general, in the initiation phase 1, the animal involved gathers information about the environment (scanning, sniffing, orientation), followed by transition to phase 2 where appetitive behavior becomes prominent (anogenital sniffing, mounting in case of sexual behavior; following, anogenital sniffing in aggression). Transition to phase 3 may follow, which is the consummatory/executive phase. In case of sexual behavior, this includes mounting, intromission, and finally, ejaculation; in aggression, this includes lateral threat, biting, jump attacks, keeping down, and chasing [9].

Both sexual and aggressive behavior in male rats can be described by a "funnel"-like pattern of behavior [49–51]. By manipulations such as electrical stimulation or lesions in the (ventro)medial hypothalamus, this pattern of behavioral funneling can be interrupted, e.g., electrical stimulation in the VMH in a resident-intruder situation [49] strongly reduces the chance on full aggression, because the stimulation strongly promotes return to phase 1 (scanning and initiation phase). Remarkably, stimulation (either electrically or optogenetically) of the VMHvl in mice can evoke both aggressive and sexual behavior [25, 52–54]. Extensive studies indicate that intermingled, antagonistic brain circuits for aggressive and sexual behavior are present in the VMHvl [15, 55].

Administration of 5-HT_{1A}-receptor agonists (e.g., 8-OH-DPAT, flesinoxan, buspirone, ipsapirone, and others [31]) dose-dependently increases the number of ejaculations and reduces the ejaculation latencies during a certain test duration (e.g., 30 min). Moreover, the number of mounts and intromissions during the successive ejaculation series decrease (**Figure 2**). This whole profile has been described as "pro-sexual" and can be aligned with the funnel-model hypothesis, assuming that 5-HT_{1A}-receptor activation strongly drives the direction of sexual behavior toward the final consummatory phase, ejaculation.

Recently, we tested some new 5-HT_{1A}-receptor agonists on male rat sexual behavior [56]. They are so-called "biased" or "functionally selective" high potency 5-HT_{1A}-receptor agonists, F15599 and F13714, and have distinct pre- and postsynaptic agonistic activity [57]. However, like in aggression (see later), both "biased" agonists had potent pro-sexual activity, comparable to "classic" 5-HT_{1A}-receptor agonists such as 8-OH-DPAT or flesinoxan (similar activation of 5-HT_{1A} auto- and heteroreceptors). However, S-15535, primarily considered a 5-HT_{1A}-autoreceptor agonist and heteroreceptor antagonist, had no pro-sexual activity at all, and also no sexual inhibitory activity either [56]. This strongly suggests that "pro-sexual" activity induced by 5-HT_{1A} receptor agonists is primarily caused by activation of postsynaptic 5-HT_{1A} heteroreceptors.

5-HT_{1B}-receptor agonists inhibit male sexual behavior in the rat [58–60] and in the mouse [61]. Eltoprazine, a mixed 5-$HT_{1A/1B}$ receptor (partial) agonist [62], dose-dependently reduced male rat sexual behavior; at no dose tested, pro-sexual effects were seen, indicating that the putative 5-HT_{1A} receptor activating effects of eltoprazine were "overshadowed" by the 5-HT_{1B}-receptor agonistic effects and that the behavioral effects were caused by 5-HT_{1B}-receptor activation. A comparable mixed 5-$HT_{1A/1B}$-receptor agonistic profile in other putative 5-HT_{1B} receptor agonists such as mCPP, TFMPP, RU24969, and anpirtoline, which all have inhibitory sexual effects in male rats, points to the dominance of 5-HT_{1B} receptors over 5-HT_{1A} receptors upon concomitant activation. In mice, in contrast to rats, 5-HT_{1A}-receptor agonists (8-OH-DPAT) have an inhibitory effect in male sexual behavior [61] (**Figure 3**).

In our studies on 5-HT_{1A}-receptor knockout mice [64–66], we tested three strains of mice (the background strains used to produce the gene knockouts; 129Sv/Ev, C57Bl/6, and Swiss Webster) in male sexual behavior. **Figure 4** shows the data on number of mounts, intromission, and ejaculations and intromission and mount latencies during male/estrus female tests of 1500 s duration (25 min). In 129Sv/Ev and C57Bl/6 strains, wild-type (WT) mice had significant higher sexual behavior levels than the respective 5-HT_{1A}-receptor knockout mice. Swiss Webster mice hardly showed any sexual behaviors, neither in WT, nor in KO animals, making conclusions impossible.

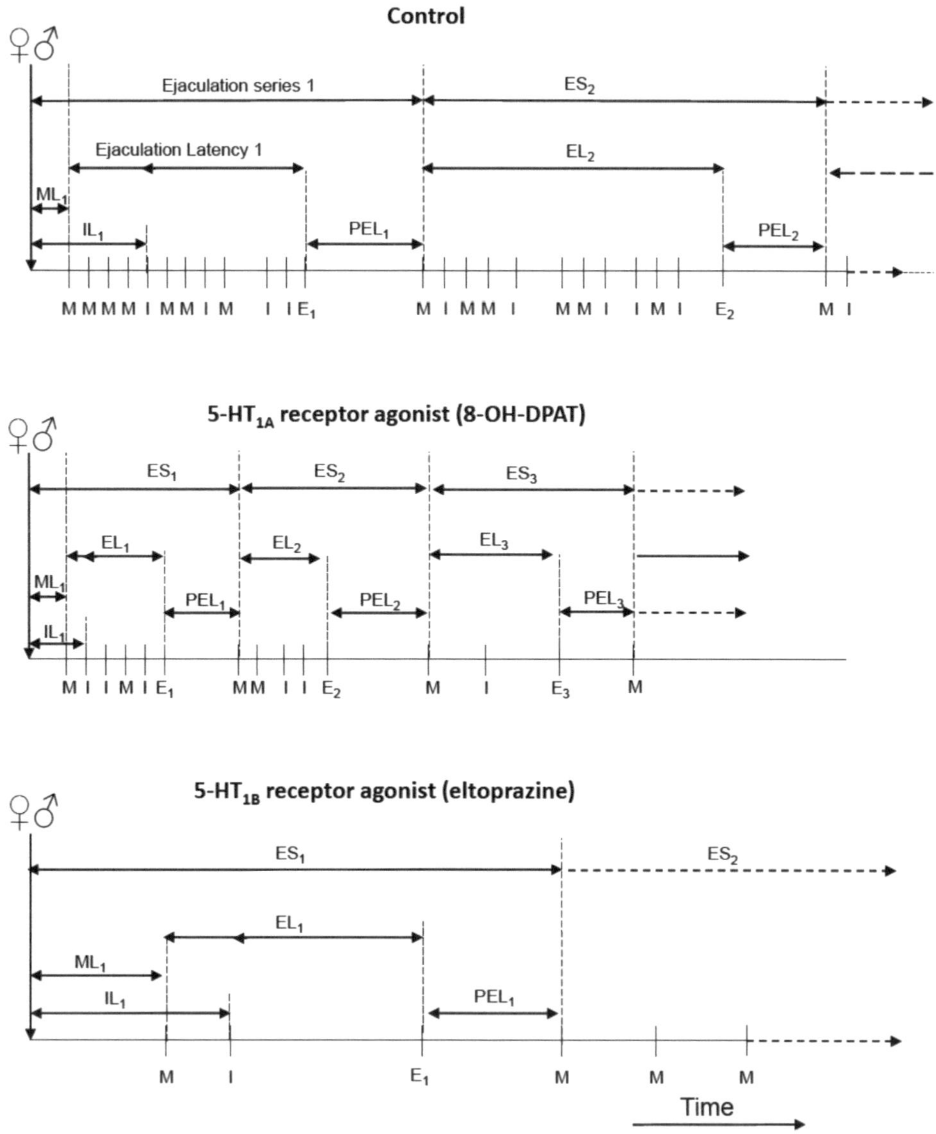

Figure 2.
Time course of sexual behavior of male rats treated with vehicle (top), (±)-8-OH-DPAT (middle), and eltoprazine (bottom) at behaviorally active dosages. M = mount, I = intromission, PEL = post-ejaculatory interval, ES = ejaculation series, EL = ejaculation latency, ML = mount latency, IL = intromission latency. Numbers (1, 2, 3, ...) indicate in which ejaculation series (ES) the behavior parameter is scored.

5-HT$_{1B}$-receptor knockout mice (in 129/SV-ter strain) have a lower baseline of sexual behavior than the corresponding wild-type mice [61]. TFMPP, a 5-HT$_{1B}$-receptor agonist had no behavioral effects in 5-HT$_{1B}$ receptor knockout mice, whereas it dose-dependently decreased male sexual behavior in wild-type mice. Intriguingly, 8-OH-DPAT also dose-dependently decreased male sexual behavior in WT and had, at these doses, no effect in the KO mice. In another mouse strain (NMRI), 8-OH-DPAT had also inhibitory effects on male mouse sexual behavior [67].

There appears a clear species difference between mice and rats regarding 5-HT$_{1A}$-receptor modulation of male sexual behavior. In contrast, such a species difference is not present in 5-HT$_{1B}$-receptor modulation. 5-HT$_{1B}$-receptor agonists inhibit both male aggression and sexual behavior in mice and rats. Selective 5-HT$_{1A}$-

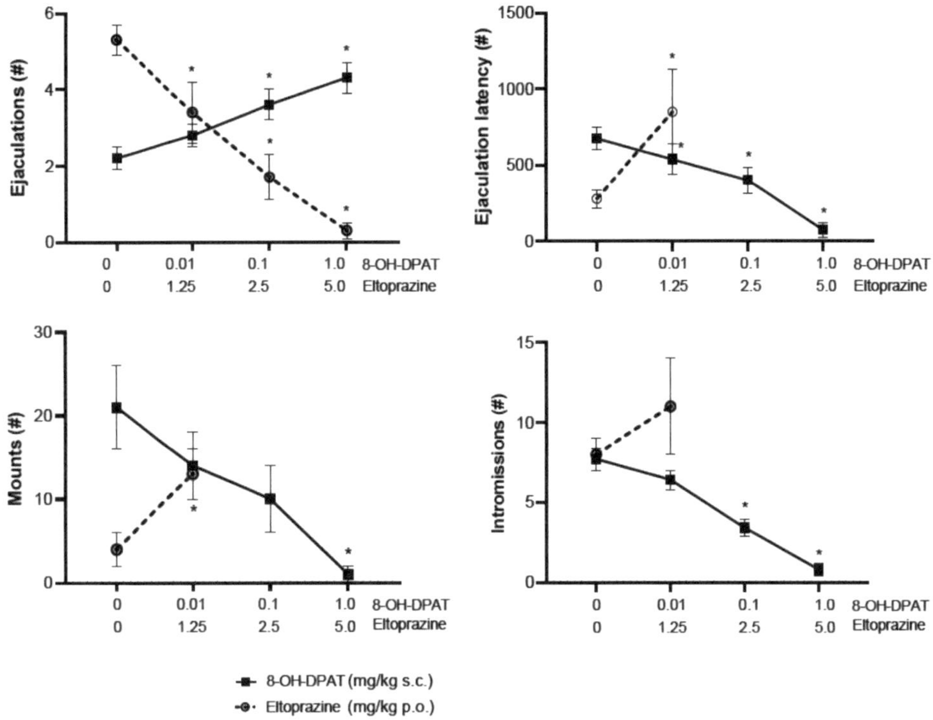

Figure 3.
*Effects of a 5-HT$_{1A}$-receptor agonist ((±)-8-OH-DPAT) and a 5-HT$_{1B}$-receptor agonist (eltoprazine) on male sexual behavior of Wistar rats. The number of ejaculations (top left), mounts (left bottom), and intromissions (right bottom) and the ejaculation latency (top right-in seconds) are shown. 8-OH-DPAT was subcutaneously administered 30 min before testing; eltoprazine orally 60 min before testing. * indicates significant difference ($p < 0.05$) from vehicle (0 mg/kg). In the figures of ejaculation latency and number of mounts and intromission, at higher doses of eltoprazine, no data are available because of absence of sexual behavior. Data are derived from [63] and Olivier-unpublished 1991.*

receptor antagonists (e.g., WAY100,635) have no intrinsic behavioral effects in either sexual or aggressive behavior, either in mice or rats [68–76]. No studies have been published on effects of 5-HT$_{1A}$-receptor antagonists on male aggression or sexual behavior in 5-HT$_{1A}$ or 5-HT$_{1B}$-receptor knockout mice.

There are limited data on chronic treatment with 5-HT$_{1A}$- or 5-HT$_{1B}$-receptor agonists on male sexual behavior. Flesinoxan, a classic 5-HT$_{1A}$-receptor agonist, was given twice daily for 14 days at 2.5 mg/kg, IP. Animals were tested acutely, subchronically (after 7 days) and chronically (after 14 days) on sexual behavior against an estrus female. Acutely, flesinoxan had pro-sexual effects, but no effects were observed after chronic administration, suggesting some tolerance [77]. The effects of a selective 5-HT$_{1B}$-receptor agonist CP-94253 (injected subcutaneously four times daily with 5 mg/kg) were also tested acutely and after 7 and 14 days. CP-94253 inhibited sexual behavior at all time points, showing that it did not induce tolerance [77].

Removing (gene knockout) 5-HT$_{1A}$ receptors from all neurons normally bearing them (serotonergic somatodendritic autoreceptors) and non-serotonergic neurons with 5-HT$_{1A}$ heteroreceptors [29] has behavioral consequences for male sexual behavior but not for male aggressive behavior. Removing 5-HT$_{1B}$ receptors from serotonergic synapses (inhibitory autoreceptors) and inhibitory postsynaptic 5-HT$_{1B}$ heteroreceptors) has contrasting effects on male sexual and aggressive behavior: male 5-HT$_{1B}$ receptor knockout mice have reduced sexual behavior, whereas male aggressive behavior is enhanced [78, 79].

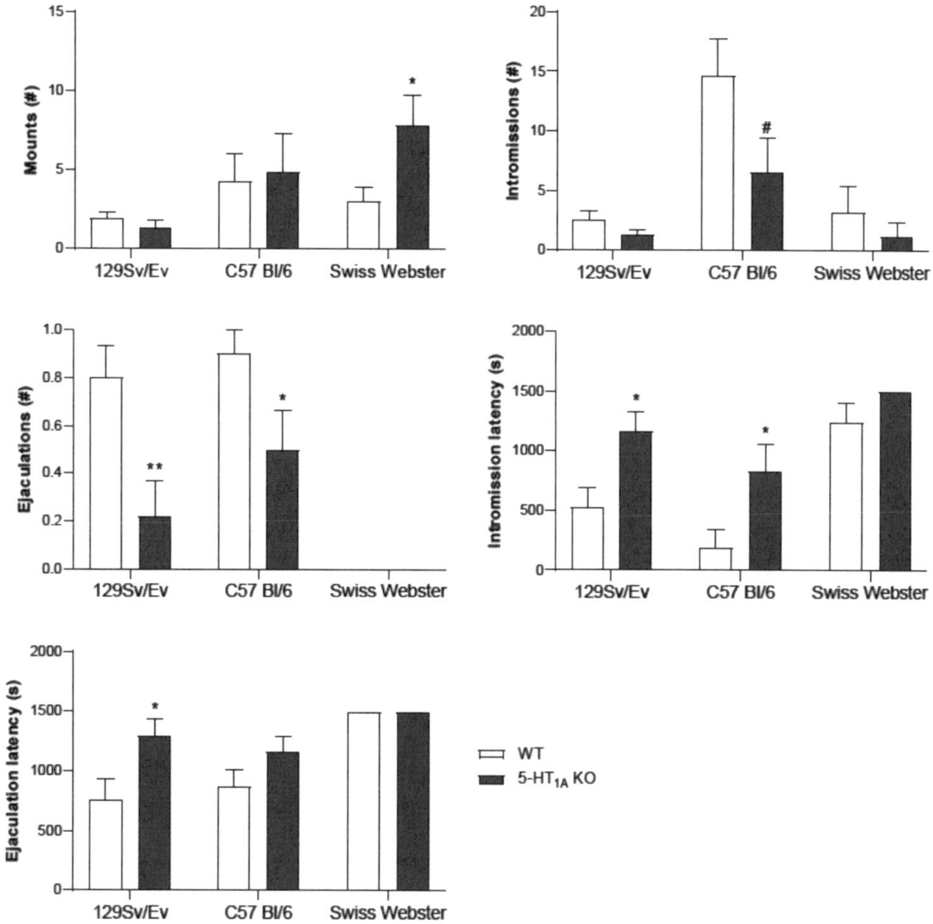

Figure 4.
*Sexual behavior parameters of 5-HT$_{1A}$-receptor knockout (5-HT$_{1A}$KO) and wild-type (WT) mice of three different strains. Latencies are expressed in seconds. Statistics: Repeated measures analysis with two time points. * $P < 0.05$; ** $P < 0.005$; # $P = 0.07$.*

Development of a tissue-specific and temporally conditional 5-HT$_{1B}$-receptor mouse model [80] brought more insight. It was shown that aggressive behavior is mediated by developmental expression of 5-HT$_{1B}$ heteroreceptors. Whole-life, whole-brain elimination of 5-HT$_{1B}$ receptors led to enhanced aggression, like present in constitutive knockout mice [78, 79]. Rescue of 5-HT$_{1B}$-receptor expression in early postnatal development, but not in adulthood, ameliorated aggression. It was shown that forebrain 5-HT$_{1B}$ heteroreceptors mediated this aggression phenotype, while reduction of 5-HT$_{1B}$ autoreceptors had no effect on aggression. Apparently, a developmental sensitive period exists, during which the presence of serotonin affects the development of adult aggression.

4. Are effects of 5-HT$_{1A}$-receptor agonists and 5-HT$_{1B}$-receptor agonists on male aggression and sexual behavior mediated by presynaptic (autoreceptor) or postsynaptic (heteroreceptor) serotonin receptors?

The big question is whether specific effects induced by activating very heterogeneous 5-HT$_{1\ (A\ or\ B)}$ receptors on very specific behavioral systems (aggression and sexual behavior) that are functioning via specific and localized neural circuitry in the brain can be influenced via the extremely nonspecific influence of autoreceptors on the serotonergic cell bodies (5-HT$_{1A}$ autoreceptors) or the serotonergic synaptic endings (5-HT$_{1B}$ autoreceptors). Remarkable is at least that selective 5-HT$_{1A}$-receptor antagonists, blocking somatodendritic autoreceptors and basically leading to enhanced 5-HT release in serotonergic synapses, do not induce behavioral effects (at least in aggression and sexual behavior). Of course, the enhanced 5-HT levels are also not able to stimulate 5-HT$_{1A}$ heteroreceptors because 5-HT$_{1A}$ receptor antagonists block these too, but other 5-HT receptors are not blocked and could be instrumental in emerging behaviors. This apparently does not happen: 5-HT$_{1A}$ receptor antagonists are generally intrinsically silent, i.e., they do not exert intrinsic behavioral effects [51, 71, 74]. Whether 5-HT$_{1B}$ autoreceptors plus serotonin transporters completely compensate for the effects of blocking 5-HT$_{1A}$ receptors on 5-HT release is largely unknown, but seems less likely. Although certainly not conclusive, we postulate that the pro-sexual effects of 5-HT$_{1A}$-receptor agonists on male sexual behavior are mediated via postsynaptic 5-HT$_{1A}$ heteroreceptors. Abundant presence of 5-HT$_{1A}$ receptors in areas containing (parts of) neural circuitry involved in all aspects of sexual behavior (e.g., the hypothalamic circuitries [52, 55]) makes this a likely hypothesis, although microinjection of selective 5-HT$_{1A}$ receptor ligands in nodes of these circuits is badly needed.

In aggression, the role of 5-HT$_{1A}$ receptors is also not evident. Although 5-HT$_{1A}$-receptor agonists have strong anti-aggressive effects in various aggression models in rodents (intermale aggression, resident-intruder aggression, colony aggression, isolation-induced aggression, and others [62, 81], these anti-aggressive effects often coincide with associated nonspecific behavioral effects such as sedation or motor retardation [29, 71, 76]. The selective but low efficacy 5-HT$_{1A}$-receptor agonist S-15535, acting preferentially as a 5-HT$_{1A}$-receptor autoreceptor agonist and as a (partial) 5-HT$_{1A}$-heteroreceptor antagonist, rather selectively decreased aggressive behavior [76], suggesting that the "classical" 5-HT$_{1A}$-receptor agonists (that activate auto- and heteroreceptors) induce the "nonspecific" anti-aggressive effects via heteroreceptor activation.

The emergence of so-called "biased" or "functionally selective" 5-HT$_{1A}$-receptor agonists yielded the possibility to study selectively presynaptic 5-HT$_{1A}$-autoreceptors versus postsynaptic 5-HT$_{1A}$-heteroreceptors. F15599 is an extremely effective 5-HT$_{1A}$-heteroreceptor agonist, with relatively low activity at autoreceptors [57, 82]. F13714 is also an effective 5-HT$_{1A}$-receptor agonist, but primarily activates 5-HT$_{1A}$-autoreceptors [57, 82]. Both "biased" agonists have anti-aggressive effects in extremely aggressive (violent) semi-wild rats [72]: no difference in their anti-aggressive profile was found, making conclusions about specific roles of pre- versus postsynaptic 5-HT$_{1A}$ receptors in aggression more complex.

Although all 5-HT$_{1A}$-receptor agonists upon acute administration seem to inhibit aggressive behavior in mice and rats, classic 5-HT$_{1A}$-receptor agonists such as 8-OH-DPAT and flesinoxan do not inhibit aggression induced by electrical stimulation in the hypothalamic attack area (HAA) in male rats [6, 12, 81, 83]. It is remarkable and unexpected that direct activation of "aggression neurons or circuitry" in the HAA (including the VMHvl) cannot be inhibited by activation of 5-HT$_{1A}$ receptors in the brain. This sharply contrasts by 5-HT$_{1B}$-receptor activation (e.g., by eltoprazine, fluprazine, or TFMPP) that dose-dependently decreases attacks (measured by enhanced stimulation thresholds), but does not influence locomotion thresholds (or even decrease them) and also dose-dependently reduces teeth chattering, an associated (autonomic) aggressive element [6, 12, 81, 83].

5-HT$_{1B}$-receptor agonists inhibit offensive aggression in mice, rats, and other species (e.g., monkeys and pigs) [29, 62, 84]. Other groups have confirmed that activation of 5-HT$_{1B}$ receptors leads to reduction of aggression [71, 85]. Support for an important role of postsynaptic 5-HT$_{1B}$ receptors has been found by the Miczek group [86, 87] and several other sources [88]. Overwhelming evidence suggests that postsynaptic (heteroreceptor) 5-HT$_{1B}$ receptors are involved in the mediation of specific anti-offensive aggression (serenic) activity [29]. Considerable efforts still need to be made to unravel the neural localization of these postsynaptic 5-HT$_{1B}$ receptors, because several conflicting data exist.

A weak and underreported aspect of aggression (and sexual behavior) research is that studies are almost only performed after acute administration. No chronic aggression studies with 5-HT$_{1A}$-receptor agonists have been performed as far as we are aware. For 5-HT$_{1B}$-receptor agonists, some chronic aggression studies in mice and rats were performed. Fluprazine, an early serenic [90, 91], was tested in wild house mice that were selected for a high level of aggression, measured by the attack latency when confronted with a male opponent [89]. Sixteen wild male mice of the SAL-line were selected for Short Attack Latencies (<100 s) and were trained in three successive 10-min trials to reach a stable short attack latency (**Figure 5A**-pre value). In the fourth trial, eight mice received saline (IP) and eight mice received fluprazine (20 mg/kg IP, 30 min before testing). **Figure 5A** shows the strong anti-aggressive activity of acutely administered fluprazine. Chronic administration was performed using osmotic minipumps. Saline had no effects on the latency time, whereas after 7 days of 400 mg/kg/day via minipump administration, fluprazine had strong anti-aggressive activity (**Figure 5B**). Although the chronic effects of fluprazine seemed diminished compared with acute dosing, it was unknown whether a dose of 400 mg/kg/day led to comparable plasma levels of fluprazine than after acute administration, although some tolerance (desensitization of 5-HT$_{1B}$ receptors) might be possible. However, this seems unlikely seen the results of a chronic study with eltoprazine in male Tryon Maze Dull (TMD-S3) rats, a strain

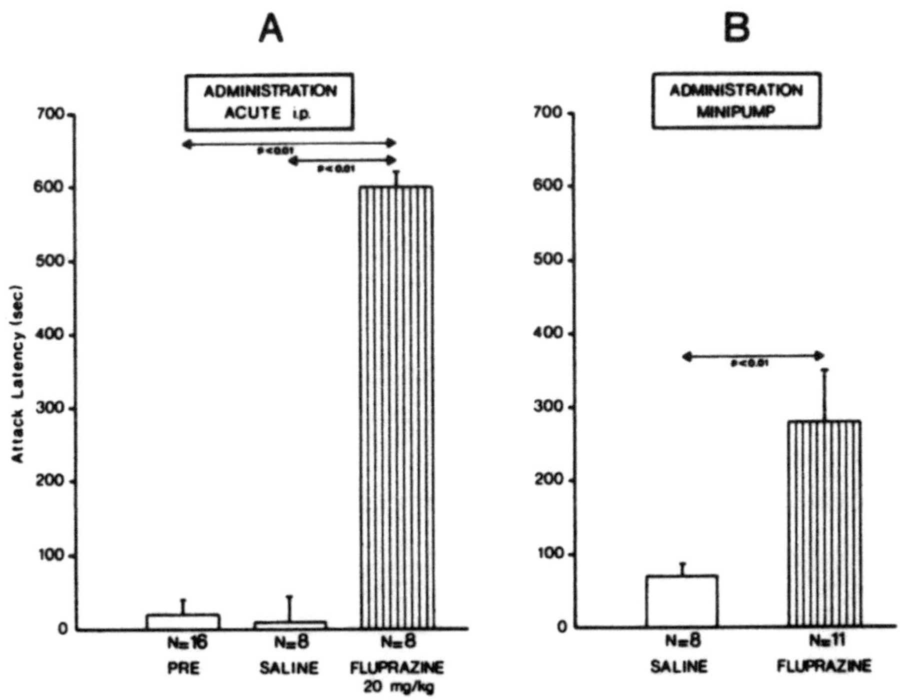

Figure 5.
Effects of fluprazine on attack latencies (sec) of wild house mice selected for aggressive behavior. Panel A shows the acute effects of vehicle and fluprazine 20 mg/kg IP. Panel B shows the effects after 7 days treatment of chronic vehicle or chronic fluprazine (200 mg/kg SC) administered via Alzet® osmotic minipumps [89].

with a high level of residential aggression [92]. After initial training, male rats were used for the resident-intruder test during a 4-week treatment period. Eltoprazine (0, 1, and 3 mg/kg PO) was given 60 min before a 10-min aggression test. Acutely, eltoprazine reduced offensive aggression without any effects on social and nonsocial behaviors. Subsequently, eltoprazine or vehicles were daily administered for 4 weeks, and a resident-intruder test was performed once weekly. The anti-aggressive effects of eltoprazine remained stable over the 4-week period, whereas exploration was enhanced, but no adverse effects were found. After a washout of 1-week aggressive behavior returned to baseline. These data showed no tolerance for the anti-aggressive effects of eltoprazine [93]. In a comparable study using osmotic minipumps for 7 days with 20-mg/kg/day eltoprazine, also no evidence was found for tolerance to the anti-aggressive activity confirming the specificity of the effects [94].

5. Overview of serotonin, sexual behavior, and aggression

Table 1 summarizes effects of 5-HT_{1A} and 5-HT_{1B}-receptor agonists on male sexual and aggressive behavior in mice and rats. 5-HT_{1A}-receptor agonists enhance male sexual behavior in the rat, but decrease it in the mouse. In contrast, 5-HT_{1A}-receptor agonists decrease male aggression in most offensive aggression models in mice and rats, although not in a very essential model, HAA stimulation in rats and behavioral effects are often not very specific, and induced side effects such as sedation or sensoric-motor disturbances might be (co)-causative in the reduction of offensive behavior.

In contrast, 5-HT_{1B}-receptor agonists show highly specific anti-aggressive effects in all offensive aggression models and also reduce male sexual behavior. Neither 5-HT_{1A}-receptor antagonists, nor 5-HT_{1B}-receptor antagonists exert any behavioral effects in either male aggression or male sexual behavior models. Chronic administration of 5-HT_{1A}-receptor agonists seems to induce tolerance, whereas 5-HT_{1B}-receptor agonists do not.

These profiles favor 5-HT_{1B}-receptor agonists over 5-HT_{1A}-receptor agonists with regard to anti-aggressive activity, whereas 5-HT_{1A}-receptor agonists may have a role in pro-sexual effects that may be useful in certain male human sexual dysfunctions, e.g., delayed ejaculation.

In the following part, the history of the development of specific anti-aggressive (offensive) drugs is depicted (**Box 1**).

		5-HT_{1A} receptor	**5-HT_{1A} receptor**	**5-HT_{1B} receptor**	**5-HT_{1B} receptor**
Ligand	**Species**	**Sexual behavior**	**Aggression**	**Sexual behavior**	**Aggression**
Agonist	Rat	↑	↓O?	↓	↓
Agonist	Mouse	↓	↓	↓	↓
Antagonist	Rat	O	O	O	O
Antagonist	Mouse	nt	O	O	O
Knockout	Mouse	↓	O	↓	↑

↑ = *increase;* ↓ = *decrease;* O = *no effect;* ***nt*** = *not tested.*

Table 1.
Summary of effects of 5-HT receptor ligands on male aggressive and sexual behavior in mice and rats.

The discovery and development of drugs, specifically aimed at reduction of pathological aggression and destructive behavior in psychiatric patients, were started halfway the seventies of last century by Philips-Duphar in the Netherlands. It was already at that time clear that pathological destructive behavior, sometimes named "aggressive," "violent," "agitated," or "dysfunctional," is widely present in psychiatric and neurological disorders and cannot, even up to this time, adequately be treated with psychotropic drugs. A striking variety of drugs were and are used in patients with these severely troubled behavioral disturbances, including neuroleptics or hypnotics, mainly used for their sedative properties, benzodiazepines, lithium, beta-blockers antidepressants and anticonvulsants [95].

In the mid-seventies, Philips-Duphar started a search for specific anti-aggressive drugs. At that time, the pre-molecular era, there was no clue for which target to search, and consequently, the quest for anti-aggressive drugs was steered by animal aggression models and tests [96]. One of the authors (BO) was hired by Philips-Duphar because of their expertise and background in aggression models and brain mechanisms involved in aggression [29]. Throughout the sixties and seventies, pharmacological laboratories used simple but often unnatural animal models involving various aspects of agonistic behaviors (offense, defense, flight) to detect psycho-activity of newly synthesized drugs; the aim was not to detect "anti-aggressive" drugs as therapeutics but merely a read-out for psychoactive effects. For example, neuroleptic activity in a molecule could be easily detected using isolation-induced fighting in male mice [97]. Such models are functionally simple to run and score and therefore extremely suitable for screening, but they do not reveal the mechanism of action and do not predict the specificity of the observed effect and cannot distinguish the compound tested from any other compound that shows pharmacological activity in the model or test.

Because we had no clue about a mode of action to pursue specific anti-aggressive activity in a molecule at that time, a behavioral cascade of animal models of aggressive behavior was created. The "isolation-induced aggression" test in male mice was the primary screening test to determine an ED_{50} (in mg/kg orally) for aggression reduction. As this measure did not reveal the specificity of the anti-aggressive activity, further tests were developed to measure the behavioral specificity of the aggression reducing effects of psychoactive drugs. By using ethological methods in mice and rats [94] and combined lead-finding and screening of more than 2000 new chemical structures, some phenylpiperazine analogues were found that fulfilled primary pharmacological criteria for a non-sedative anti-aggressive structure. In 1980, after a dedicated search for optimal anti-aggressive activity, DU27716 (fluprazine) was selected for further development. Fluprazine and its later successors (eltoprazine, batoprazine) showed the specific anti-aggressive profile in which offensive aggression was reduced, whereas social behavior and exploration were not affected. This profile has been depicted as SERENIC [98]. Eltoprazine was taken into clinical development up to phase 2B, but for several reasons, no phase 3 studies were initiated. Unfortunately, since then (1994), no new developments in the search for serenics have been undertaken.

Serenics were found and developed based on a purely translational basis: animal models of aggression predicting human (pathological) aggression [62]. Although a risky approach, no target-specific search was possible, as the putative underlying mechanisms of action were unknown. In the course of time, however, it became clear that serenics interacted with central serotonergic (5-HT) systems. In the 1980s, the rapid development of receptor binding techniques and the discovery of subtype receptors of various neurotransmitters played an increasing role in the unraveling of the mode of action of drugs. The most prominent feature of serenics was their affinity for serotonergic receptors. Over time [62] it became clear that serenics (eltoprazine) have high affinity for 5-HT$_1$ receptors, specifically for 5-HT$_{1A}$ and 5-HT$_{1B}$ receptors. Further research has shown that eltoprazine exerts its serenic activity because of its (partial) agonistic activity at 5-HT$_{1A}$ and 5-HT$_{1B}$ receptors. There is evidence [88, 99, 100] that serenic activity is mediated postsynaptically via 5-HT$_{1B}$ receptors [84], although a role for 5-HT$_{1A}$ receptors cannot be excluded [71].

Although serotonin has been considered for a long time as a very important neurotransmitter in the modulation of aggression and impulsivity [101], it does not work in isolation; other neurotransmitters clearly play an important role too [86, 102]. Apparently, however, serotonin is a key player in modulation of aggression mechanism and circuitry; a PUBMED search (March 22, 2021) on "aggression" coupled to "serotonin" yields 3010 hits, with "dopamine" 1627 hits, with "noradrenaline" 849 hits, with "GABA" 705 hits, whereas with other neurotransmitters yields lower hits.

The specific search for serenics, independent of the underlying molecular target, has not been pursued after the development stop of eltoprazine in 1994. Since then, fundamental research on aggression has dwindled for some time although many relevant studies in man and animal are still pursued. Verhoeven and Tuinier [103] pleaded for continued research into serenics, strongly supported by Coccaro et al. [101] who "hoped that new insights into the neurobiology of aggression will reveal novel avenues for treatment of this destructive and costly behavior." The recent surge in applying new techniques in neurobiology has also brought exciting findings in the circuitry and genetics of aggression that might facilitate future search for new serenics.

Box 1.
Serenics: Drugs with specific anti-aggressive activity.

Author details

Berend Olivier[1,2,3*] and Jocelien D.A. Olivier[3]

1 Department of Psychopharmacology, Utrecht Institute for Pharmaceutical Sciences, Utrecht University, Utrecht, The Netherlands

2 Department of Psychiatry, Yale School of Medicine, New Haven, USA

3 Neurobiology, Groningen Institute for Evolutionary Life Sciences (GELIFES), Rijksuniversiteit Groningen, Groningen, The Netherlands

*Address all correspondence to: b.olivier@uu.nl

References

[1] Hess WR. Stammganglien-Reizversuchen. Berichten der gesamten. Physiologie. 1927;**42**:554-555

[2] Panksepp J. Aggression elicited by electrical stimulation of the hypothalamus in albino rats. Physiology & Behavior. 1971;**6**:321-329. DOI: 10.1016/0031-9384(71)90163-6

[3] Woodworth CH. Attack elicited in rats by electrical stimulation of the lateral hypothalamus. Physiology & Behavior. 1971;**6**:345-353. DOI: 10.1016/0031-9384(71)90166-1

[4] Koolhaas JM. Hypothalamically induced intraspecific aggressive behaviour in the rat. Experimental Brain Research. 1978;**32**:365-375. DOI: 10.1007/BF00238708

[5] Kruk MR, van der Poel AM, de Vos-Frerichs TP. The induction of aggressive behaviour by electrical stimulation in the hypothalamus of male rats. Behaviour. 1979;**70**:292-322. DOI: 10.1163/156853979x00106

[6] Siegel A, Roeling TA, Gregg TR, Kruk MR. Neuropharmacology of brain-stimulation-evoked aggression. Neuroscience and Biobehavioral Reviews. 1999;**23**:359-389. DOI: 10.1016/s0149-7634(98)00040-2

[7] Olivier B, Wiepkema PR. Behaviour changes in mice following electrolytic lesions in the median hypothalamus. Brain Research. 1974;**65**:521-5244. DOI: 10.1016/0006-8993(74)90241-8

[8] Olivier B. The ventromedial hypothalamus and aggressive behavior in the rat. Aggressive Behavior. 1977;**3**: 47-56

[9] Olivier B, Olivier-Aardema R, Wiepkema PR. Effect of anterior hypothalamic and mammillary area lesions on territorial aggressive behaviour in male rats. Behavioural Brain Research. 1983;**9**:59-81. DOI: 10.1016/0166-4328(83)90014-1

[10] Olivier B. Behavioural fuctions of the medial hypothalamus in the rat [PhD-thesis]. Rijksuniversiteit Groningen; 1977. pp. 1-220

[11] Van den Berg MJ, ter Horst GJ, Koolhaas JM. The nucleus premammillaris ventralis (PMV) and aggressive behavior in the rat. Aggressive Behavior. 1983;**9**:41-47

[12] Kruk MR. Ethology and pharmacology of hypothalamic aggression in the rat. Neuroscience and Biobehavioral Reviews. 1991;**15**:527-538. DOI: 10.1016/s0149-7634(05)80144-7

[13] Hrabovszky E, Halász J, Meelis W, Kruk MR, Liposits Z, Haller J. Neurochemical characterization of hypothalamic neurons involved in attack behavior: Glutamatergic dominance and co-expression of thyrotropin-releasing hormone in a subset of glutamatergic neurons. Neuroscience. 2005;**133**:657-666. DOI: 10.1016/j.neuroscience.2005.03.042

[14] Kruk MR, Van der Laan CE, Mos J, Van der Poel AM, Meelis W, Olivier B. Comparison of aggressive behaviour induced by electrical stimulation in the hypothalamus of male and female rats. Progress in Brain Research. 1984;**61**: 303-314

[15] Lee H, Lein ES, Perona P, Anderson DJ. Functional identification of an aggression locus in the mouse hypothalamus. Nature. 2011;**470**: 221-226

[16] de Boer SF, Olivier B, Veening J, Koolhaas JM. The neurobiology of offensive aggression: Revealing a modular view. Physiology & Behavior. 2015;**146**:111-127. DOI: 10.1016/j.physbeh.2015.04.040

[17] Yamaguchi T, Lin D. Functions of medial hypothalamic and mesolimbic dopamine circuitries in aggression. Current Opinion in Behavioral Sciences. 2018;**24**:104-112. DOI: 10.1016/j.cobeha.2018.06.011

[18] Newman SW. The medial extended amygdala in male reproductive behavior. A node in the mammalian social behavior. Annals. New York Academy of Sciences. 1999;**877**:242-257

[19] Kumar A, Dudley CA, Moss RL. Functional dichotomy within the vomeronasal system: Distinct zones of neuronal activity in the accessory olfactory bulb correlate with sex specific behaviors. The Journal of Neuroscience. 1999;**19**:RC32. DOI: 10.1523/JNEUROSCI.19-20-j0003.1999

[20] Veening JG, Coolen LM, de Jong TR, Joosten HW, de Boer SF, Koolhaas JM, et al. Do similar neural systems subserve aggressive and sexual behaviour in male rats? Insights from c-Fos and pharmacological studies. European Journal of Pharmacology. 2005;**526**:226-239. DOI: 10.1016/j.ejphar.2005.09.041

[21] Yamaguchi T, Wei D, Song SC, Lim B, Tritsch NX, Lin D. Posterior amygdala regulates sexual and aggressive behaviors in male mice. Nature Neuroscience. 2020;**23**:1111-1124. DOI: 10.1038/s41593-020-0675-x

[22] Falkner AL, Grosenick L, Davidson TJ, Deisseroth K, Lin D. Hypothalamic control of male aggression-seeking behavior. Nature Neuroscience. 2016;**19**:596-604. DOI: 10.1038/nn.4264

[23] Yu Q, Teixeira CM, Mahadevia D, Huang Y, Balsam D, Mann JJ, et al. Dopamine and serotonin signaling during two sensitive developmental periods differentially impact adult aggressive and affective behaviors in mice. Molecular Psychiatry. 2014;**19**:688-698. DOI: 10.1038/mp.2014.10

[24] Lee H, Kim DW, Remedios R, Anthony TE, Chang A, Madisen L, et al. Scalable control of mounting and attack by Esr1+ neurons in the ventromedial hypothalamus. Nature. 2014;**509**:627-632. DOI: 10.1038/nature13169

[25] Chen P, Hong W. Neural circuit mechanisms of social behavior. Neuron. 2018;**98**:16-30. DOI: 10.1016/j.neuron.2018.02.026

[26] Hashikawa Y, Hashikawa K, Falkner AL, Lin D. Ventromedial hypothalamus and the generation of aggression. Frontiers in Systems Neuroscience. 2017;**11**:94. DOI: 10.3389/fnsys.2017.00094

[27] Krzywkowski P, Penna B, Gross CT. Dynamic encoding of social threat and spatial context in the hypothalamus. eLife. 2020;**9**:e57148. DOI: 10.7554/eLife.57148

[28] Sharp T. Serotonergic feedback control. In: Muller CP, Jacobs BL, editors. Handbook of Behavioral Neurobiology of Serotonin. Amsterdam: Elsevier; 2010. pp. 233-258

[29] Olivier B. Serotonin: A never-ending story. European Journal of Pharmacology. 2015;**753**:2-18. DOI: 10.1016/j.ejphar.2014.10.031

[30] Murphy DI, Lerner A, Rudnick G, Lesch KP. Serotonin transporter: Gene, genetic disorders and pharmacogenetics. Molecular Interventions. 2004;**4**:109-123

[31] Snoeren EM, Veening JG, Olivier B, Oosting RS. Serotonin 1A receptors and sexual behavior in male rats: A review. Pharmacology, Biochemistry, and Behavior. 2014;**121**:102-114. DOI: 10.1016/j.pbb.2013.11.007

[32] Marson L, McKenna KE. A role for 5-hydoxytryptamine in descending inhibition of spinal sexual reflexes. Experimental Brain Research. 1992;**88**:313-320

[33] Marson L, Gravitt K. Spinal neurons activated with the urethrogenital reflex in the male rat. Brain Research. 2004; **1026**:108-115

[34] Marson L, McKenna KE. Stimulation of the hypothalamus initiates the urethrogenital reflex in male rats. Brain Research. 1994;**638**: 103-108

[35] Kippin TE, Sotiropoulos V, Badih J, Pfaus JG. Opposing roles of the nucleus accumbens and anterior lateral hypothalamic area in the control of sexual behaviour in the male rat. The European Journal of Neuroscience. 2004;**19**:698-704

[36] Lorrain DS, Matuszewich L, Friedman RD, Hull EM. Extracellular serotonin in the lateral hypothalamic area is increased during the postejaculatory interval and impairs copulation in male rats. The Journal of Neuroscience. 1997;**17**:9361-9366

[37] Vertes RP. A PHA-L analysis of ascending projections of the dorsal raphe nucleus in the rat. The Journal of Comparative Neurology. 1991;**313**: 643-668

[38] Vertes RP, Fortin WJ, Crane AM. Projections of the median raphe nucleus in the rat. The Journal of Comparative Neurology. 1999;**407**:555-582

[39] Uphouse L. Pharmacology of serotonin and female sexual behavior. Pharmacology, Biochemistry, and Behavior. 2014;**121**:31-42

[40] Uphouse L, Guptarak J. Serotonin and sexual behavior. In: Muller CP, Jacobs BL, editors. Handbook of Behavioral Neurobiology of Serotonin. Amsterdam: Elsevier; 2010. pp. 347-365

[41] Olivier JDA, Olivier B. Antidepressants and sexual dysfunction; translational aspects. Current Sexual Health Reports. 2019;**11**:156-166

[42] Barnes NM, Ahern GP, Becamel C, Bockaert J, Camilleri M, Chaumont-Dubel S, et al. International union of basic and clinical pharmacology. CX. Classification of receptors for 5-hydroxytryptamine; pharmacology and function. Pharmacology Review. 2021; **73**:310-520

[43] Youdim MB, Edmondson D, Tipton KF. The therapeutic potential of monoamine oxidase inhibitors. Nature Reviews: Neuroscience. 2006;**7**:295-309. DOI: 10.1038/nrn1883

[44] Artigas F. Serotonin receptors involved in antidepressant effects. Pharmacology & Therapeutics. 2013; **137**:119-131

[45] Artigas F. Future direction for serotonin and antidepressants. ACS Chemical Neuroscience. 2013;**4**:5-8

[46] Adell A, Celada P, Abellan MT, Artigas F. Origin and functional role of the extracellular serotonin in the midbrain raphe nuclei. Brain Research Reviews. 2002;**39**:154-180

[47] Ahlenius S, Larsson K, Svensson L, Hjorth S, Carlsson A, Lindberg P, et al. Effects of a new type of 5-HT receptor agonist on male rat sexual behavior. Pharmacology, Biochemistry, and Behavior. 1981;**15**:785-792. DOI: 10.1016/0091-3057(81)90023-x

[48] Veening JG, Coolen LM. Neural mechanisms of sexual behavior in the male rat: Emphasis on ejaculation-related circuits. Pharmacology, Biochemistry, and Behavior. 2014;**121**: 170-183. DOI: 10.1016/j.pbb.2013.12.017

[49] Veening J. Behavioural functions of the VMH in the rat: An ethological approach [PhD thesis]. Rijksuniversiteit Groningen; 1975. pp. 1-127

[50] Veening JG. Brain and behaviour: Morphological and functional aspects of the hypothalamus in the rat.

European Journal of Morphology. 1992; **30**:53-66

[51] Olivier JDA, Janssen J, Pattij T, de Prètre S, Olivier B. Antidepressant, sexual behavior and translational models for male sexual dysfunctions: Development of animal models, pharmacology and genetics. In: Kim Y-K, Amidfur M, editors. Translational Research Methods for Major Depressive Disorder. Neuromethods, vol. 179. NewYork: Humana Press; 2021

[52] Anderson DJ. Optogenetics, sex, and violence in the brain: Implications for psychiatry. Biological Psychiatry. 2012; **71**(12):1081-1089. DOI: 10.1016/j.biopsych.2011.11.012

[53] Hashikawa K, Hashikawa Y, Falkner A, Lin D. The neural circuits of mating and fighting in male mice. Current Opinion in Neurobiology. 2016; **38**:27-37. DOI: 10.1016/j.conb.2016.01.006

[54] Yang CF, Chiang MC, Gray DC, Prabhakaran M, Alvarado M, Juntti SA, et al. Sexually dimorphic neurons in the ventromedial hypothalamus govern mating in both sexes and aggression in males. Cell. 2013;**153**:896-909. DOI: 10.1016/j.cell.2013.04.017

[55] Anderson DJ. Circuit modules linking internal states and social behaviour in flies and mice. Nature Reviews. Neuroscience. 2016;**17**: 692-704. DOI: 10.1038/nrn.2016.125

[56] Esquivel-Franco DC, de Boer SF, Waldinger M, Olivier B, Olivier JDA. Pharmacological studies on the role of 5-HT1A receptors in male sexual behavior of wildtype and serotonin transporter knockout rats. Frontiers in Behavioral Neuroscience. 2020;**14**:40. DOI: 10.3389/fnbeh.2020.00040

[57] Newman-Tancredi A. Biased agonism at serotonin 5-HT1A receptors: Preferential postsynaptic activity for improved therapy of CNS disorders. Neuropsychiatry. 2011;**1**:149-164

[58] Fernández-Guasti A, Escalante A, Agmo A. Inhibitory action of various 5-HT1B receptor agonists on rat masculine sexual behaviour. Pharmacology, Biochemistry, and Behavior. 1989;**34**: 811-816. DOI: 10.1016/0091-3057(89)90279-7

[59] Fernández-Guasti A, Rodríguez-Manzo G. Further evidence showing that the inhibitory action of serotonin on rat masculine sexual behavior is mediated after the stimulation of 5-HT1B receptors. Pharmacology, Biochemistry, and Behavior. 1992;**42**: 529-533. DOI: 10.1016/0091-3057(92)90150-e

[60] Hillegaart V, Ahlenius S. Facilitation and inhibition of male rat ejaculatory behaviour by the respective 5-HT1A and 5-HT1B receptor agonists 8-OH-DPAT and anpirtoline, as evidenced by use of the corresponding new and selective receptor antagonists NAD-299 and NAS-181. British Journal of Pharmacology. 1998;**125**:1733-1743. DOI: 10.1038/sj.bjp.0702239

[61] Rodríguez-Manzo G, López-Rubalcava C, Hen R, Fernández-Guasti A. Participation of 5-HT(1B) receptors in the inhibitory actions of serotonin on masculine sexual behaviour of mice: Pharmacological analysis in 5-HT(1B) receptor knockout mice. British Journal of Pharmacology. 2002;**136**:1127-1134. DOI: 10.1038/sj.bjp.0704827

[62] Olivier B, Mos J, Raghoebar M, de Koning P, Mak M. Serenics. Progress in Drug Research. 1994;**42**:167-308. DOI: 10.1007/978-3-0348-7153-2_6

[63] Chan JS, Snoeren EM, Cuppen E, Waldinger MD, Olivier B, Oosting RS. The serotonin transporter plays an important role in male sexual behavior: A study in serotonin transporter knockout rats. The Journal of Sexual

Medicine. 2011;**8**:97-108. DOI: 10.1111/j.1743-6109.2010.01961.x

[64] Groenink L, Pattij T, De Jongh R, Van der Gugten J, Oosting RS, Dirks A, et al. 5-HT1A receptor knockout mice and mice overexpressing corticotropin-releasing hormone in models of anxiety. European Journal of Pharmacology. 2003;**463**:185-197. DOI: 10.1016/s0014-2999(03)01281-0

[65] Pattij T, Broersen LM, van der Linde J, Groenink L, van der Gugten J, Maes RA, et al. Operant learning and differential-reinforcement-of-low-rate 36-s responding in 5 HT1A and 5-HT1B receptor knockout mice. Behavioural Brain Research. 2003;**141**:137-145. DOI: 10.1016/s0166-4328(02)00345-5

[66] Vinkers CH, Oosting RS, van Bogaert MJ, Olivier B, Groenink L. Early-life blockade of 5-HT(1A) receptors alters adult anxiety behavior and benzodiazepine sensitivity. Biological Psychiatry. 2010;**67**:309-316. DOI: 10.1016/j.biopsych.2009.08.013

[67] Svensson K, Larsson K, Ahlenius S, Arvidsson LE, Carlsson A. Evidence for a facilitatory role of central 5-HT in male mouse sexual behavior. In: Dourish CT, Ahlenius S, Hutson PH, editors. Brain 5-HT$_{1A}$ Receptors: Behavioural and Neurochemical Pharmacology. Chichester: Ellis Horwood; 1987. pp. 199-210

[68] Schijven D, Sousa VC, Roelofs J, Olivier B, Olivier JD. Serotonin 1A receptors and sexual behavior in a genetic model of depression. Pharmacology, Biochemistry, and Behavior. 2014;**121**:82-87. DOI: 10.1016/j.pbb.2013.12.012

[69] Ahlenius S, Larsson K. Evidence for an involvement of 5-HT1B receptors in the inhibition of male rat ejaculatory behavior produced by 5-HTP. Psychopharmacology. 1998;**137**:374-382. DOI: 10.1007/s002130050633

[70] Ahlenius S, Larsson K. Synergistic actions of the 5-HT1A receptor antagonist WAY-100635 and citalopram on male rat ejaculatory behavior. European Journal of Pharmacology. 1999;**379**:1-6. DOI: 10.1016/s0014-2999(99)00483-5

[71] de Boer SF, Koolhaas JM. 5-HT1A and 5-HT1B receptor agonists and aggression: A pharmacological challenge of the serotonin deficiency hypothesis. European Journal of Pharmacology. 2005;**526**:125-139. DOI: 10.1016/j.ejphar.2005.09.065

[72] de Boer SF, Newman-Tancredi A. Anti-aggressive effects of the selective high-efficacy 'biased' 5-HT$_1$A receptor agonists F15599 and F13714 in male WTG rats. Psychopharmacology. 2016;**233**:937-947. DOI: 10.1007/s00213-015-4173-x

[73] Bell R, Hobson H. 5-HT1A receptor influences on rodent social and agonistic behavior: A review and empirical study. Neuroscience and Biobehavioral Reviews. 1994;**18**:325-338. DOI: 10.1016/0149-7634(94)90046-9

[74] Bell R, Lynch K, Mitchell P. Lack of effect of the 5-HT(1A) receptor antagonist WAY-100635 on murine agonistic behaviour. Pharmacology, Biochemistry, and Behavior. 1999;**64**:549-554. DOI: 10.1016/s0091-3057(99)00105-7

[75] de Boer SF, Lesourd M, Mocaer E, Koolhaas JM. Selective antiaggressive effects of alnespirone in resident-intruder test are mediated via 5-hydroxytryptamine1A receptors: A comparative pharmacological study with 8-hydroxy-2-dipropylaminotetralin, ipsapirone, buspirone, eltoprazine, and WAY-100635. The Journal of Pharmacology and Experimental Therapeutics. 1999;**288**:1125-1133

[76] de Boer SF, Lesourd M, Mocaër E, Koolhaas JM. Somatodendritic 5-HT(1A)

autoreceptors mediate the anti-aggressive actions of 5-HT(1A) receptor agonists in rats: An ethopharmacological study with S-15535, alnespirone, and WAY-100635. Neuropsychopharmacology. 2000;**23**: 20-33. DOI: 10.1016/S0893-133X(00) 00092-0

[77] Li Y, Pehrson AL, Oosting RS, Gulinello M, Olivier B, Sanchez C. A study of time- and sex-dependent effects of vortioxetine on rat sexual behavior: Possible roles of direct receptor modulation. Neuropharmacology. 2017;**121**:89-99. DOI: 10.1016/j.neuropharm.2017.04.017

[78] Bouwknecht JA, Hijzen TH, van der Gugten J, Maes RA, Hen R, Olivier B. Absence of 5-HT(1B) receptors is associated with impaired impulse control in male 5-HT(1B) knockout mice. Biological Psychiatry. 2001;**49**: 557-568. DOI: 10.1016/s0006-3223(00) 01018-0

[79] Saudou F, Amara DA, Dierich A, LeMeur M, Ramboz S, Segu L, et al. Enhanced aggressive behavior in mice lacking 5-HT1B receptor. Science. 1994; **265**:1875-1878. DOI: 10.1126/ science.8091214

[80] Nautiyal KM, Tanaka KF, Barr MM, Tritschler L, Le Dantec Y, David DJ, et al. Distinct circuits underlie the effects of 5-HT1B receptors on aggression and impulsivity. Neuron. 2015;**86**:813-826. DOI: 10.1016/j. neuron.2015.03.041

[81] Olivier B, Mos J, Tulp M, Schipper J, den Daas S, van Oortmerssen G. Serotonergic involvement in aggressive behavior in animals. In: van Praag H, Plutchik R, Apter A, editors. Violence and Suicidality: Perspectives in Clinical and Psychobiological Research. New York, Brunner/Mazel, 1990. 79-137.

[82] Garcia-Garcia AL, Newman-Tancredi A, Leonardo ED. 5-HT(1A) receptors in mood and anxiety: Recent insights into autoreceptor versus heteroreceptor function. Psychopharmacology. 2014;**231**: 623-636. DOI: 10.1007/s00213-013-3389-x.(Berl)

[83] Olivier B, Mos J, Rasmussen D. Behavioural pharmacology of the serenic, eltoprazine. Drug Metabolism and Drug Interactions. 1990;**8**:31-83. DOI: 10.1515/dmdi.1990.8.1-2.31

[84] Olivier B, van Oorschot R. 5-HT1B receptors and aggression: A review. European Journal of Pharmacology. 2005;**526**:207-217. DOI: 10.1016/j. ejphar.2005.09.066

[85] Olivier B, Mos J, van Oorschot R, Hen R. Serotonin receptors and animal models of aggressive behavior. Pharmacopsychiatry. 1995;**28**(Suppl 2): 80-90. DOI: 10.1055/s-2007-979624

[86] Takahashi A, Quadros IM, de Almeida RM, Miczek KA. Brain serotonin receptors and transporters: Initiation vs. termination of escalated aggression. Psychopharmacology. 2011; **213**:183-212. DOI: 10.1007/s00213-010-2000-y

[87] Centenaro LA, Vieira K, Zimmermann N, Miczek KA, Lucion AB, de Almeida RM. Social instigation and aggressive behavior in mice: Role of 5-HT1A and 5-HT1B receptors in the prefrontal cortex. Psychopharmacology. 2008;**201**:237-248. DOI: 10.1007/ s00213-008-1269-6

[88] Sijbesma H, Schipper J, de Kloet ER, Mos J, van Aken H, Olivier B. Postsynaptic 5-HT1 receptors and offensive aggression in rats: A combined behavioural and autoradiographic study with eltoprazine. Pharmacology, Biochemistry, and Behavior. 1991;**38**:447-458. DOI: 10.1016/ 0091-3057(91)90305-l

[89] Van Oortmerssen GA, Benus I, Dijk GJ. Studies in wild house mice: Genotype-environment interactions for

attack latency. Netherland Journal of Zoology. 1985;**35**:155-169

[90] Olivier B, van Dalen. Social behavior in rats and mice: An ethological based model for differentiating psychoactive drugs. Aggressive Behavior. 1982;**8**:163-168

[91] van der Poel AM, Olivier B, Mos J, Kruk MR, Meelis W, van Aken JH. Anti-aggressive effect of a new phenylpiperazine compound (DU27716) on hypothalamically induced behavioural activities. Pharmacology, Biochemistry, and Behavior. 1982;**17**:147-153. DOI: 10.1016/0091-3057(82)90277-5

[92] Olivier B. Selective anti-aggressive properties of DU 27725: Ethological analyses of intermale and territorial aggression in the male rat. Pharmacology, Biochemistry, and Behavior. 1981;**14**(Suppl. 1):61-77. DOI: 10.1016/s0091-3057(81)80012-3

[93] Mos J, van Aken HH, van Oorschot R, Olivier B. Chronic treatment with eltoprazine does not lead to tolerance in its anti-aggressive action, in contrast to haloperidol. European Neuropsychopharmacology. 1996;**6**:1-7. DOI: 10.1016/0924-977x(95)00051-p

[94] Olivier B, Rasmussen D, Raghoebar M, Mos J. Ethopharmacology: A creative approach to identification and characterisation of novel psychotropics. Drug Metabolism and Drug Interactions. 1990;**8**:11-29. DOI: 10.1515/dmdi.1990.8.1-2.11

[95] Rasmussen DL, Olivier B, Raghoebar M, Mos J. Possible clinical applications of serenics and some implications of their preclinical profile for their clinical use in psychiatric disorders. Drug Metabolism and Drug Interactions. 1990;**8**:159-186. DOI: 10.1515/dmdi.1990.8.1-2.159

[96] Olivier B, Raghoebar M, Mos J, Hartog J. Rasmussen D. Serenics: An introduction. Drug Metabolism and Drug Interactions. 1990;**8**:1-9

[97] Janssen PAJ, Jageman AH, Niemegeers JE. Effects of various drugs on isolation-induced fighting behavior of male mice. The Journal of Pharmacology and Experimental Therapeutics. 1959;**125**:471-475

[98] Olivier B, van Dalen D, Hartog J. A new class of psychoactive drugs: Serenics. Drugs of the Future. 1986;**11**: 473-499

[99] Mos J, Olivier B, Poth M, van Aken H. The effects of intraventricular administration of eltoprazine, 1-(3-trifluoromethylphenyl)piperazine hydrochloride and 8-hydroxy-2-(di-n-propylamino)tetralin on resident intruder aggression in the rat. European Journal of Pharmacology. 1992;**212**: 295-298. DOI: 10.1016/0014-2999(92)90348-8

[100] Mos J, Olivier B, Poth M, Van Oorschot R, Van Aken H. The effects of dorsal raphe administration of eltoprazine, TFMPP and 8-OH-DPAT on resident intruder aggression in the rat. European Journal of Pharmacology. 1993;**238**:411-415. DOI: 10.1016/0014-2999(93)90877-k

[101] Coccaro EF, Fanning JR, Phan KL, Lee R. Serotonin and impulsive aggression. CNS Spectrums. 2015;**20**: 295-302. DOI: 10.1017/S1092852915000310

[102] Rosell DR, Siever LJ. The neurobiology of aggression and violence. CNS Spectrums. 2015;**20**: 254-279. DOI: 10.1017/S109285291500019X

[103] Verhoeven WMA, Tuinier S. Serenics: Anti-aggression drugs throughout history. Clinical Neuropsychiatry. 2007;**4**:135-143

Chapter 6

Experimental Serotonin Syndrome: Effects of GABA-ergic Medications and 5-HT_2-Antagonists

Rumen Nikolov and Kalina Koleva

Abstract

Serotonin syndrome (SS) is a potentially life-threatening adverse drug effect that occurs after an overdose or combined administration of two or more drugs that increase the serotonin levels. In humans, SS is represented by a triad of symptoms including mental status changes, neuromuscular hyperactivity and autonomic dysfunction. The manifestations of the syndrome observed in rodents resemble the symptoms of SS in humans. Theoretically, SS can occur as a result of stimulation of any of the seven families of the serotonin receptors. However, most data support the involvement of 5-HT_{1A} and 5-HT_{2A} receptors. A number of studies indicate the effectiveness of 5-HT_2 antagonists and GABA-ergic agents in the treatment of the hyperthermia and other symptoms of SS in rats. Therefore, animal models of SS may help to further elucidate the mechanism of its development and the possibilities for its treatment.

Keywords: 5-HT_2 antagonists, GABA-ergic agents, serotonin syndrome, rats

1. Introduction

Serotonin syndrome is a drug-induced condition caused by medications that increase intrasynaptic serotonin levels. It is characterized by a triad of symptoms that includes neuromuscular hyperactivity, altered mental status and autonomic dysfunction.

The syndrome was first described in 1960 as "Indolamine syndrome" in patients on therapy with monoamine oxidase inhibitors (MAOIs) who develop symptoms of serotonin syndrome after taking tryptophan – a serotonin precursor [1]. Since then, the number of reported cases of serotonin syndrome has increased significantly. The medical community's attention to serotonin syndrome was drawn in 1984 by the unusual death of 18-year-old Libby Zion in a New York City hospital, which may have been linked to the development of serotonin syndrome after concomitant use of an MAOI and opioid analgesic. The opioid analgesic pethidine was administered to the girl suffering from depression and taking the antidepressant phenelzine, which led to the development of a fatal serotonin syndrome [2, 3].

Of all serotonergic drugs, antidepressants are the most common cause of serotonin syndrome, and recent data suggest that the most common drug combination associated with serotonin syndrome is that between selective serotonin reuptake inhibitors (SSRIs) and opioids [2]. As a relatively rare adverse drug reaction, the incidence of serotonin syndrome is difficult to be calculated during randomized controlled trials [4]. Moreover, it is estimated that over 85% of physicians are unaware of the condition [5]. The non-specific manifestation of the syndrome leads to its difficult recognition and underreporting, which further complicates the determination of its incidence. It is considered that serotonin syndrome occurs in 15% of patients who overdose on selective serotonin reuptake inhibitors. The actual incidence of serotonin syndrome is thought to be significantly higher than reported [6–8].

2. Molecular mechanism of serotonin syndrome development

Serotonin syndrome results from an increase in intrasynaptic serotonin levels caused by overstimulation of both central and peripheral serotonin receptors [9, 10]. Theoretically, serotonin syndrome can occur as a result of stimulation of any receptor of all seven serotonin receptor families [11]. However, the role of 5-HT_{1A} and 5-HT_{2A} is most often mentioned [6, 7, 11, 12]. Moreover, the 5-HT_{2A} receptor is thought to mediate the most serious consequences of the serotonin syndrome (**Table 1**).

Some authors suggest that the development of serotonin syndrome requires the accumulation of a critical amount of serotonin. However, studies show that this level of serotonin is probably different for each patient. Experimental studies in animal models of serotonin syndrome have shown that other neurotransmitters such as noradrenaline (NA), N-methyl-D-aspartate (NMDA), gamma-aminobutyric acid (GABA) and dopamine may also play a role in the development of serotonin syndrome but their role is not fully understood [6, 13].

It is shown that in serotonin syndrome CNS serotonin levels increase between 40 and 140 times. At the same time, dopamine levels are increased 10 to 44 times [14, 15]. Other studies indicate overactivation of the noradrenergic system with a rise in NA levels up to 15.9 times in serotonin syndrome, but the cause remains unknown. Some authors explain this increase in NA levels with activation of 5-HT2A receptors. This is supported by the fact that no significant increase in NA was observed with prior administration of ritanserin and pipamperone which act as antagonists of these receptors. On the other hand, there is evidence of the involvement of 5-HT1A receptors, although the administration of 5-HT1A antagonists does not prevent the increase in NA levels [14, 15]. The degree of NA increase may

Receptor		Function related to serotonin toxicity
Type	**Subtype**	
5-HT_1	5-HT_{1A}	neuronal inhibition, thermoregulation, hyperactivity associated with anxiety, hypoactivity associated with depression
	5-HT_{1D}	locomotion, muscle tone
5-HT_2	5-HT_{2A}	neuronal excitation, vasoconstriction, platelet aggregation
	5-HT_{2B}	smooth muscle contraction
5-HT_3	—	nausea and vomiting
5-HT_4	—	increased GIT motility

5-HT = 5-hydroxytryptamine (serotonin); GIT = gastrointestinal tract.

Table 1.
Serotonin receptors associated with the serotonin syndrome development [10–12].

be related to the prognosis of serotonin syndrome, although it is not fully understood. At the same time, some of the observed symptoms of autonomic instability may be due to an overactivated noradrenergic system [14].

3. Implicated drugs

Drugs and substances that increase serotonin levels are known as serotonergic, and a mechanism by which they do that are as follows:

- Increased serotonin synthesis
- Increased serotonin release
- Activation of serotonergic receptors
- Serotonin reuptakc inhibition
- Inhibition of serotonin metabolism

The full list of all serotonergic substances is long, but antidepressants and, in recent years, some opioids take the central place. It is important to note that

Mechanism	Implicated drugs
Increased serotonin synthesis	**Dietary supplements:** L-tryptophan
Increased serotonin release	**Illicit substances:** Amphetamines **Opioids:** Tramadol, Oxycodone, Pethidine **Antidepressants:** Mirtazapine **OTC drugs:** Dextromethorphan
Activation of serotonergic receptors	**Antidepressants:** Mirtazapine, Trazodone **Opioids:** Fentanyl, Pethidine **Anxiolytics:** Buspirone **Antimigraines:** Triptans
Serotonin reuptake inhibition	**Antidepressants:** Bupropion, Nefazodone, Trazodone; **SNRIs** (Venlafaxine, Desvenlafaxine, Duloxetine); **SSRIs** (Fluoxetine, Fluvoxamine, Paroxetine, Sertraline, Citalopram, Escitalopram); **TCAs** (Amitriptyline, Nortriptyline, Imipramine, Desipramine, Clomipramine, Amoxapine, Doxepin, Maprotiline, Trimipramine); **Opioids:** Tramadol, Pethidine, Tapentadol, Levomethorphan, Levorphanol, Methadone, Pentazocine, Dextropropoxyphen, Fentanyl, Remifentanyl **OTC drugs:** Dextromethorphan **Antiemetics:** Ondansetron, Granisetron, **Herbal supplements:** *Hypericum perforatum* (St. John's wort)
Inhibition of serotonin metabolism	**MAOIs:** Tranylcypromine, Phenelzine, Isocarboxazid, Nialamid, Iproniazid, Pargyline, Clorgiline, Moclobemide, Toloxatone **Antibiotics:** Linezolid **Dyes:** Methylene blue **Triptans:** Sumatriptan, Rizatriptan,, Zolmitriptan, Almotriptan, Eletriptan, Frovatriptan, Naratriptan **Anxiolytics:** Buspirone **Herbal supplements:** Hypericum perforatum (St. John's wort)

Table 2.
Implicated drugs [5–7, 16–19].

substances with serotonergic activity include not only antidepressants and opioids but also a number of other drugs used in everyday medical practice – some antibiotics, antiemetics, anxiolytics, antipsychotics, as well as over-the-counter drugs (OTC), dietary supplements, some illicit drugs and more [5–7, 16–19].

Some of the antidepressants, opioids, and other drugs reported in the literature causing serotonin syndrome, as well as the mechanisms by which they increase serotonin levels are listed in **Table 2**.

4. Experimental serotonin syndrome

The term "serotonin syndrome" in animals was first used in 1979 by Hwang and Van Woert [20, 21]. Manifestation of serotonin toxicity has been described in various animal species, however, most literature data, respectively most studies, are available on the development of serotonin syndrome in mice and rats [20].

In contrast to humans, in whom the symptoms of serotonin syndrome are well defined, the literature describes a wide variety of manifestations and different combinations of responses characterizing the development of serotonin syndrome in rodents.

There is considerable heterogeneity in the animal models reported in the literature. The use of different assessment methods, different response sets and different scales in assessing the effects of increased serotonergic tone limits quantitative comparisons of laboratory results. In this regard, Haberzettl et al. [20] conducted a systematic literature review of the described models of serotonin syndrome in rats and mice and evaluated the observed behavioral and autonomic manifestations. Based on the frequency of behavioral manifestations, the team divides them into traditional and additional, distinguishing those that reliably characterize the development of serotonin syndrome in rodents. The described behavioral and autonomic symptoms of serotonin syndrome in rats are presented in **Table 3**.

It is widely believed that 5-HT_{1A} receptors mediate most behavioral manifestations of serotonin syndrome in rats [22–31]. In support of this are studies demonstrating the induction of serotonin syndrome behaviors by the administration of 5-HT_{1A} agonists [26, 32, 33] and the induction of a narrower spectrum of manifestations such as hind limb abduction, a Straub phenomenon and low body posture, from the partial 5-HT_{1A}-agonist buspirone [31].

Other behavioral responses such as head weaving and wet dog shake, are mediated by 5-HT_{2A} receptors [22, 34–37]. For example, head weaving in rats induced by the administration of the non-selective MAO inhibitor phenelzine and the SSRI paroxetine was dose-dependently antagonized by 5-HT_2 antagonists [35, 37]. In addition, head weaving caused by the administration of a 5-$HT_{2A/2C}$ agonist has been antagonized by the administration of a 5-HT_{2A} antagonist, but not by a 5-$HT_{2C/2B}$ antagonist [38].

The analysis of Haberzettl et al. showed that the most common autonomic dysregulation manifestation observed in rats with serotonin syndrome is the change in the body temperature. The hyperthermic reaction observed is thought to be mainly related to the activation of 5-HT_{2A} receptors [14, 39]. Experimental studies confirmed the involvement of 5-HT_{1A} and 5-HT_{2A} receptors in thermoregulation in rats. For example, blockade of 5-HT_2 receptors by ketanserin or pirenperone causes a decrease in body temperature, while blockade of 5-HT_{1A} receptors by pindolol results in an increase in body temperature [40].

Although not a mandatory manifestation of serotonin syndrome, hyperthermia is one of the leading causes of observed mortality in experimental serotonin syndrome. In both animals and humans, it is hyperthermia that mainly causes

Behavioral manifestations		Autonomic manifestations
Traditional	**Additional**	
forepaw treading head weaving hind limb abduction low body posture Straub phenomenon tremor backward walking	body twitches chewing head shakes head twitches hyperactivity hyperreactivity locomotor activity (increased or decreased) myoclonus rearing wet dog shake	body temperature (increased or decreased) lower lip retraction penile erection pyloric erection salivation

Table 3.
Serotonin syndrome manifestation in rats.

complications. Such complications in humans could include seizures, rhabdomyolysis, myoglobinuria, metabolic acidosis, renal failure, acute respiratory distress syndrome, respiratory failure, disseminated intravascular coagulation (DIC syndrome), coma and death [6].

The manifestation of serotonin syndrome observed in rodents resembles the manifestation of serotonin syndrome in humans (**Table 4**). For example, neuromuscular manifestations such as tremor and muscle rigidity have been observed in both humans and rodents. Myoclonus, which is a clinical symptom of serotonin syndrome in humans, in rodents may manifest as head twitches and forepaw treading. The Straub phenomenon observed in rodents may refer to the muscle rigidity observed in humans [21]. According to autonomic dysregulation manifestation, changes in body temperature occur in both rodents and humans.

The most difficult to differentiate in animals is the third group of symptoms typical for the manifestation of serotonin syndrome in humans - mental status changes. However, hyperactivity and to some extent the hyperreactivity observed in rodents are associated with agitation observed in humans. Moreover, it is important

Symptoms/manifestations of serotonin syndrome	Humans	Rodents
Neuromuscular disorders	clonus tremor hyperreflexia muscle rigidity myoclonus	head weaving tremor hind limb abduction Straub phenomenon low body posture backward walking
Autonomic dysfunction	diaphoresis hyperthermia (>38 °C) diarrhea shivering	change in body temperature (increase or decrease)
Mental status changes	agitation confusion hyperactivity hypomania anxiety	hyperactivity hyperreactivity

Table 4.
Symptoms and manifestations of serotonin syndrome in humans and rodents – Comparison.

to note that the current criteria for diagnosing serotonin syndrome in humans, Hunter's criteria, do not include as a mandatory diagnostic criterion changes in mental status, which confirms the validity and applicability of the animal model of serotonin syndrome [21].

Two classical models of serotonin syndrome in rats have been described in the literature induced by concomitant administration of serotonergic substances with different mechanisms of action: 5-HTP (100 mg/kg i.p.) - a precursor of serotonin and clorgyline (2 mg/kg i.p.) - selective MAO-A inhibitor [14] and fluoxetine (10 mg/kg i.p.) - a selective serotonin reuptake inhibitor and tranylcypromine (3.5 mg/kg, i.p.) - a non-selective MAO inhibitor [12].

5. Effect of GABA-ergic drugs on experimental models of serotonin syndrome

Many central neurotransmitters, such as serotonin, norepinephrine, dopamine, acetylcholine, GABA and glutamate, are involved in the thermoregulation. GABA is a major central inhibitory neurotransmitter involved in thermoregulatory processes. The role of GABA as a thermoregulatory neurotransmitter or modulator is suggested by the good distribution of the mediator in the hypothalamus, confirmed by autoradiographic and immunohistochemical studies [41–43] and its central action. In addition, GABA-ergic neurons, as well as postsynaptic $GABA_A$-ergic receptors have been identified in PO/AH (preoptic area/anterior hypothalamus) [44–46].

Potentiation of the central inhibitory effect of GABA is achieved by several different mechanisms, including allosteric modulation of GABA receptors (benzodiazepines, barbiturates, Z-hypnotics, propofol and fospropofol), direct GABA- or GABA-receptor agonist action (respectively muscimol, baclofen), increased synthesis of GABA (e.g., gabapentin, pregabalin, sodium valproate), inhibition of enzymatic degradation of GABA (e.g., vigabatrin, sodium valproate) and inhibition of neuronal or glial uptake of GABA (e.g., tiagabine).

Benzodiazepines mediate their pharmacological effects by enhancing the inhibitory effect of GABA on the CNS by binding to a specific modulating site on $GABA_A$-ergic receptors containing 1, 2, 3 or 5 alpha-subunits. Benzodiazepines have no affinity for receptor complexes containing 4 or 6 alpha-subunits [47]. Activation of specific benzodiazepine receptors by diazepam or other benzodiazepines increase the frequency of $GABA_A$-associated chloride channel opening [48].

The pharmacological activity of valproic acid is expressed in potentiation of GABA-ergic neurotransmission and prolongation of the inactivation of voltage-dependent neuronal sodium channels [49]. Sodium valproate is thought to increase brain GABA concentration by the following mechanisms: (1) inhibition of GABA-transaminase enzyme activity and decreased GABA degradation [50] 2) stimulating GAD activity [51] and increasing GABA synthesis; (3) decreased GABA turnover [52]. Vigabatrin (gamma-vinyl GABA) is a vinyl-substituted analogue of GABA that selectively and irreversibly inhibits the activity of the enzyme GABA-transaminase (GABA-T) and significantly increases the concentration of GABA in the brain [53].

After central and systemic administration of diazepam, sodium valproate, and vigabatrin dose-dependent decreases of body temperature in rats is observed [54–57]. GABA-induced hypothermia has been suggested to be mediated by $GABA_A$ and/or $GABA_B$ receptor activation [58, 59]. The hypothermic effect of sodium valproate and vigabatrin occurs later than diazepam-induced hypothermia, which can be explained by their indirect mechanism of potentiation of GABA-ergic mediation.

These results are further confirmed in our studies, where we found that substances with a GABA-ergic mechanism of action such as diazepam, sodium valproate and vigabatrin effectively reduced the hyperthermic response in experimental serotonin syndrome in rats induced by concomitant administration of 5-HTP (100 mg/kg i.p.) - a precursor of serotonin and clorgyline (2 mg/kg i.p.) - selective MAO-A inhibitor [14]. The reduction in serotonergic-induced hyperthermia with pretreatment of GABA-mimetic drugs is most likely due to an increase in central GABA-ergic neurotransmission through activation of $GABA_A$ receptors (e.g., diazepam) as well as through indirect action by increasing GABA concentration (e.g., sodium valproate, vigabatrin). These results on the hyperthermia associated with serotonin syndrome support the hypothesis of an interaction between the GABA-ergic and serotonincrgic systems in thermoregulatory processes.

In our studies, after the concomitant administration of 5-HTP (100 mg/kg i.p.) and clorgyline (2 mg/kg i.p.), a model of serotonin syndrome with typical behavioral and autonomic manifestations developed. Tremor occurs 10 minutes after injection, the hyperthermic reaction develops at 30 minutes, and the maximum value is observed 60 minutes after injection of the substances. All animals in this group died between 60 and 90 minutes after injection of serotonin. Pretreatment with diazepam at a dose of 5 mg/kg i.p. reduced the hyperthermic reaction at 30 and 60 min compared to the group with a model of serotonin syndrome, in which saline was administered prior to the injection of serotonergic agent. Administration of sodium valproate at a dose of 300 mg/kg i.p. reduced the hyperthermic reaction at 30 and 60 min compared to the group with a model of serotonin syndrome, in which saline was administered before the injection of serotonergic substances [56, 60]. Additionally, in another of our experiments, we used a modified model of serotonin syndrome induced by the concomitant administration of fluoxetine (10 mg/kg i.p.) - a selective serotonin reuptake inhibitor and clorgyline (2 mg/kg i.p.) - selective MAO-A inhibitor. Vigabatrin at a dose of 300 mg/kg i.p. significantly decreased the hyperthermic response between 150 and 300 min in rats with a serotonin syndrome model, compared to the group with a model of serotonin syndrome in which only saline was administered before the injection of the serotonergic substances [57, 61].

In summary pretreatment with diazepam (5 mg/kg i.p.), sodium valproate (300 mg/kg i.p.), and vigabatrin (300 mg/kg i.p.) decreased hyperthermia in different experimental models of the serotonin syndrome. These results suggest involvement of interactions between GABA-ergic and serotonergic systems in the processes of thermoregulation.

We assume that in addition to direct GABA-ergic mechanisms, interactions between neurotransmitters or mediator systems are involved in the influence of hyperthermia in serotonin syndrome by GABA-ergic substances. Presynaptic $GABA_B$ receptors affect the release of norepinephrine, dopamine, and 5-hydroxytryptamine [62]. Expression of predominantly $GABA_B$ receptors has been found in most of the serotonin and catecholamine neurons in the nuclei of the brainstem, which are involved in the regulation of autonomic functions [63]. Interactions between the GABA-ergic and serotonergic systems are mediated by presynaptic heteroreceptor $GABA_B$-inhibition of 5-HT release or by G-protein-coupled interaction between $5\text{-}HT_{1A}$ and $GABA_B$-ergic receptors [64].

6. Effect of 5-HT$_2$-antagonists on experimental models of serotonin syndrome

Hyperthermia is the most common cause of complications of life-threatening forms of serotonin syndrome in humans and is one of the leading causes of mortality reported in experimental models of serotonin syndrome [6, 7].

As already mentioned, several studies indicate the role of 5-HT_{2A} receptors in the development of a hyperthermic response in rats. In this regard, the effect of a number of 5-HT_2 antagonists in influencing the hyperthermic response in experimental serotonin syndrome has been studied. Some of the serotonin antagonists investigated are cyproheptadine, ritanserin, ketanserin, mirtazapine, some antipsychotics such as chlorpromazine, risperidone and olanzapine [8, 11–15]. Results demonstrate a significant involvement of the 5-HT_{2A} receptors in the development of hyperthermic response in experimental serotonin syndrome [65].

Studies have shown that cyproheptadine effectively affects the hyperthermic response in an experimental model of serotonin syndrome. Moreover, a comparative study demonstrates that, unlike other 5-HT_2 antagonists, it prevents both the development of serotonin syndrome and the mortality of experimental animals [14, 66].

The role of atypical antipsychotics in the treatment of serotonin syndrome has been increasingly discussed in the last few years, given that most atypical antipsychotics work primarily by blocking 5-HT_2 receptors [67].

Moreover, temperature dysregulation is a documented side effect of antipsychotic drugs [68–72]. That most often manifests in the development of hyperthermia, a life-threatening symptom characteristic of the malignant neuroleptic syndrome (MNS). Data from various clinical cases, summarized in recent years by van Marum [68] and Zonnenberg [69, 70], show that the use of classical or atypical antipsychotics carries the risk of developing another, less well-documented adverse drug reaction, namely hypothermia. In humans, hypothermia is defined as a body temperature below 35 ° C, distinguishing three degrees: mild (33–35 ° C), moderate (28–33 ° C) and severe (<28 ° C) hypothermia [69].

Although the hypothermic effect of antipsychotics is less known than the hyperthermic one expressed in MNS, analysis of the literature data shows that there are almost equal reports of hypothermia (480 cases) and hyperthermia (524 cases) associated with the use of antipsychotics. Zonnenberg et al. consider that the actual incidence of hypothermia associated with the use of antipsychotics is at least 10 times higher than the documented [69]. For the first time, the development of hypothermia after the use of antipsychotic drugs was described by Loughnane in a 26-year-old patient on chlorpromazine therapy [73].

The analyzes of van Marum et al. and Zonnenberg et al. indicate that hypothermia most often occurs one week after starting antipsychotic therapy or after increasing the dose. They also indicated that the use of atypical antipsychotics was more common (approximately 55% of cases), with risperidone being the most commonly reported [68, 69, 74]. Mild hypothermia associated with low-dose risperidone has also been observed in a child with verbal and physically aggressive behavior [75].

Analyzes by van Marum and Zonnenberg show that antipsychotics with a higher affinity for blocking 5-HT2A than D2 receptors are more often associated with the development of hypothermia [68, 69]. This is also confirmed by experimental and clinical studies which demonstrate that the atypical antipsychotics olanzapine and risperidone cause a decrease in body temperature indicating that the mechanism of hypothermic action is associated with blockade of 5-HT_2 receptors [72, 74–76].

7. Conclusion

From all data reported thus far, it can be concluded that 5-HT_2 receptors and the GABA system are strongly involved in the development of hyperthermia in serotonin syndrome and the mortality associated with it.

DOI: http://dx.doi.org/10.5772/intechopen.96362

Drug-induced hyperthermia is resistant to the action of classical antipyretics therefore their use is not recommended. The use of acetylsalicylic acid and other classical antipyretics not only has no effect in the case of drug-induced hyperthermia but may even cause a worsening of the course of the hyperthermic reaction. In our opinion, due to the proven hypothermic effect of the mentioned GABA-ergic drugs and 5-HT_2-antagonists, their use in the therapeutic regimen of hyperthermia in specific hyperthermic syndromes is appropriate.

The similarity in the manifestation of the syndrome in rats and humans can serve as a basis for further elucidation of the mechanism of development of serotonin syndrome in humans. The animal model of serotonin syndrome can be used to study drugs and drug combinations that pose a potential risk of developing serotonin syndrome in humans and the possibilities for its prevention.

Author details

Rumen Nikolov* and Kalina Koleva
Department of Pharmacology and Toxicology, Medical Faculty, Medical University, Sofia

*Address all correspondence to: rnikolov@medfac.mu-sofia.bg

References

[1] Oates, J. A., & Sjoerdsma, A. (1960). Neurologic effects of tryptophan in patients receiving a monoamine oxidase inhibitor. Neurology, 10, 1076-1078.

[2] Abadie, D., Rousseau, V., Logerot, S., Cottin, J., Montastruc, J. L., & Montastruc, F. (2015). Serotonin Syndrome: Analysis of Cases Registered in the French Pharmacovigilance Database. Journal of clinical psychopharmacology, 35(4), 382-388.

[3] Arora, B., & Kannikeswaran, N. (2010). The serotonin syndrome-the need for physician's awareness. International journal of emergency medicine, 3(4), 373-377.

[4] Werneke, U., Jamshidi, F., Taylor, D. M., & Ott, M. (2016). Conundrums in neurology: diagnosing serotonin syndrome - a meta-analysis of cases. BMC neurology, 16, 97.

[5] Watson, W. A., Litovitz, T. L., Klein-Schwartz, W., Rodgers, G. C., Jr, Youniss, J., Reid, N., Rouse, W. G., Rembert, R. S., & Borys, D. (2004). 2003 annual report of the American Association of Poison Control Centers Toxic Exposure Surveillance System. The American journal of emergency medicine, 22(5), 335-404.

[6] Volpi-Abadie, J., Kaye, A. M., & Kaye, A. D. (2013). Serotonin syndrome. The Ochsner journal, 13(4), 533-540.

[7] Boyer, E. W., & Shannon, M. (2005). The serotonin syndrome. The New England journal of medicine, 352(11), 1112-1120.

[8] Ables, Adrienne & Nagubilli, Raju. (2010). Prevention, Diagnosis, and Management of Serotonin Syndrome. American family physician. 81. 1139-42.

[9] Francescangeli, J., Karamchandani, K., Powell, M., & Bonavia, A. (2019). The Serotonin Syndrome: From Molecular Mechanisms to Clinical Practice. International journal of molecular sciences, 20(9), 2288.

[10] Scotton, W. J., Hill, L. J., Williams, A. C., & Barnes, N. M. (2019). Serotonin Syndrome: Pathophysiology, Clinical Features, Management, and Potential Future Directions. International journal of tryptophan research: IJTR, 12, 1178646919873925.

[11] Racz, R., Soldatos, T. G., Jackson, D., & Burkhart, K. (2018). Association Between Serotonin Syndrome and Second-Generation Antipsychotics via Pharmacological Target-Adverse Event Analysis. Clinical and translational science, 11(3), 322-329.

[12] Sun-Edelstein, C., Tepper, S. J., & Shapiro, R. E. (2008). Drug-induced serotonin syndrome: a review. Expert opinion on drug safety, 7(5), 587-596.

[13] Nisijima, K., Shioda, K., Yoshino, T., Takano, K., & Kato, S. (2004). Memantine, an NMDA antagonist, prevents the development of hyperthermia in an animal model for serotonin syndrome. Pharmacopsychiatry, 37(2), 57-62.

[14] Nisijima, K., Yoshino, T., Yui, K., & Katoh, S. (2001). Potent serotonin (5-HT)(2A) receptor antagonists completely prevent the development of hyperthermia in an animal model of the 5-HT syndrome. Brain research, 890(1), 23-31.

[15] Sleight, A. J., Marsden, C. A., Martin, K. F., & Palfreyman, M. G. (1988). Relationship between extracellular 5-hydroxytryptamine and behaviour following monoamine

oxidase inhibition and L-tryptophan. British journal of pharmacology, 93(2), 303-310.

[16] Bronstein, A. C., Spyker, D. A., Cantilena, L. R., Jr, Rumack, B. H., & Dart, R. C. (2012). 2011 Annual report of the American Association of Poison Control Centers' National Poison Data System (NPDS): 29th Annual Report. Clinical toxicology (Philadelphia, Pa.), 50(10), 911-1164.

[17] Logan, B. K., Mohr, A. L. A., Friscia, M., Krotulski, A. J., Papsun, D. M., Kacinko, S. L., Ropero-Miller, J. D., & Huestis, M. A. (2017). Reports of adverse events associated with use of novel psychoactive substances, 2013-2016: A review. Journal of Analytical Toxicology, 41(7), 573-610.

[18] Fleckenstein AE, Volz TJ, Riddle EL, Gibb JW, Hanson GR. (2007) New insights into the mechanism of action of amphetamines. Annual Review of Pharmacology and Toxicology; 47, 681-698.

[19] Hassan, Z., Bosch, O. G., Singh, D., Narayanan, S., Kasinather, B. V., Seifritz, E., Kornhuber, J., Quednow, B. B., & Müller, C. P. (2017). Novel Psychoactive Substances-Recent Progress on Neuropharmacological Mechanisms of Action for Selected Drugs. Frontiers in psychiatry, 8, 152.

[20] Haberzettl, R., Bert, B., Fink, H., & Fox, M. A. (2013). Animal models of the serotonin syndrome: a systematic review. Behavioural brain research, 256, 328-345.

[21] Hwang, E. C., & Van Woert, M. H. (1979). Behavioral and biochemical actions of p-chlorophenylethylamine (p-CPEA) in mice. Life sciences, 24(7), 595-601.

[22] Isbister, G. K., & Buckley, N. A. (2005). The pathophysiology of serotonin toxicity in animals and humans: implications for diagnosis and treatment. Clinical neuropharmacology, 28(5), 205-214.

[23] Lucki, I., Nobler, M. S., & Frazer, A. (1984). Differential actions of serotonin antagonists on two behavioral models of serotonin receptor activation in the rat. The Journal of pharmacology and experimental therapeutics, 228(1), 133-139.

[24] Zhang, G., Krishnamoorthy, S., Ma, Z., Vukovich, N. P., Huang, X., & Tao, R. (2009). Assessment of 5-hydroxytryptamine efflux in rat brain during a mild, moderate and severe serotonin-toxicity syndrome. European journal of pharmacology, 615 (1-3), 66-75.

[25] Goodwin, G. M., De Souza, R. J., Wood, A. J., & Green, A. R. (1986). The enhancement by lithium of the 5-HT1A mediated serotonin syndrome produced by 8-OH-DPAT in the rat: evidence for a post-synaptic mechanism. Psychopharmacology, 90(4), 488-493.

[26] Goodwin, G. M., & Green, A. R. (1985). A behavioural and biochemical study in mice and rats of putative selective agonists and antagonists for 5-HT1 and 5-HT2 receptors. British journal of pharmacology, 84(3), 743-753.

[27] Goodwin, G. M., De Souza, R. J., Green, A. R., & Heal, D. J. (1987). The pharmacology of the behavioural and hypothermic responses of rats to 8-hydroxy-2-(di-n-propylamino) tetralin (8-OH-DPAT). Psychopharmacology, 91(4), 506-511.

[28] Green, A. R., Guy, A. P., & Gardner, C. R. (1984). The behavioural effects of RU 24969, a suggested 5-HT1 receptor agonist in rodents and the effect on the behaviour of treatment with antidepressants. Neuropharmacology, 23(6), 655-661.

[29] Lu, J. Q., & Nagayama, H. (1996). Circadian rhythm in the response of central 5-HT1A receptors to 8-OH-DPAT in rats. Psychopharmacology, 123(1), 42-45.

[30] Lu, J. Q., & Nagayama, H. (1997). Circadian rhythm in the function of central 5-HT1A receptors is endogenous in nature. Cellular and molecular life sciences: CMLS, 53(3), 224-226.

[31] Smith, L. M., & Peroutka, S. J. (1986). Differential effects of 5-hydroxytryptamine1a selective drugs on the 5-HT behavioral syndrome. Pharmacology, biochemistry, and behavior, 24(6), 1513-1519.

[32] Assié, M. B., Bardin, L., Auclair, A. L., Carilla-Durand, E., Depoortère, R., Koek, W., et al. (2010). F15599, a highly selective post-synaptic 5-HT(1A) receptor agonist: in-vivo profile in behavioural models of antidepressant and serotonergic activity. The international journal of neuropsychopharmacology, 13(10), 1285-1298.

[33] Forster, E. A., Cliffe, I. A., Bill, D. J., Dover, G. M., Jones, D., Reilly, Y., & Fletcher, A. (1995). A pharmacological profile of the selective silent 5-HT1A receptor antagonist, WAY-100635. European journal of pharmacology, 281(1), 81-88.

[34] Peroutka, S. J., Lebovitz, R. M., & Snyder, S. H. (1981). Two distinct central serotonin receptors with different physiological functions. Science (New York, N.Y.), 212(4496), 827-829.

[35] Yap, C. Y., & Taylor, D. A. (1983). Involvement of 5-HT2 receptors in the wet-dog shake behaviour induced by 5-hydroxytryptophan in the rat. Neuropharmacology, 22(7), 801-804.

[36] Roth BL, Hyde EG. (1997) Pharmacology of 5-HT2 receptors. In: Baumgarten HGGM, editor. Handbook of experimental pharmacology, serotonergic neurons and 5-HT receptors in the CNS. Berlin, Heidelberg, New York: Springer; p.367-94.

[37] Koshikawa, F., Koshikawa, N., & Stephenson, J. D. (1985). Effects of antidepressant drug combinations on cortical 5-HT2 receptors and wet-dog shakes in rats. European journal of pharmacology, 118(3), 273-281.

[38] Willins, D. L., & Meltzer, H. Y. (1997). Direct injection of 5-HT2A receptor agonists into the medial prefrontal cortex produces a head-twitch response in rats. The Journal of pharmacology and experimental therapeutics, 282(2), 699-706.

[39] K. M., Hill, J. L., & Murphy, D. L. (1995). Evidence that 1-(2,5-dimethoxy-4-iodophenyl)-2-aminopropane (DOI)-induced hyperthermia in rats is mediated by stimulation of 5-HT2A receptors. Psychopharmacology, 117(2), 193-199.

[40] Gudelsky, G. A., Koenig, J. I., & Meltzer, H. Y. (1986). Thermoregulatory responses to serotonin (5-HT) receptor stimulation in the rat. Evidence for opposing roles of 5-HT2 and 5-HT1A receptors. Neuropharmacology, 25(12), 1307-1313.

[41] Palacios, J. M., Wamsley, J. K., & Kuhar, M. J. (1981). High affinity GABA receptors-autoradiographic localization. Brain research, 222(2), 285-307.

[42] Vincent, S. R., Hökfelt, T., & Wu, J. Y. (1982). GABA neuron systems in hypothalamus and the pituitary gland. Immunohistochemical demonstration using antibodies against glutamate decarboxylase. Neuroendocrinology, 34(2), 117-125.

[43] Decavel, C., & Van den Pol, A. N. (1990). GABA: a dominant

neurotransmitter in the hypothalamus. The Journal of comparative neurology, 302(4), 1019-1037.

[44] Yasumatsu, M., Yazawa, T., Otokawa, M., Kuwasawa, K., Hasegawa, H., & Aihara, Y. (1998). Monoamines, amino acids and acetylcholine in the preoptic area and anterior hypothalamus of rats: measurements of tissue extracts and in vivo microdialysates. Comparative biochemistry and physiology. Part A, Molecular & integrative physiology, 121(1), 13-23.

[45] Herbison, A. E., Heavens, R. P., & Dyer, R. G. (1990). Endogenous release of gamma-aminobutyric acid from the medial preoptic area measured by microdialysis in the anaesthetised rat. Journal of neurochemistry, 55(5), 1617-1623.

[46] Fénelon, V. S., & Herbison, A. E. (1996). In vivo regulation of specific GABAA receptor subunit messenger RNAs by increased GABA concentrations in rat brain. Neuroscience, 71(3), 661-670.

[47] Möhler, H., Fritschy, J. M., & Rudolph, U. (2002). A new benzodiazepine pharmacology. The Journal of pharmacology and experimental therapeutics, 300(1), 2-8.

[48] Twyman, R. E., Rogers, C. J., & Macdonald, R. L. (1989). Differential regulation of gamma-aminobutyric acid receptor channels by diazepam and phenobarbital. Annals of neurology, 25(3), 213-220.

[49] McNamara, J.O. Pharmacotherapy of the epilepsies. (2006) In: Hardmann, J.G., Limbrid, L.E., Gilman, A.G., editors. Godmann and Gilman's the pharmacological basis of therapeutics. New York: McGraw-Hill.

[50] Löscher W. (1999). Valproate: a reappraisal of its pharmacodynamic properties and mechanisms of action. Progress in neurobiology, 58(1), 31-59.

[51] Bolaños, J. P., & Medina, J. M. (1993). Evidence of stimulation of the gamma-aminobutyric acid shunt by valproate and E-delta 2-valproate in neonatal rat brain. Molecular pharmacology, 43(3), 487-490.

[52] Owens, M. J., & Nemeroff, C. B. (2003). Pharmacology of valproate. Psychopharmacology bulletin, 37 Suppl 2, 17-24.

[53] Angehagen, M., Ben-Menachem, E., Rönnbäck, L., & Hansson, E. (2003). Novel mechanisms of action of three antiepileptic drugs, vigabatrin, tiagabine, and topiramate. Neurochemical research, 28(2), 333-340.

[54] Zarrindast, M. R., & Dibayan, M. (1989). Involvement of GABAA receptor sites in diazepam hypothermia. General pharmacology, 20(6), 855-859.

[55] Swiader, M. J., Luszczki, J. J., Zwolan, A., Wierzchowska-Cioch, E., Wielosz, M., & Czuczwar, S. J. (2004). Is a hypothermic effect of LY300164, valproate and phenobarbital evident in mice?. Roczniki Akademii Medycznej w Bialymstoku (1995), 49, 270-274.

[56] Nikolov R, Yakimova K. (2008). Effects of GABA-acting drugs diazepam and sodium valproate on thermoregulation in rats. Journal of Thermal Biology, 33(8): 459-463.

[57] Nikolov, R. P., & Yakimova, K. S. (2011). Effects of GABA-transaminase inhibitor Vigabatrin on thermoregulation in rats. Amino acids, 40(5), 1441-1445

[58] Zarrindast, M. R., & Oveissi, Y. (1988). GABAA and GABAB receptor sites involvement in rat thermoregulation. General pharmacology, 19(2), 223-226.

[59] Rawls SM, Tallarida RJ, Kon DA et al. (2004). GABAA-receptors modulate cannabinoid evoked hypothermia. Pharmacology Biochemistry and Behavior, 78 (1): 83-91.

[60] Nikolov, R. (2014). Effects of sodium valproate on the hyperthermic reaction in experimental serotonin syndrome. Meditsinski pregled, 50, № 2, 45-48.

[61] Nikolov, R.P., K.N. Koleva, M.H. Hristov, K.S. Yakimova. (2020). Hyperthermia in experimental models of serotonin syndrome: influence of vigabatrin. Bulgarian chemical comminications, 52(1), 138-141.

[62] Clark, W. G., & Lipton, J. M. (1985). Changes in body temperature after administration of amino acids, peptides, dopamine, neuroleptics and related agents: II. Neuroscience and biobehavioral reviews, 9(2), 299-371.

[63] Burman, K. J., Ige, A. O., White, J. H., Marshall, F. H., Pangalos, M. N., Emson, P. C., Minson, J. B., & Llewellyn-Smith, I. J. (2003). GABAB receptor subunits, R1 and R2, in brainstem catecholamine and serotonin neurons. Brain research, 970(1-2), 35-46.

[64] Mannoury la Cour, C., Hanoun, N., Melfort, M., Hen, R., Lesch, K. P., Hamon, M., & Lanfumey, L. (2004). GABA(B) receptors in 5-HT transporter- and 5-HT1A receptor-knock-out mice: further evidence of a transduction pathway shared with 5-HT1A receptors. Journal of neurochemistry, 89(4), 886-896.

[65] Porcelli, S., Drago, A., Fabbri, C., Gibiino, S., Calati, R., & Serretti, A. (2011). Pharmacogenetics of antidepressant response. Journal of psychiatry & neuroscience: JPN, 36(2), 87-113.

[66] Gillman P. K. (1999). The serotonin syndrome and its treatment. Journal of psychopharmacology (Oxford, England), 13(1), 100-109.

[67] Kasper, S., Praschak-Rieder, N., Tauscher, J., & Wolf, R. (1997). A risk-benefit assessment of mirtazapine in the treatment of depression. Drug safety, 17(4), 251-264.

[68] van Marum, R. J., Wegewijs, M. A., Loonen, A. J., & Beers, E. (2007). Hypothermia following antipsychotic drug use. European journal of clinical pharmacology, 63(6), 627-631.

[69] Zonnenberg, C., Bueno-de-Mesquita, J. M., Ramlal, D., & Blom, J. D. (2017). Hypothermia due to Antipsychotic Medication: A Systematic Review. Frontiers in psychiatry, 8, 165.

[70] Zonnenberg, C., Bueno-de-Mesquita, J. M., Ramlal, D., & Blom, J. D. (2019). Antipsychotic-Related Hypothermia: Five New Cases. Frontiers in psychiatry, 10, 543.

[71] Ajayi, O. O., & Holroyd, S. (2017). Severe recurrent hypothermia in an elderly patient with refractory mania associated with atypical antipsychotic, valproic acid and oxcarbazepine therapy. BMJ case reports, 2017, bcr2017222462.

[72] Oerther, S., & Ahlenius, S. (2000). Atypical antipsychotics and dopamine D(1) receptor agonism: an in vivo experimental study using core temperature measurements in the rat. The Journal of pharmacology and experimental therapeutics, 292(2), 731-736.

[73] Loughnane T. (1968). Hypothermia in a young adult. Lancet (London, England), 2(7565), 455-456.

[74] Razaq, M., & Samma, M. (2004). A case of risperidone-induced

hypothermia. American journal of therapeutics, 11(3), 229-230.

[75] Grau, K., Plener, P. L., Gahr, M., Denzer, C., & Freudenmann, R. W. (2017). Mild Hypothermia in a Child with Low-Dose Risperidone. Zeitschrift fur Kinder- und Jugendpsychiatrie und Psychotherapie, 45(4), 335-337.

[76] Rasnayake, L. R., Wimalarathne, H., Jayapala, R. K., Gamage, C. D., Dassanayake, D. L., Ratnayake et al. (2011). An unusual case of hypothermia associated with therapeutic doses of olanzapine: a case report. Journal of medical case reports, 5, 189.

Chapter 7

Role of 5-HT in Cerebral Edema after Traumatic Brain Injury

Priya Badyal, Jaspreet Kaur and Anurag Kuhad

Abstract

The pathogenesis of edema after traumatic brain injury is complex including the destruction of micro-vessels and alterations in microcirculation around the primary injury and leakage of plasma constituents into the tissue, due to permeability changes of the vessel walls. Many functional molecules like histamine, serotonin, arachidonic acid, prostaglandins and thromboxane have been shown to induce blood–brain barrier (BBB) disruption or cell swelling. It is believed that released 5-HT binds to 5-HT_2 receptors stimulating cAMP and prostaglandins in vessels that cause more vesicular transport in endothelial cells leading to serum component's extravasation. The additional amount of serotonin into the tissue due to injury maintains the state of increased vascular permeability that ultimately causes edema. Serotonin is clearly involved in early cytotoxic edema after TBI. Reduction of serotonin in the nervous tissue reduces swelling and the milder cell changes in the brain or spinal cord of traumatized rats. Inhibition of serotonin synthesis before closed head injury (CHI) in rat models or administration of serotonin antiserum after injury attenuates BBB disruption and brain edema volume swelling, and brain pathology. Maintaining low serotonin levels immediately after injury may show neuroprotection and combat various secondary outcomes that occur after traumatic brain injury.

Keywords: TBI, 5-HT (5-Hydroxytryptamine), cerebral edema, BBB permeability, brain damage, neuroprotection

1. Introduction

Traumatic brain injury (TBI), the principal cause of morbidity and mortality is a serious medical problem in people under 40 years of age. As a major cause of death, it is a major worldwide concern and due to lifetime disability it also puts a huge burden on society [1]. Despite the scale of this public health crisis, no effective TBI therapies currently exist [2]. The hope for effective treatment is derived from the fact that much of the post-traumatic damage to the injured brain is caused by a secondary injury cascade of consecutive pathophysiological events, including opening of the blood–brain barrier (BBB), formation of edema, excitotoxicity, inflammatory response activation, oxidative stress and ultimately cell death, which exacerbates the primary injury [3]. While a variety of factors lead to elevated TBI-related mortality and morbidity, the occurrence of cerebral edema with brain swelling remains the most important outcome that contributes to morbidity and mortality [4]. In the first week after traumatic brain injury, considering the prevalence of cytotoxic (or cellular) edema, brain swelling can only occur with the addition of water from the vasculature to the cranial vault. As such, blood–brain barrier permeability control has been a subject of recent research that aims to treat brain edema [4]. Many functional molecules like histamine, serotonin, arachidonic acid, prostaglandins and thromboxane have been shown to induce BBB disruption or cell swelling. It is believed that released 5-HT binds to 5-HT_2 receptors stimulating cAMP and prostaglandins in vessels that cause more vesicular transport in endothelial cells and also leading to serum components extravasation [5].

It is well known that serotonin (5-hydroxytryptamine, 5-HT) is involved in emotional disorders, such as depression and schizophrenia [6]. 5-HT has a role in cerebral edema after TBI [7]. Serotonin has been reported to increase nitrogenoxide (NO) tissue levels, and NO contributes to inflammation by increasing vascular permeability, which leads to edema formation [8, 9]. Activation of the 5-HT_{2B} receptor induces endothelium-dependent NO release [10]. Increased calcium levels in endothelium lead to NO formation through the eNOS pathway, followed by a cGMP-dependent mechanism to increase vascular permeability [11]. Therefore, it seems likely that 5-HT may play a significant role in edema after traumatic insults to the brain. Therefore, in the present chapter the role of endogenous 5-HT in BBB breakdown and in edema formation is discussed as a pharmacological approach to alleviate cerebral edema after TBI.

2. Pathophysiology of cerebral edema

After brain injury, secondary complications like cerebral edema are a pressing medical problem and can increase mortality to nearly 80% if severe [12]. Cerebral edema and brain swelling are estimated to account for up to 50% of patient mortality following traumatic brain injury [4]. Cerebral edema is now understood to develop in stages, where each stage is marked by distinct morphological and molecular changes [13]. Minutes after acute central nervous system (CNS) injury, cytotoxic edema or cellular swelling manifests itself. After cytotoxic edema, ionic edema, an extracellular edema that arises in the presence of an intact blood brain barrier (BBB), forms immediately. Hours after the initial insult, vasogenic edema, an extracellular edema which involves extravasation of plasma proteins manifested [13]. Neurons are considered as fragile cells and cannot survive without support from other cell types. So, in addition to provide neuroprotection, a new aim for acute brain injury research is to investigate and attenuate mechanisms of endothelial, astrocytic, and microglial dysfunction and, thereby, create an environment permissible to neuronal survival. It follows that cerebral edema, a phenomenon arising from astrocyte and endothelium dysfunction, is an important subject for fundamental research and therapeutic intervention [13].

The term BBB refers to an organization of different cell types that separates the luminal contents of the cerebral vasculature from the brain interstitium. Brain ISF, which interacts openly with cerebrospinal fluid (CSF), is designed for neuronal activity and differs from blood serum because it includes higher levels of Cl^- and Mg^{2+} and lower concentrations of K^+, Ca^{2+} and HCO^{3-} [14]. The Virchow Robin space and the astrocyte endfeet that are part of BBB are recognised as important anatomical components of the so-called "cerebral glymphatic system" [15]. This system is designed to account for CSF movements observed in the healthy brain that can operate from the parenchyma to clear solutes such as amyloid beta and promote the transport of tiny lipophilic molecules, particularly during sleep [15–17].

A pathological rise in the water mass contained by the interstitial space of the brain is cerebral edema. Cytotoxic edema is swelling of oncotic cells, resulting in fluid accumulation intracellular rather than extracellular and is best considered as a precursor to extracellular ionic edema. A mass effect that exerts pressure on the surrounding shell of tissue is caused by brain swelling. The rigid enclosure of the skull magnifies this pressure rise, which puts an upper limit on the volume to which the brain can expand. It exerts mechanical forces on the skull interior as the brain swells, thereby increasing intracranial tissue pressure. Capillary lumens collapse as tissue pressure reaches capillary pressure, precipitating a feed forward phase in which the surrounding shell ischemia induces more edema development and further swelling in the next shell [18].

Two key theories exist about the immediate source of the new water mass required for brain swelling. In one theory, water, driven by osmotic forces, travels from the capillary lumen into the parenchyma and is transmitted through capillary endothelial cells. In support of the first theory, local blood perfusion status is closely correlated with the formation of ionic edema [19]. Magnetic resonance imaging (MRI) reveals that edema is first observed in regions of peri-infarction that are actively perfused in human stroke [20]. However, acceptance of this theory is not universal, as there are doubts about the levels of expression of widely cited molecular mechanisms for influx of ions and water via endothelium in the brain [21]. A recent explanation of the glymphatic system has led to the formulation of a second theory, in which CSF is the immediate source of water and ions. In this theory, swelling occurs when the influx of CSF into the parenchyma is increased and/or interstitial fluid (ISF)efflux is impaired, a condition that precipitates the parenchymatic relative accumulation of ISF [21]. The two theories do not account well for the formation of vasogenic edema.

Cytotoxic edema is a premorbid cellular process also known as cellular edema, whereby extracellular Na^+ and other cations enter into neurons and astrocytes and accumulate intracellularly due to failure of energy-dependent mechanisms of extrusion. This process takes place following CNS injury in all CNS cell types, but is especially prevalent in astrocytes. Astrocyte swelling tends to be a response of astrocytes to injury and occurs rapidly following a number of forms of CNS injury, including ischemia, trauma, hypoglycemia, epileptic status, and fulminant hepatic failure [14]. In the development of cerebral edema and swelling, cytotoxic edema is an important initial stage, as it generates the driving force for the influx of ionic and vasogenic edema, which induces swelling. As a consequence of primary active transport or secondary active transport, osmolite cellular influx may occur. A continuous supply of adenosine triphosphate (ATP) is needed for primary active transport to provide energy for "pumps" such as the Na^+/K^+-ATPase and Ca^{2+}ATPase [13]. Secondary active transport utilises the potential energy stored in transmembrane ionic gradients that was previously generated through primary active transport. Secondary active transporters include ion channels and cotransporters such as the $Na^+/K^+/Cl^-$ co-transporter (NKCC) [1, 22] and the Na^+/Ca^{2+} exchanger. After many types of CNS injury, intracellular ATP becomes depleted and due to that mechanism independent of intracellular ATP, like secondary active transport, are more likely to be involved in the formation of ionic edema [13]. NKCC1 is constitutively expressed by astrocytes in all region of the adult brain [22–24]. In vitro experiments using cultured primary astrocytes is shown that NKCC1 leads to cell swelling in conditions of high extracellular potassium [25, 26]. In vivo, swelling is decreased by the NKCC1 inhibitor bumetanide after trauma and ischemia [27–29].

Acute CNS injury activates a program of molecular changes in the neurovascular unit before and after transcription that leads to the development of endothelial "permeability pores" and subsequent loss of BBB integrity. Based on the key substances undergoing transcapillary motion, progressive endothelial dysfunction can be organised into three stages, i.e. ionic edema, vasogenic edema, and hemorrhagic conversion [13].

Vasogenic edema is a type of extracellular edema characterized by BBB breakdown, in which a pore of transendothelial permeability develops that allows the interstitial brain compartment to extravasation of water and plasma proteins such as albumin and IgG. Capillary structural integrity, unlike hemorrhage, is maintained during vasogenic edema in such a way that erythrocyte passage is prevented [30]. It is thought that the three phases of endothelial dysregulation occur sequentially, although the speed of change between phases possibly depends on the form and severity of injury. In addition, since many etiologies of brain endothelial dysregulation and cerebral edema are focal in nature, brain tissue typically displays a complex spatiotemporal pattern of the various stages of endothelial dysregulation. Significant gaps still remain in our understanding of how specific proteins contribute to cerebral edema [13].

3. Serotonergic role in development of cerebral edema

In many brain disorders, edema is a severe complication, including traumatic injury. Traumatic brain edema pathogenesis is complex and involves physical disruption of microvessels, microcirculatory changes in and around the primary injury, and changes in the permeability of the vessel walls that contribute to plasma constituents leaking into the tissue [31]. There are reasons to assume that many of these events are caused by a variety of chemical mediators, such as biogenic amines, arachidonic acid, leucotrienes, histamine and free radicals, that are released or activated in and around the primary lesion [32]. However, the role of serotonin (5-hydroxytryptamine, 5-HT) is not well understood in traumatic brain edema. In multiple neurological disorders and in pathological conditions, several lines of recent evidence suggest a presumptive function of this amine [7]. Major changes in the synthesis of serotonin occur in important brain injuries such as stroke, ischemia and trauma, as well as in experimental cold injury lesions and other neurological diseases [7]. Increased serotonin content occurs after traumatic brain insults in the walls of the cerebral vessels, cerebrospinal fluid and brain [5]. In a wide range of psychiatric disorders and mental disturbances, irregular serotonin levels in the blood and brain have been identified [33]. In cerebral vessels, serotonergic receptors are present and intracarotid, intravenous or intracerebroventricular serotonin infusion substantially affects the cerebral circulation and metabolism as well as increasing the permeability of the blood–brain barrier (BBB) [7, 32, 34]. Therefore, various studies were conducted to examine the function of endogenous 5-HT in BBB breakdown, edema formation and early cellular changes in experimental models of traumatic brain injury. Therefore, it seems probable that 5-HT could play an important role in edema formation and cellular changes following traumatic insults to the brain.

Studies show that endogenous depletion of 5-HT before acute insult to the brain substantially thwarts the production of edema and early cellular changes, suggesting that this amine plays an important role in the pathophysiology of traumatic brain injury [35]. Clearly, physical damage to the brain can initiate a cascade of biochemical and structural events in and around the primary injury [36]. Edema is one of those secondary events that may aggravate a primary injury, and studies suggest that serotonin could be involved in edema-causing micro vascular reactions [7]. Serotonin is present in many neuronal pathways arising from the nuclei of the dorsal raphe and leptomeninges mast cells and in blood platelets [33]. Changes in the concentration of serotonin most possibly occur during the progression of the injury. At the same time as edema is produced, additional quantities of serotonin may be brought in from the blood or from neurons. However, biochemical determinations suggest a rise in the serotonin content of the traumatized brain [37]. Serotonin is a powerful chemical micro vascular response mediator to cerebral edema [32]. Results of para-chlorophenylalanine (pCPA) pretreatment before trauma induction are consistent with the notion that serotonin plays a role as a vascular permeability-increasing compound that contributes to early edema [7, 38]. Para-chlorophenylalanine (pCPA), acts as a selective and irreversible inhibitor of tryptophan hydroxylase, which is a rate-limiting enzyme in the biosynthesis of serotonin. This is further demonstrated by the fact that the degree of cell changes in the periphery of the initial lesion is lower in pCPA pretreated rats than in non-treated animals with the same type of injury [7]. Therefore, it seems obvious that the decrease in the content of serotonin in the nervous tissue is somehow reflected in the decreased swelling and milder changes in the brain of traumatized rats. Nevertheless, apart from the effects of serotonin, arachidonic acid release, prostaglandins and thromboxane can synergistically contribute to edema formation.

The microdialysis technique was used in the popular carotid artery for intra-arterial recordings. This new application was found to be a genuinely acceptable and effective method that allows direct measurements of HPLC plasma serotonin without any further extraction process [39]. Studies show a significant increase in downstream plasma serotonin concentrations in response to acute non-occlusive common carotid artery thrombosis (CCAT) that appears to be caused solely by endothelium photochemical and not photo thermal impact. As a mediator of blood brain barrier disturbance and/or irregular cerebral blood flow and/or neuronal impairment in ischemic stroke and transient ischemic attacks (TIA's), the rise in serotonin may be of significant importance [39].

3.1 Role of 5-HT2 receptors in formation of edema

5-HT$_2$-receptor antagonists, ketanserin [40] and LY 53857 [41] prevent capsaicin-induced mouse ear edema [42]. Antagonists of the 5-HT$_1$-receptor and 5-HT$_3$-receptor ICS 205–930 and MDL 72222 [43] respectively, had no effect on edema caused by capsaicin [42]. The findings clearly indicate that 5-HT is partially involved in the development of edema via 5-HT$_2$ receptors. 5-HT is known to induce plasma extravasation by direct action on rat microvasculature [44] and to produce vasodilation on peripheral blood vessels through 5-HT$_1$ receptors [44]. A recent study indicated that endogenous nitric oxide, in addition to 5-HT receptors, is involved in a 5-HT-induced increase in vascular permeability in mouse skin [45]. In addition to activation of 5-HT$_2$ receptors, 5-HT plays a role of releasing neuropeptides including SP as the second mediator of increased vascular permeability at inflammatory sites [46]. Mediators like SP, bradykinin and prostaglandins, on the other hand, can release tachykinins from primary afferent terminals [47]. Many functional molecules like histamine, serotonin, arachidonic acid, prostaglandins and thromboxane have been confirmed to induce BBB disruption or cell swelling. It is believed that released 5-HT binds to 5-HT$_2$ receptors that stimulate cAMP and prostaglandins in vessels that cause more vesicular transport in endothelial cells and leading to serum components extravasation. The additional amount of serotonin into the tissue due to injury maintains the state of increased vascular permeability that ultimately causes edema. Changes in serotonin concentration were detected early after focal traumatic injury to the rat spinal cord and were associated with edema formation and alterations in blood flow [35]. Compared to controls, the serotonin concentration in the traumatised section increased more than 100 percent in five hours after the injury. The water content of the traumatised section estimated 5 h after the injury was also gradually increased whereas para-chlorophenylalamine, serotonin synthesis inhibitor, impeded the elevation in water content measured 5 h after the trauma [35].

3.2 Effect of antibodies to serotonin in closed head injury

Closed head injury (CHI) is a serious clinical issue that leads to immediate death for most patients [48]. Swelling of the brain in a closed cranial compartment that results in compression of the brain's vital centers tends to be primarily responsible for instant deaths [49]. CNS microhemorrhage, blood–brain barrier (BBB) permeability breakdown, and brain edema development, alone or in combination, are primarily responsible for cell damage and long-term neurodegenerative changes following CHI [37, 50, 51]. Unfortunately, so far, no effective validated therapies are accessible. Efforts to understand the molecular mechanisms of early pathophysiological events in an animal model of CHI are therefore urgently required to explore the possible therapeutic potential of different neuroprotective agents in order to reduce the development of edema and cell death.

In brain or spinal cord injuries increased plasma and brain levels of serotonin following CHI is seen in previous studies [50, 51]. There was a strong link between this rise in tissue serotonin levels and BBB breakdown and edema formation [52]. This is further reinforced by the fact that previous inhibition by p-chlorophenylalanine (pCPA) of serotonin biosynthesis greatly attenuated the formation of brain edema, BBB damage, and cell injury in brain and spinal cord injury [50, 51, 53]. Taken together, these findings strongly indicate an important role for serotonin in CNS trauma pathophysiology. Subsequent trials of CNS damage using serotonin receptor blocker drugs showed controversial results, however [34, 54, 55]. Blocking of 5-HT_{2c} and 5-HT_{1A} serotonin receptors improves cognitive function and reduces the formation of brain edema at low doses [52, 56, 57], other serotonin receptor antagonists, in fact, exacerbated the pathological outcome following brain injury [58, 59]. Thus, further research is needed into the role of serotonin receptors in mediating brain pathology in CNS injuries. Since serotonin has more than seven receptor types with several subtypes of receptors [52, 56, 58]. There can be no clear view on this topic of amine involvement using a few unspecific receptor antagonists. In addition, the dosage response and time schedule of drug therapy can further affect the final outcome [60].

Results from studies demonstrate that intracerebroventricular administration of monoclonal serotonin antibodies either 30 min before or 30 min after CHI induced profound neuroprotection. Therefore, after CHI, marked decreases in BBB disruption, brain edema formation, and cell injury were noted in serotonin antiserum-treated animals. Such novel results indicate that early intervention in CHI with serotonin antiserum is neuroprotective [60]. Taken together, these findings suggest the active participation of this amine during the early stages of CHI, in the cellular and molecular pathways of brain edema formation and BBB breakdown. The neuroprotective effects of antiserum serotonin in CHI are dose-dependent. This indicates that to induce neuroprotection, enough serotonin antiserum is required to block in vivo brain serotonin. On the other hand, when given 60 min after CHI, even a high concentration of serotonin antiserum was ineffective. This means that serotonin involvement is important for brain pathology within 30 minutes of CHI [60].

Elevation in plasma and brain serotonin concentration by intravenous injection of serotonin (10 to 20 g/kg/min) in animals without CHI disrupts the BBB function within 10 min [52, 59, 60]. This effect of the serotonin on BBB interruption is reversible. To measure BBB disruption, many approaches are used. Extravasation of Evans blue (EB) dye is the most commonly used procedure. Normally, Evans blue does not move through the BBB and hence its presence in brain tissue suggests permeability alterations. Thus, when the same dye was administered 2 to 3 hours after serotonin administration, BBB permeability to Evans blue dye was no longer observed. This means that the dosage and length of exposure to serotonin play a significant role in development of brain pathology. This principle is further confirmed by the prevention of BBB breakdown by previous serotonin synthesis inhibition, which attenuated an increase in plasma and brain serotonin in CHI [60].

BBB permeability breakdown is associated with vasogenic brain edema formation and cell injury [61–63]. Protein leakage from the vascular compartment via the blood–brain interface into the neuronal microenvironment will alter osmotic balance. A change in osmotic balance will allow the bulk flow of water from the vascular compartment to the cerebral compartments. Furthermore, the release of neurochemical mediators of brain edema, e.g. serotonin, prostaglandin, histamine and neuropeptides, via particular receptor-mediated pathways, will further affect water transfer from blood to the brain. These neurochemicals also cause the BBB process to break down. This hypothesis is consistent with a close relationship between the development of brain edema, the amount of serotonin and BBB disruption in CHI [60].

3.3 Serotonergic receptors in brain edema

Tissue collected after ischemic insult in gerbils showed two binding sites for ketanserin, one with a lower and one with a higher affinity than that found in sham-operated and ischemic animal brains. Ketanserin, a quinazoline derivative, is a selective 5-HT2 serotonin receptor antagonist with weak adrenergic receptor blocking properties. The results strongly suggest that the properties of binding sites for the S2 receptor are altered in ischemia-induced cerebral edema [64]. The demonstrated regulation of the binding sites of ketanserin appears to correlate with the observed attenuated metabolic rate (= increased release) but not with the abnormal brain 5-HT levels. Studies indicate that the variations in 5-HT ischemic patterns are most likely related to the type and model of ischemia and/or brain structure examined, as well as to the 5-HT detection system used [64]. However, in the brains of gerbils subjected to 15 min bilateral carotid artery occlusion without recirculation, 5-HT metabolism is unquestionably disturbed [65–67]. Therefore, there may be numerous explanations for the lack of apparent changes in the kinetic characteristics of 5-HT_2 receptor binding sites, especially if the presynaptic region is considered to be the primary site of the ischemically disrupted 5-HT pathway. The most critical of these are: (a) the insufficient lapse of time (15 min of ischemia) and/or the absence of recirculation required for the production of post-synaptic changes; and/or (b) the presence in the subcellular compartment of altered 5-HT_2 receptor properties obscured by the analysis of the entire cortical homogenate rather than the relevant fraction [64].

In neuronal and/or glial and/or vascular postsynaptic membranes, the modified 5-HT_2 receptors may be localized. Desensitization and hypersensitization of the receptor sites are demonstrated by the detection of 5-HT_2 postsynaptic binding sites with lower and higher affinities (indicated by apparent higher K_D and lower K_D) after 1 h of recirculation than those seen in the ischemic and control cortex. Due to increased release, reduced uptake and reuptake of 5-HT in the presynaptic regions, this could be the result of inappropriately accessible 5-HT at the postsynaptic receptor sites [64]. In general, this phenomenon is consistent with the well-known agonist-specific desensitization of high levels of hormones and neurohormones exposed to cell membranes, whereas their depletion results in supersensitization [68]. In addition, in the recovery period (recirculation of 1 and 2 h), the observed 5-HT_2 binding sites with a higher affinity (lower K_D) than those seen in ischemic and control brains may indicate either an unmasked pre-existing site or an additional binding site. It can be assumed that the existing disruptions of the 5-HT pathway and its adverse effects are not limited to the presynaptic, but also include the postsynaptic subcellular compartments, based on the observed changes in the properties of S2 receptor binding sites [64].

In addition, it is conceivable that the presynaptically released 5-HT into the synaptic cleft is also able to directly impact the membrane. In this way, unmetabolized 5-HT overflow can lead to increased permeability of the membrane, allowing for more pronounced passive ion transfer and water accumulation in the cells [64]. This inference is confirmed by the additional increase in Na^+ observed, a decrease in K^+ concentration and a decrease in Na^+-K^+-ATPase activity at the time of most marked cell swelling. In particular, the concomitant occurrence of changes in the kinetic properties of S2 receptors and the activity of Na^+K^+-ATPase is of concern, since an increase in PGF2a levels was also observed after the same period of ischemia and recirculation. 5-HT can stimulate the development of PGF_{2a}, since this amine increases the formation of PGF1a in cultured cerebrovascular elements. Nevertheless, it remains to be clarified if 5-HT affects directly or indirectly Na^+K^+-ATPase operation [64] list Nevertheless, at the time of the most conspicuously increased cellular water in the brain of gerbils subjected to ischemia and recirculation, the observed alteration of 5-HT_2 receptors strongly supports the argument of 5-HT involvement in edema formation and/or progression [64].

4. Neuroprotective role of serotonin after TBI

4.1 In cerebral ischemia

The severity of secondary TBI mechanisms depends on the severity of the injury or the primary insult location. Reductions in cerebral blood flow [69, 70] have been reported to exceed ischemic levels in conditions of extreme TBI. Cerebral ischemia is therefore addressed as one secondary cause of injury that may be involved in brain trauma [69, 71]. There is a massive increase in the concentration of both excitatory and inhibitory neurotransmitters in the extracellular space during cerebral ischemia [72–75]. It has been proposed that over-excitation of neurons triggered by excitatory amino acid neurotransmitters plays a major role in the pathogenesis of ischemic neuronal destruction [76]. Glutamate induces an influx of Ca^{2+} and Na^+ into the neuron by acting on N-methyl-D-aspartate (NMDA) and non NMDA receptors. The neuronal membrane depolarizes strongly and can allow Ca^{2+} to reach the cell through additional pathways. These events can lead to a neurotoxic accumulation of intracellular Ca^{2+} [77]. In addition to glutamate antagonists, agents that induce neuronal membrane hyperpolarisation may be able to reduce the influx of Ca^{2+} via these ionophores and may exert neuroprotective effects. 5-HydroxytryptaminelA (5-HT_{1A}) receptors through Ca^{2+}-independent K^+-conductance mediate an inhibitory, hyperpolarizing effect on cortical and hippocampal neurons [78–80]. It has been shown that 5-HT_{1A} receptor agonists imitate 5-HT's hyperpolarizing activity on the resting membrane potential, increase the firing threshold, and decrease the firing rate of hippocampal CA_l, cortical, and dorsal raphe neurons [81]. The complexity of 5-HT's function in cerebral ischemia is probably due to the multiplicity within the brain of 5-HT receptors and their distinct distribution and densities. 5-HT_{1A} receptors mediate the inhibitory effect on neurons, as mentioned above. However, 5-HT also stimulates hippocampal and cortical neurons via 5-HT_2 receptors [80, 82].

4.2 In neurocognitive and neuropsychiatric disorders following traumatic brain injury

Due to variable diagnostic criteria, the prevalence of post-TBI depression varies from 6–77% [83], and up to 53% in the first year after injury [84]. The association between TBI and the development of neuropsychiatric disorders is well documented

[85, 86]. Disruption of the serotonergic system is one unifying factor that underlies acquired neuropsychiatric disorders following TBI. As the blood–brain barrier cannot be crossed by serotonin, synthesis must occur de novo in the brain. The shearing of brain stem axons during TBI effectively interferes with pontine and medullary serotonergic projections, resulting in decreased serotonin metabolism and production [87–90]. Selective serotonin reuptake inhibitors (SSRIs) are a class of antidepressant agents which inhibit serotonin reuptake by presynaptic cell monoamine transporters and increase extracellular concentration of serotonin, enabling increased serotonin availability in the synaptic cleft and increase activation of postsynaptic serotonergic receptors, resulting in increased synaptic signaling. SSRIs are involved in regulation of neuronal cell survival and neuroplasticity for the treatment of psychiatric disorders, including depression, obsessive–compulsive disorder, bulimia, and panic disorder [91]. Serotonin modulates mood, arousal, emotion, and working memory, and thus constitute SSRIs an attractive, treatable, and potentially long-term pharmacological intervention for neurocognitive and neuropsychiatric deficits post-TBI [92]. Consequently, the judicious use of SSRIs in post-TBI depression treatment is of great importance and impact.

5. Pharmacological interventions after TBI related to serotonin

A growing number of patients are surviving with residual neurological impairments due to improvements in the treatment of head trauma. A commission of the National Institute of Health reports that there are currently 2.5 to 6.5 million Americans with TBI-related disabilities [93]. Information from various disciplines and professions beginning at the time of injury and continuing through the recovery process is required for successful treatment of TBI. In both the sub-acute (less than 1 month post TBI) and chronic (more than 1 month post TBI) stages, pharmacotherapy is used. Selective serotonin reuptake inhibitors (SSRIs) have been found to be helpful in the treatment of behavioral syndromes in patients with TBI, especially in the sub-acute recovery phases [94], but also in chronic settings. Most studies indicate that SSRIs enhance neurobehavioral, neurocognitive, and neuropsychiatric deficits, especially agitation, depression, psychomotor retardation, and recent memory loss, but most of the information comes from non-randomized studies. Similarly, bupropion boosts the levels of both dopamine and norepinephrine and is a weak serotonin reuptake inhibitor. This agent has been effective in treating restlessness at 150 mg per day [95]. For anxiety, depressed mood, and deficits in psychomotor pace and recent memory, sertraline administered at an average dose of 100 mg daily for 8 weeks was found to be beneficial but shorter treatment durations have shown no benefit [94]. There was a strong link between the rise in tissue serotonin levels and BBB breakdown and edema formation [52]. This is further reinforced by the fact that previous inhibition by p-chlorophenylalanine (pCPA) of serotonin biosynthesis greatly attenuated the formation of brain edema, BBB damage, and cell injury in brain and spinal cord injury [53]. Blocking of 5-HT_{2c} and 5-HT_{1A} serotonin receptors improves cognitive function and reduces the formation of brain edema at low doses [52, 56]. Thus, 5-HT_2 receptor functions need to be explored more in the development of cerebral edema and this can be used as pharmacological intervention to reduce cerebral edema.

6. Conclusion

Due to permeability changes in the vessel walls, the pathogenesis of edema after traumatic brain injury is complex, including disruption of micro vessels and changes in microcirculation around the primary injury and leakage of plasma constituents into the tissue. To cause BBB disruption or cell swelling, several functional molecules such as histamine, serotonin, prostaglandins and thromboxane are involved. The 5-HT released is believed to bind to 5-HT2 receptors stimulating cAMP and prostaglandins in vessels that trigger further vesicular transport in endothelial cells, leading to extravasation of the serum portion. Serotonin is involved in early cytotoxic edema after TBI. Reduction of serotonin in the nervous tissue is shown to reduce swelling and the milder cell changes in the brain or spinal cord of traumatized rats. Inhibition of serotonin synthesis before CHI in rat models or administration of serotonin antiserum after injury attenuates BBB disruption and brain edema, volume swelling, and brain pathology. BBB disturbance and brain edema, volume swelling, and brain pathology are attenuated by inhibition of serotonin production before CHI in rat models or the administration of serotonin antiserum after injury. Immediately after injury, maintaining low serotonin levels can demonstrate neuroprotection and fight various secondary outcomes that occur after traumatic brain injury.

Author details

Priya Badyal, Jaspreet Kaur and Anurag Kuhad*
Pharmacology Research Laboratory, University Institute of Pharmaceutical Sciences, Panjab University, Chandigarh, India

*Address all correspondence to: anurag_pu@yahoo.com; anurag.kuhad@pu.ac.in

References

[1] Jin Y, Lin Y, Feng JF, Jia F, Gao G, Jiang JY. Attenuation of Cell Death in Injured Cortex after Post-Traumatic Brain Injury Moderate Hypothermia: Possible Involvement of Autophagy Pathway. World Neurosurg. 2015; 84(2):420-30

[2] Li Q, Wu X, Yang Y, Zhang Y, He F, Xu X, et al. Tachykinin NK1 receptor antagonist L-733,060 and substance P deletion exert neuroprotection through inhibiting oxidative stress and cell death after traumatic brain injury in mice. Int J Biochem Cell Biol. 2019;

[3] Bayir H, Kochanek PM, Kagan VE. Oxidative stress in immature brain after traumatic brain injury. Developmental Neuroscience. 2006. 28:420-31

[4] Donkin JJ, Vink R. Mechanisms of cerebral edema in traumatic brain injury: Therapeutic developments. Current Opinion in Neurology. 2010. 23(3):293-9.

[5] Pappius HM, Dadoun R, McHugh M. The effect of p-chlorophenylalanine on cerebral metabolism and biogenic amine content of traumatized brain. J Cereb Blood Flow Metab. 1988; 8(3):324-334

[6] S.M. Hung A, Y.M. Tsui T, C.Y. Lam J, S.M. Wai M, M. Chan W, T. Yew D. Serotonin and its Receptors in the Human CNS with New Findings - A Mini Review. Curr Med Chem. 2011; 18(34):5281-8

[7] Olsson Y, Sharma HS, Pettersson CÅ V. Effects of p-chlorophenylalanine on microvascular permeability changes in spinal cord trauma - An experimental study in the rat using 131I-sodium and lanthanum tracers. Acta Neuropathol. 1990; 79(6):595-603

[8] Chiavegatto S, Nelson RJ. Interaction of nitric oxide and serotonin in aggressive behavior. In: Hormones and Behavior. 2003. 44(3):233-41

[9] Fukumura D, Gohongi T, Kadambi A, Izumi Y, Ang J, Yun CO, et al. Predominant role of endothelial nitric oxide synthase in vascular endothelial growth factor-induced angiogenesis and vascular permeability. Proc Natl Acad Sci U S A. 2001; 98 (5) 2604-2609

[10] Manivet P, Mouillet-Richard S, Callebert J, Nebigil CG, Maroteaux L, Hosoda S, et al. PDZ-dependent activation of nitric-oxide synthases by the serotonin 2B receptor. J Biol Chem. 2000; 275(13):9324-31

[11] Borgdorff P, Fekkes D, Tangelder GJ. Hypotension caused by extracorporeal circulation: Serotonin from pump-activated platelets triggers nitric oxide release. Circulation. 2002; 106:2588-2593

[12] Kochanek KD, Xu J, Murphy SL, Miniño AM, Kung HC. Deaths: final data for 2009. Natl Vital Stat Rep. 2011; 60(3):1-116

[13] Stokum JA, Gerzanich V, Simard JM. Molecular pathophysiology of cerebral edema. Journal of Cerebral Blood Flow and Metabolism. 2016. 36(3):513-38

[14] Di Terlizzi R, Platt S. The function, composition and analysis of cerebrospinal fluid in companion animals: Part I - Function and composition. Vet J. 2006; 172(3):422-31

[15] Iliff JJ, Wang M, Liao Y, Plogg BA, Peng W, Gundersen GA, et al. A paravascular pathway facilitates CSF flow through the brain parenchyma and the clearance of interstitial solutes, including amyloid β. Sci Transl Med. 2012; 4(147):147ra111

[16] Thrane VR, Thrane AS, Plog BA, Thiyagarajan M, Iliff JJ, Deane R, et al. Paravascular microcirculation facilitates rapid lipid transport and astrocyte

signaling in the brain. Sci Rep. 2013; 3:2582

[17] Iliff JJ, Nedergaard M. Is there a cerebral lymphatic system? In: Stroke. 2013. 44:S93–S95

[18] Hossmann KA, Schuier FJ. Experimental brain infarcts in cats. I. Pathophysiological observations. Stroke. 1980; 11(6):583-92

[19] Bell BA, Symon L, Branston NM. CBF and time thresholds for the formation of ischemic cerebral edema, and effect of reperfusion in baboons. J Neurosurg. 1985; 62(1):31-41

[20] Quast MJ, Huang NC, Hillman GR, Kent TA. The evolution of acute stroke recorded by multimodal magnetic resonance imaging. Magn Reson Imaging. 1993; 11(4):465-71

[21] Thrane AS, Rangroo Thrane V, Nedergaard M. Drowning stars: Reassessing the role of astrocytes in brain edema. Trends in Neurosciences. 2014. 37(11):620-8

[22] Yan Y, Dempsey RJ, Sun D. Expression of Na+-K+-Cl- cotransporter in rat brain during development and its localization in mature astrocytes. Brain Res. 2001; 911(1):43-55

[23] Yan Y, Dempsey RJ, Sun D. Na+-K+-Cl- cotransporter in rat focal cerebral ischemia. J Cereb Blood Flow Metab. 2001; 21(6):711-21

[24] Jayakumar AR, Norenberg MD. The Na-K-Cl Co-transporter in astrocyte swelling. In: Metabolic Brain Disease. 2010. 25(1):31-8

[25] Hamann S, Herrera-Perez JJ, Zeuthen T, Alvarez-Leefmans FJ. Cotransport of water by the Na+-K+-2Cl cotransporter NKCC1 in mammalian epithelial cells. J Physiol. 2010; 588(21):4089-101

[26] Su G, Kintner DB, Sun D. Contribution of Na+-K+-Cl- cotransporter to high-[K+]o- induced swelling and EAA release in astrocytes. Am J Physiol - Cell Physiol. 2002; 282(5):C1136-46

[27] Lu KT, Cheng NC, Wu CY, Yang YL. NKCC1-mediated traumatic brain injury-induced brain edema and neuron death via Raf/MEK/MAPK cascade. Crit Care Med. 2008; 36(3):917-22

[28] O'Donnell ME, Tran L, Lam TI, Liu XB, Anderson SE. Bumetanide inhibition of the blood-brain barrier Na-K-Cl cotransporter reduces edema formation in the rat middle cerebral artery occlusion model of stroke. J Cereb Blood Flow Metab. 2004; 24(9):1046-56

[29] Yan Y, Dempsey RJ, Flemmer A, Forbush B, Sun D. Inhibition of Na+-K+-Cl- cotransporter during focal cerebral ischemia decreases edema and neuronal damage. Brain Res. 2003; 961(1):22-31

[30] Vorbrodt AW, Lossinsky AS, Wisniewski HM, Suzuki R, Yamaguchi T, Masaoka H, et al. Ultrastructural observations on the transvascular route of protein removal in vasogenic brain edema. Acta Neuropathol. 1985; 66(4):265-73

[31] Unterberg AW, Stover J, Kress B, Kiening KL. Edema and brain trauma. Neuroscience. 2004; 129(4):1021-9

[32] Wahl M, Unterberg A, Baethmann A, Schilling L. Mediators of blood-brain barrier dysfunction and formation of vasogenic brain edema. Journal of Cerebral Blood Flow and Metabolism. 1988. 8(5):621-34

[33] McEntee WJ, Crook TH. Serotonin, memory, and the aging brain. Psychopharmacology. 1991. 103(2):143-9

[34] Sharma HS, Olsson Y, Kumar Dey P. Changes in blood-brain barrier and cerebral blood flow following elevation of circulating serotonin level in anesthetized rats. Brain Res. 1990; 517(1-2):215-23

[35] Sharma HS, Olsson Y, Dey PK. Early accumulation of serotonin in rat spinal cord subjected to traumatic injury. Relation to edema and blood flow changes. Neuroscience. 1990;

[36] Nag S, Manias JL, Stewart DJ. Pathology and new players in the pathogenesis of brain edema. Acta Neuropathologica. 2009. 118(2):197-217

[37] Day PK, Sharma HS. Ambient temperature and development of traumatic brain oedema in anaesthetized animals. Indian J Med Res. 1983;

[38] Sharma HS, Olsson Y. Edema formation and cellular alterations following spinal cord injury in the rat and their modification with p-chlorophenylalanine. Acta Neuropathol. 1990; 79(6):604-10.

[39] Dietrich WD. The Role of Neurotransmitters in Brain Injury. Vol. 10, Journal of Cerebral Blood Flow & Metabolism. 1990. 758-758 p.

[40] Leysen JE, Awouters F, Kennis L, Laduron PM, Vandenberk J, Janssen PAJ. Receptor binding profile of R 41 468, A novel antagonist at 5-HT2 receptors. Life Sci. 1981; 28(9)1015-22

[41] Cohen ML, Fuller RW, Kurz KD. LY53857, a selective and potent serotonergic (5-HT2) receptor antagonist, does not lower blood pressure in the spontaneously hypertensive rat. J Pharmacol Exp Ther. 1983; 227(2):327-32.

[42] Inoue H, Nagata N, Koshihara Y. Participation of Serotonin in Capsaicin-Induced Mouse Ear Edema. Jpn J Pharmacol. 1995; 69(1):61-8

[43] Fozard JR. MDL 72222: a potent and highly selective antagonist at neuronal 5-hydroxytryptamine receptors. Naunyn Schmiedebergs Arch Pharmacol. 1984; 326(1):36-44

[44] Arvier PT, Chahl LA, Ladd RJ. Modification by capsaicin and compound 48/80 of dye leakage induced by irritants in the rat. Br J Pharmacol. 1977; 59(1):61-8

[45] Fujii E, Irie K, Uchida Y, Tsukahara F, Muraki T. Possible role of nitric oxide in 5-hydroxytryptamine-induced increase in vascular permeability in mouse skin. Naunyn Schmiedebergs Arch Pharmacol. 1994; 350(4):361-4

[46] Mantione CR, Rodriguez R. A bradykinin (BK)1 receptor antagonist blocks capsaicin-induced ear inflammation in mice. Br J Pharmacol. 1990; 99(3): 516-518.

[47] Holzer P. Capsaicin: Cellular targets, mechanisms of action, and selectivity for thin sensory neurons. Pharmacological Reviews. 1991. 43(2):143-201

[48] Ommaya AK, Goldsmith W, Thibault L. Biomechanics and neuropathology of adult and paediatric head injury. British Journal of Neurosurgery. 2002. 16(3):220-42

[49] Goyal K, Yadav R. Traumatic brain injury. In: Acute Neuro Care: Focused Approach to Neuroemergencies. 2020.

[50] Vannemreddy P, Ray AK, Patnaik R, Patnaik S, Mohanty S, Sharma HS. Zinc protoporphyrin IX attenuates closed head injury-induced edema formation, blood-brain barrier disruption, and serotonin levels in the rat. Acta Neurochir Suppl. 2006; 96:151-6.

[51] Dey PK, Sharma HS. Influence of ambient temperature and drug treatments on brain oedema induced by impact injury on skull in rats. Indian J Physiol Pharmacol. 1984; 28(3):177-86

[52] Sharma HS. Influence of Serotonin on the Blood-Brain and the Blood-Spinal Cord Barriers. In: Blood-Spinal Cord and Brain Barriers in Health and Disease. 2004.

[53] Sharma HS, Winkler T, Stålberg E, Mohanty S, Westman J. p-Chlorophenylalanine, an inhibitor of serotonin synthesis reduces blood-brain barrier permeability, cerebral blood flow, edema formation and cell injury following trauma to the rat brain. Acta Neurochir Suppl. 2000; 76:91-5

[54] Nichols CD. Serotonin. In: Encyclopedia of the Neurological Sciences. 2014.

[55] Sharma HS, Westman J, Cervós Navarro J, Dey PK, Nyberg F. Probable involvement of serotonin in the increased permeability of the blood-brain barrier by forced swimming. An experimental study using Evans blue and 131I-sodium tracers in the rat. Behav Brain Res. 1995; 189-196

[56] Salzman SK, Kelly G, Chavin J, Wang L, Puniak MA, Agresta CA, et al. Characterization of mianserin neuroprotection in experimental spinal trauma: Dose/route response and late treatment. J Pharmacol Exp Ther. 1994; 269(1):322-8

[57] Salzman SK, Puniak MA, Liu Z -j, Maitland-Heriot RP, Freeman GM, Agresta CA. The serotonin antagonist mianserin improves functional recovery following experimental spinal trauma. Ann Neurol. 1991; 30(4):533-41

[58] Faden AI, Salzman S. Pharmacological strategies in CNS trauma. Trends in Pharmacological Sciences. 1992. 13:29-35

[59] Sharma HS, Winkler T, Stålberg E, Olsson Y, Dey PK. Evaluation of traumatic spinal cord edema using evoked potentials recorded from the spinal epidural space. An experimental study in the rat. J Neurol Sci. 1991; 102(2):150-62

[60] Sharma HS, Patnaik R, Patnaik S, Mohanty S, Sharma A, Vannemreddy P. Antibodies to serotonin attenuate closed head injury induced blood-brain barrier disruption and brain pathology. In: Annals of the New York Academy of Sciences. 2007. 1122:295-312

[61] Sharma HS, Westman J, Nyberg F. Pathophysiology of brain edema and cell changes following hyperthermic brain injury. Progress in Brain Research. 1998. 115:351-412

[62] Sharma HS, Westman J, Nyberg F, Cervos-Navarro J, Dey PK. Role of serotonin and prostaglandins in brain edema induced by heat stress. An experimental study in the young rat. Acta Neurochir Suppl (Wien). 1994; 60:65-70.

[63] Sharma HS, Olsson Y, Nyberg F, Dey PK. Prostaglandins modulate alterations of microvascular permeability, blood flow, edema and serotonin levels following spinal cord injury: An experimental study in the rat. Neuroscience. 1993; 443-449

[64] Wroblewska B, Ueki Y, Mršulja BB, Djuričić BM, Spatz M. Serotonin Receptors in Ischemic Brain Edema. Brain Edema. 1985;178-84.

[65] Maruki C, Merkel N, Rausch WD, Spatz M. Brain Monoamines in Cerebral Ischemic Edema, the Effect of Gamma-Hydroxy-Butyrate. In: Recent Progress in the Study and Therapy of Brain Edema. 1984.

[66] Mršulja BB, Djuričić BM, Cvejić V, Mićić D V. Pharmacological Approach to Postischemic Brain Edema in Gerbils. In:

Recent Progress in the Study and Therapy of Brain Edema. 1984.

[67] Mršulja BB, Mršulja BJ, Spatz M, Klatzo I. Monoamines in Cerebral Ischemia in Relation to Brain Edema. Dyn Brain Edema. 1976;187-92.

[68] Iyengar R, Birnbaumer L. Agonist-specific desensitization: molecular locus and possible mechanism. Adv Cyclic Nucleotide Res. 1981;14:93-100.

[69] Marion DW, Darby J, Yonas H. Acute regional cerebral blood flow changes caused by severe head injuries. J Neurosurg. 1991; 74(3):407-14

[70] Zauner A, Bullock R, Kuta AJ, Woodward J, Young HF. Glutamate Release and Cerebral Blood Flow after Severe Human Head Injury. Acta Neurochir Suppl. 1996; 67:40-4

[71] Bouma GJ, Muizelaar JP, Choi SC, Newlon PG, Young HF. Cerebral circulation and metabolism after severe traumatic brain injury: The elusive role of ischemia. J Neurosurg. 1991; 75(5):685-93

[72] Benveniste H, Drejer J, Schousboe A, Diemer NH. Elevation of the Extracellular Concentrations of Glutamate and Aspartate in Rat Hippocampus During Transient Cerebral Ischemia Monitored by Intracerebral Microdialysis. J Neurochem. 1984; 43(5):1369-74

[73] Hagberg H, Andersson P, Lacarewicz J, Jacobson I, Butcher S, Sandberg M. Extracellular Adenosine, Inosine, Hypoxanthine, and Xanthine in Relation to Tissue Nucleotides and Purines in Rat Striatum During Transient Ischemia. J Neurochem. 1987; 49(1):227-31

[74] Globus MY-., Busto R, Dietrich WD, Martinez E, Valdes I, Ginsberg MD. Effect of Ischemia on the In Vivo Release of Striatal Dopamine, Glutamate, and γ-Aminobutyric Acid Studied by Intracerebral Microdialysis. J Neurochem. 1988; 51(5):1455-64

[75] Sarna GS, Obrenovitch TP, Matsumoto T, Symon L, Curzon G. Effect of Transient Cerebral Ischaemia and Cardiac Arrest on Brain Extracellular Dopamine and Serotonin as Determined by In Vivo Dialysis in the Rat. J Neurochem. 1990; 55(3):937-40

[76] Jørgensen MB, Diemer NH. Selective neuron loss after cerebral ischemia in the rat: Possible role of transmitter glutamate. Acta Neurol Scand. 1982; 66(5):536-46

[77] Choi DW. Glutamate neurotoxicity and diseases of the nervous system. Neuron. 1988. 1(8):623-34

[78] Beck SG, Clarke WP, Goldfarb J. Spiperone differentiates multiple 5-hydroxytryptamine responses in rat hippocampal slices in vitro. Eur J Pharmacol. 1985; 116(1-2):195-7

[79] Andrade R, Malenka RC, Nicoll RA. A G protein couples serotonin and GABAB receptors to the same channels in hippocampus. Science (80-). 1986; 234(4781):1261-5

[80] Colino A, Halliwell J V. Differential modulation of three separate K-conductances in hippocampal ca1 neurons by serotonin. Nature. 1988; 328(6125):73-7

[81] Basse-Tomusk A, Rebec G V. Ipsapirone depresses neuronal activity in the dorsal raphe nucleus and the hippocampal formation. Eur J Pharmacol. 1986; 130(1-2):141-3

[82] Davies MF, Deisz RA, Prince DA, Peroutka SJ. Two distinct effects of 5-hydroxytryptamine on single cortical neurons. Brain Res. 1987; 2):347-52

[83] Jorge RE, Robinson RG, Moser D, Tateno A, Crespo-Facorro B, Arndt S. *Major* Depression Following Traumatic

Brain Injury. Arch Gen Psychiatry. 2004; 61(1):42-50

[84] Bombardier CH, Fann JR, Temkin NR, Esselman PC, Barber J, Dikmen SS. Rates of major depressive disorder and clinical outcomes following traumatic brain injury. JAMA - J Am Med Assoc. 2010; 303(19): 1938-45

[85] Koponen S, Taiminen T, Portin R, Himanen L, Isoniemi H, Heinonen H, et al. Axis I and II psychiatric disorders after traumatic brain injury: A 30-year follow-up study. Am J Psychiatry. 2002; 159(8):1315-21

[86] Koponen S, Taiminen T, Hiekkanen H, Tenovuo O. Axis I and II psychiatric disorders in patients with traumatic brain injury: A 12-month follow-up study. Brain Inj. 2011; 25(11):1029-34

[87] Markianos M, Seretis A, Kotsou A, Christopoulos M. CSF neurotransmitter metabolites in comatose head injury patients during changes in their clinical state. Acta Neurochir (Wien). 1996; 138(1):57-9

[88] Tsuiki K, Yamamoto YL, Diksic M. Effect of Acute Fluoxetine Treatment on the Brain Serotonin Synthesis as Measured by the α-Methyl-l-Tryptophan Autoradiographic Method. J Neurochem. 1995; 65(1):250-6

[89] Tsuiki K, Takada A, Nagahiro S, Grdiša M, Diksic M, Pappius HM. Synthesis of Serotonin in Traumatized Rat Brain. J Neurochem. 1995; 64(3):1319-25

[90] Kline AE, Yu J, Horváth E, Marion DW, Dixon CE. The selective 5-HT1A receptor agonist repinotan HCl attenuates histopathology and spatial learning deficits following traumatic brain injury in rats. Neuroscience. 2001; 106(3):547-55.

[91] Schneier FR, Campeas R, Carcamo J, Glass A, Lewis-Fernandez R, Neria Y, et al. COMBINED MIRTAZAPINE and SSRI TREATMENT of PTSD: A PLACEBO-CONTROLLED TRIAL. Depress Anxiety. 2015; 32(8): 570-579

[92] Mostert JP, Koch MW, Heerings M, Heersema DJ, De Keyser J. Therapeutic potential of fluoxetine in neurological disorders. CNS Neuroscience and Therapeutics. 2008. 14(2):153-164

[93] Iaccarino MA, Bhatnagar S, Zafonte R. Rehabilitation after traumatic brain injury. In: Handbook of Clinical Neurology. 2015. 127:411-22

[94] Meythaler JM, Depalma L, Devivo MJ, Guin-Renfroe S, Novack TA. Sertraline to improve arousal and alertness in severe traumatic brain injury secondary to motor vehicle crashes. Brain Inj. 2001; 15(4):321-31

[95] Teng CJ, Bhalerao S, Lee Z, Farber J, Morris H, Foran T, et al. The use of bupropion in the treatment of restlessness after a traumatic brain injury. Brain Inj. 2001; 15(5):463-7

Chapter 8

Serotonin Pathway in Neuroimmune Network

Giada Mondanelli and Claudia Volpi

Abstract

Once considered merely as a neurotransmitter, serotonin (5-HT) now enjoys a renewed reputation as an interlocutor in the dense and continuous dialogue between neuroendocrine and immune systems. In the last decades, a role has been depicted for serotonin and its derivatives as modulators of several immunological events, due to the expression of specific receptors or enzymes controlling 5-HT metabolism in diverse immune cell types. A growing body of evidence suggests that the effects of molecules belonging to the 5-HT pathways on the neuroimmune communication may be relevant in the clinical outcome of autoimmune/inflammatory pathologies of the central nervous system (CNS), such as multiple sclerosis, but also in Alzheimer's disease, or in mood disorders and major depression. Moreover, since the predominance of 5-HT is produced by enterochromaffin cells of the gastrointestinal tract, where 5-HT and its derivatives are important mucosal signalling molecules giving rise to the so-called "brain-gut axis", alterations in brain-gut communication are also involved in the pathogenesis and pathophysiology of several psychiatric and neurologic disorders. Here we illustrate how functional interactions between immune and neuronal cells are crucial to orchestrate tissue homeostasis and integrity, and the role of serotonin pathway components as pillars of the neuroimmune system.

Keywords: neuroimmune system, tryptophan metabolism, serotonin, N-acetylserotonin, melatonin, indoleamine 2,3-dioxygenase

1. Introduction

It's now widely accepted that the immune system and neuroendocrine system function in close association of each other, to such an extent that it's possible to refer to them as "neuroimmune system" [1]. The interactions that take place within the neuroimmune system involve the production and use of immune factors, as well as neuroendocrine mediators, in a role-playing game where it's impossible to trace the belonging of specific molecules exclusively in one of the two systems. The constant dialogue between the participants to the neuroimmune communication in the CNS and in the periphery not only allows the fine tuning of the immune response, but also the synaptic plasticity, and alterations in the propagation of neuroimmune messages may account for several immune-mediated and psychiatric diseases.

Here we examine the role of serotonin and its derivatives in the neuroimmune communication and we highlight the importance of an appropriate balance between the production of tryptophan metabolites for the maintenance of the neuroimmune homeostasis. Moreover, we give a perspective on how the regulation of the metabolic pathways leading to different tryptophan metabolites, including serotonin and derived molecules, could represent a significant pharmacological target for the treatment of various CNS diseases.

2. Serotonin pathway in the neuroimmune system: an overview

Under physiological conditions, the majority of Tryptophan (Trp) is degraded along the kynurenine pathway (KP) and only about 1% is metabolized into serotonin (5-HT) in the so-called methoxyindoles pathway (**Figure 1**). This metabolic route begins with the transformation of Trp into 5-hydroxytryptophan and then into serotonin through two consecutive reactions catalyzed by the enzymes tryptophan hydroxylase (TPH) and 5-hydroxytryptophan decarboxylase (AADC). Subsequently, the rate-limiting enzyme arylalkylamine N-acetyltransferase (AANAT) promotes the acetylation of serotonin into N-acetylserotonin (NAS), which, in turn, serves as a substrate for the hydroxyindole-O-methyl transferase (HIOMT or acetylserotonin O-methyltransferase, ASMT) to generate melatonin. Then, melatonin can be cleaved by indoleamine 2,3-dioxygenase 1 (IDO1) in a non-specific reaction and transformed into N-acetyl-N-formyl-5-methoxykynurenamine (AFMK). Additional enzymatic or oxidative pathways other than IDO1 are responsible for the generation of AFMK from the common precursor. Specifically, AFMK can arise from reaction of melatonin with hydroxyl radical and the subsequent interaction of the new-born melatonyl species with superoxide anion [2]. Moreover,

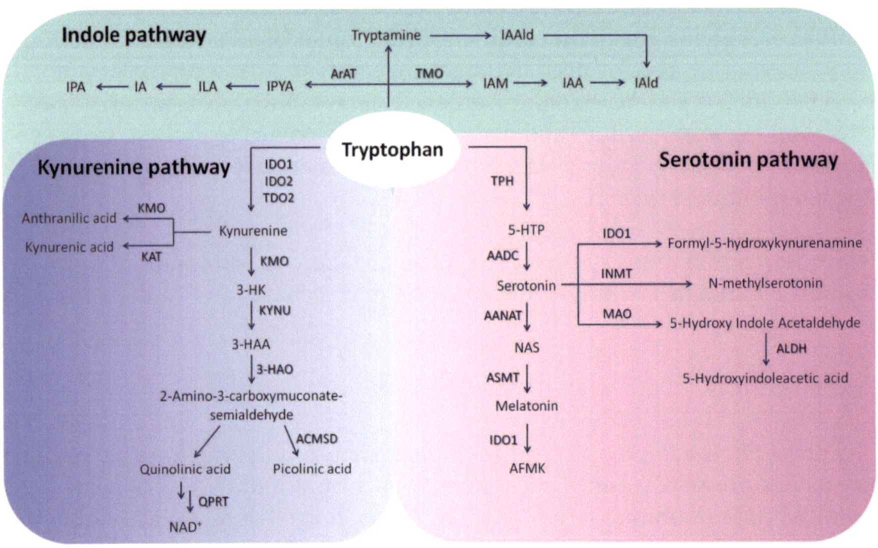

Figure 1.
Tryptophan metabolism along the kynurenine, serotonin and indole pathways. The majority of tryptophan is converted into kynurenine, whereas only about 1% is metabolized into serotonin. A small amount of tryptophan is used by the gut microbiota to produce indole derivatives. AADC, aromatic amino acid decarboxylase; AANAT, arylalkylamine N-acetyltransferase; ALDH, aldehyde dehydrogenase; AFMK, acetyl-N-formyl-5-methoxykynurenamine; ArAT, acromatic amino acid aminotransferase; ASMT, N-acetylserotonin O-methyltransferase; 3-HAA, 3-hydroxyanthranilic acid; 3-HK, 3-hydroxykynurenine; 5-HTTP, 5-hydroxytryptophan; IA, indoleacrylic acid; IAA, indoleacetic acid; Iald, indole-3-aldehyde; IAAld, indole-3-acetaldehyde; IAM, indole-3-acetamide; IDO1, indoleamine 2–3-dioxygenase 1; ILA, indolelactic acid; INMT, indolethylamine-N-methyltransferase; IPA, indole-3-propionic acid; IPYA, Indole-3-pyruvate; KAT, kynurenine aminotransferase; KMO, kynurenine-3-monooxygenase; KYNU, kynureninase; MAO, monoamine oxidase; NAD+, nicotinamide adenine dinucleotide; NAS, Nacetylserotonin; TDO2, tryptophan 2,3-dioxygenase; TMO, tryptophan 2-monooxygenase; TPH, tryptophan hydroxylase.

melatonin can yield to AFMK either by directly scavenging hydrogen peroxide or serving as a substrate of neutrophils' myeloperoxidase [3, 4].

Serotonin is a double life metabolite acting as neurotransmitter and peripheral hormone [5]. As a matter of fact, about 5% of the total serotonin is synthesized by serotoninergic neurons and operates within the CNS, while the majority of human body's serotonin is produced by enterochromaffin cells (EC) located in the gastrointestinal tract (GI). A significant amount of gut serotonin is released in the bloodstream where it is rapidly absorbed and stored by platelets and, to a lesser extent, by immune cells [6]. Although both TPH and AADC are necessary for the production of serotonin, TPH is the rate-limiting enzyme, as demonstrated by its weak affinity for any other amino acid and by the reduced serotonin levels upon pharmacologic or genetic ablation of the enzyme [7]. TPH exists into two isoforms that mainly differ in terms of cellular localization, i.e. TPH1- expressed by EC cells - and TPH2, found in central neurones [8].

The balance between the biosynthesis and the metabolism affects the bioavailability of serotonin. Indeed, besides the main branch of methoxyindoles pathway that yields to AFMK as end product, three additional catabolic reactions are responsible for the biotransformation of serotonin into metabolites mainly excreted with the urine [9]. In particular, through the catalysis mediated by IDO1, monoamine oxidases (MAO) or indolethylamine-N-methyltransferase (INMT), serotonin is converted into formyl-5-hydroxykynurenamine, 5-hydroxyindoleacetic acid and N-methylserotonin, respectively. Although rapidly metabolized, serotonin can be taken up by serotonin reuptake transporters (SERT) expressed in the CNS, platelets, GI and peripheral vasculature; once in the cytosol, the metabolite is immediately packaged into vesicles by vesicular monoamine transporter (VMAT) that prevents further degradation by mitochondrial MAO. Calcium-dependent exocytosis, such as that triggered during an inflammatory response or vascular injury, is responsible for the release of serotonin from the storing vesicles.

As an archetype of chronobiological hormone, melatonin is mainly produced by the pineal gland in response to circadian rhythm, i.e. the concentration of melatonin rises in the darkness and decreases in the daytime [10]. Along with melatonin, pineal NAS levels are higher at night than during the day, as opposed to pineal serotonin whose concentration peaks with the lightering. The rhythmic rotation between daily and nightly profiles of pineal indoles is controlled by the circadian clock located in the suprachiasmatic nuclei of the hypothalamus [11]. In homeostatic conditions during the darkness, the norepinephrine-mediated activation of adrenergic receptors results in an increase of cytosolic calcium and cAMP, which activate the protein kinase A (PKA) with the consequent phosphorylation of the cAMP response element binding protein (CREB). Phosphorylated CREB migrates into the nucleus and induces the transcription of *Aanat* gene, thus fuelling the synthesis of NAS and melatonin. Moreover, PKA phosphorylates AANAT, protecting the enzyme from the proteasomal degradation.

This central clock not only ensures the adaptation of living organisms to the cyclic and seasonal environmental changes, but also allows the efficient handling of immune responses [12]. If on one hand, pineal melatonin can regulate the immune responses and rhythmically vary the immune system's components, on the other hand signals sent by immune cells can be perceived by pineal gland as feedback for the regulation of melatonin production [13, 14]. This back and forward switch in melatonin biosynthesis, namely immune-pineal axis, is considered the cornerstone of the neuroendocrine-immune network that allows the communication between immune, nervous and endocrine systems [15].

Pathogen-associated molecular patterns (PAMPs, such as bacterial lipopolysaccharide and viral double stranded RNA) as well as danger-associated molecular patterns (DAMPs; including tissue debris and amyloid β peptide) trigger the shift between pineal and extra-pineal melatonin synthesis. By interacting with their cognate receptors, PAMPs and DAMPs promote the nuclear translocation of the transcription factor nuclear factor κ-light-chain-enhancer of activated B cells (NF-κB), which binds to the promoter of target genes coding for pro-inflammatory mediators as well as of anti-inflammatory factors involved in the later recovery phase. *Aanat* is one of the genes whose transcription is regulated by NF-κB either positively or negatively, depending on cellular microenvironment. Specific NF-κB dimers allow the activation of the immune system in synch with the relocation of melatonin production from the pineal gland to the activated immune cells and vice versa. In the pinealocytes, the homodimer p50/p50 inhibits *Aanat* transcription, while in macrophages the heterodimer RelA/c-Rel induces Aanat gene expression and thus fuels the local melatonin production [16]. Whilst macrophages-derived melatonin promotes their migration to damaged tissue and enhances their phagocytic capacity, it is the indole metabolite itself that directly ends the process through the inhibition of NF-κB activity [17, 18]. The blockage of NF-κB re-establishes the homeostatic conditions and shifts the synthesis of melatonin from immune cells to pinealocytes. Moreover, during the recovery phase, melatonin is assisted by the adrenal cortex hormones (namely corticosteroids) in reducing the nuclear content of pineal p50/p50 homodimer, leading to an increase of *Aanat* transcription and thus more feed for melatonin synthesis [19].

3. Serotonin and its metabolites in immune cells

In the guise of both neurotransmitter and hormone, serotonin contributes to the regulation of several physiologic processes, such as central and peripheral functions, including sleep, mood and appetite as well as heart functionality, intestinal mobility and vascular tone among the most relevant. Accumulating evidences suggest that non-neuronal serotonin is also endowed with immunoregulatory properties. As a matter of fact, several immune cells possess the machinery to synthesize, store, respond to and take serotonin up from the microenvironment [20]. Changes in serotonin levels have been reported in patients with chronic inflammation and autoimmune dysfunctions, including multiple sclerosis (MS), rheumatoid arthritis and inflammatory bowel disease [21]. Drugs that modulate serotonin signalling, such as the selective serotonin reuptake inhibitors (SSRIs), appear to affect peripheral immunity. By blocking the reuptake of serotonin, SSRIs have found a place as anti-depressant in the clinical practice and only recently their ability to influence T lymphocytes proliferation, apoptosis and cytokines' production has emerged [22].

3.1 Serotonin receptors expression in cells of the innate immune system

In mammals, seven families of serotonin receptor (5-HTRs) have been identified (**Table 1**) [23]. All 5-HTRs belong to the G-protein coupled receptor (GPCR) superfamily, with the exception of 5-HT$_3$R, which is a ligand-gated ion channel permeable to calcium, sodium and potassium, whose activation leads to a rapid depolarization of the plasma membrane. The members of the GPCR-like serotonin receptors activate an intracellular signaling cascade that involves Adenylyl cyclase (AC) and phospholipase C (PLC) as effector systems [23]. 5-HT$_1$R and 5-HT$_5$R are negatively coupled with AC and thus their activation results in a reduced cAMP. Conversely, 5-HTRs 4, 6 and 7 are positively associated with AC with the consequent raise of cAMP levels. Upon serotonin binding, 5-HT$_2$R signals through

Target	Subtype	Ligand	Type of immune cells expressed on
5-HT_1R	A	Serotonin	Mast cells, Monocytes, Macrophages, NK cells, T and B cells
	B		Immature DCs, T cells
	E		Immature DCs, Monocytes
5-HT_2R	A		Monocytes, Macrophages, Eosinophils, T and B cells
	B		Monocytes, Macrophages, immature DCs
	C		Macrophages
5-HT_3R			Monocytes, Macrophages, DCs, T and B cells
5-HT_4R			Monocytes, Macrophages, mature DCs
5-HT_5R			Unknown
5-HT_6R			Unknown
5-HT_7R			Monocytes, Macrophages, mature DCs, T and B cells
MT1		Melatonin	Monocytes, Macrophages, Nk cells, T cells
MT2			
MT3		Melatonin, NAS	Neutrophils
RORα/RORβ		Melatonin	T cells
Free radicals		Melatonin, AFMK	Macrophages, Neutrophil
COX-2			
iNOS			
TrKB		NAS	Neutrophils, Macrophages, DCs
IDO1			DCs

Table 1.
Molecular targets of serotonin and metabolites thereof, and their expression on immune cells.

PLC-mediated release of inositol triphosphate and diacylglycerol, which increases intracellular calcium levels.

By virtue of the ubiquitous expression of the 5-HTRs and the different intracellular pathways activated, the biology of serotonin appears to be somewhat intricate and this accounts for its pleiotropic functions. 5-HTRs have been identified on murine and human innate immune cells, including neutrophils, monocytes, macrophages, dendritic cells (DCs), mast cells and natural killer cells [24]. The modulatory effects of serotonin on DCs depends on their maturity state, as 5-HTRs are differentially located on mature (mainly expressing 5-HT_4R and 5-HT_7R) and immature (expressing 5-HT_1BR and 5-HT_2BR) cells [25]. The overall literature agrees on the role of serotonin in modulating migration, morphology and cytokines' production by human and murine DCs. Through the activation of 5-HT_4R and 5-HT_7R, indeed, the monoamine affects the differentiation capacity of human monocytes to DCs, and increases the release of the anti-inflammatory cytokine IL-10, meanwhile the engagement of 5-HT_7R results in increased expression of C-C chemokine receptor type 7 (CCR7), an important receptor involved in DCs migration [25, 26].

Although the expression of several 5-HTRs has been described in both human macrophages (5-HT_1AR, 5-HT_2AR, 5-HT_2BR, 5-HT_3R and 5-HT_7R) and monocytes (5-HT_2AR, 5-HT_3R, 5-HT_4R and 5-HT_7R) at transcriptional level, only specific subtypes have been confirmed by molecular and functional studies. Indeed, through 5-HT_1AR, serotonin can induce the secretion of pro-inflammatory cytokines by peritoneal macrophages as well as boosts their phagocytic activity. Contrarily, by the engagement of 5-HT_2BR and 5HT_7R, serotonin promotes the polarization of human macrophages toward the anti-inflammatory phenotype [27]. The 5-HT_1AR is the prevailing receptor involved in inducing mast cells adhesion to fibronectin and thus in promoting their recruitment to the inflammatory bed. Unlike to other innate immune cells, mast cells express TPH1 enzyme, thus they are able to deplete Trp from the microenvironment and de novo synthesise serotonin [28]. Thanks to the presence of SERT, mast cells, macrophages and DCs are able to take serotonin up, store it in vesicles and subsequently release it in a calcium-dependent manner, in response to danger signals and inflammatory stimuli.

3.2 Serotonin receptors expression in cells of the adaptive immune system

Serotonin can shape the course of not only innate, but also adaptive immune responses, as demonstrated by its co-stimulatory role in the immunological synapse between DCs and T lymphocytes. By activating the 5-HT_2BR expressed on inflammatory monocyte-derived DCs (moDCs), serotonin alters their cytokines' profile and thus interferes with the differentiation of moDCs primed-$CD4^+$ T cells toward the inflammatory Th1 and Th17 lymphocytes [29]. Besides indirectly affecting the activation of T cells, serotonin can activate the 5-HTRs expressed on T and B cells and thus directly influence their phenotype and functions. Pioneering studies have proposed that the stimulation of 5-HT_1AR and 5-HT_3R promotes T cells proliferation, while the blockage of 5-HT_1BR with a specific antagonist decreases the cytokines' production by T lymphocytes and their cell-mediated immunity [30]. In naive-T cells, signalling through the 5-HT_7R induces the phosphorylation of the kinase ERK1/2 and activates the transcription factor NF-κB, converging in IL-2 synthesis and T-cell proliferation [31].

In addition to 5-HTRs, T cells express the high affinity transporter SERT, whose modulation with the selective inhibitors (SSRIs) suppresses T cells proliferation and induces apoptosis [32]. Moreover, T lymphocytes possess all the machinery to store, produce and degrade serotonin, suggesting an autocrine and paracrine role of the monoamine in modulating T cells proliferation and function [33]. As in platelets, the secretory ability of T cells can be affected by intracellular serotonin via a process known as serotonylation, which is the covalent linking of serotonin to glutamine residues of small intracellular GTPases involved in the exocytosis. This process occurs right after the monoamine transport into the cell, involves the enzyme transglutaminase for the creation of glutamyl-amide bonds, and results into a constitutive activation of the G-protein dependent signalling cascade [34].

The complexity of peripheral serotonin has emerged since 1999, i.e. since, when applied to intestinal preparations, opposite effects appeared depending on the conditions [35]. The variety of serotonin functions outside the CNS seems to apply also to the role of the monoamine in the regulation of immune responses. Although numerous investigations have attempted to fill the gaps in such direction, the knowledge in this field remains yet incomplete [20].

3.3 Distribution of receptors for serotonin-derived metabolites in immune cells

Likewise serotonin, melatonin exhibits a functional versatility as it regulates several biologic processes, ranging from sleep and circadian rhythm to oxidative stress, age and immune function [10, 36, 37]. Mechanistically, the physiologic effects of melatonin can be achieved through the binding of membrane and nuclear receptor as well as via receptor-independent pathways; the latter involving the interaction with cytoplasmic and mitochondrial proteins [38]. Three different subtypes of membrane receptor have been identified, i.e. melatonin receptor type 1a (MT1), type 1b (MT2) and type 1c (MT3) (**Table 1**). With the exception of MT3 (which is quinone reductase-2 enzyme), the melatonin membrane receptors belong to the GPCRs superfamily and are distributed in the CNS and, to a less extent, in cardiovascular system, colon, skin and immune cells. MT1 and MT2 are negatively coupled with AC and thus their activation results in a reduced production of cAMP and the consequent failure of PKA activation. The nuclear receptor signalling of melatonin is mediated via the transcription factor retinoid Z receptors and retinoid orphan receptors (RZR/ROR). RZR/ROR is an orphan member of the nuclear receptor superfamily, which encompasses the product of three genes: RORα, RORβ and RORγ. In immunocompetent cells, specific nuclear melatonin-binding sites have been reported, including RORα and RORβ in human lymphocytes, and RORα in both thymus and spleen of mice [39, 40].

Whilst the MT1/MT2 receptors are mainly responsible for the neuronal functions of melatonin, the activation of both nuclear and membrane receptors appears to be primarily involved in the imunomodulatory and anti-tumor effects of the hormone [41]. The exogenous administration of melatonin stimulates monocyte as well as macrophage production in both bone marrow and spleen of mice, by activating MT receptor and increasing the sensitivity of progenitors to stimulants such as IL-4 and GM-CSF [42]. Human monocytes express both membrane and nuclear melatonin receptor, whose activation stimulates the production of the pro-inflammatory cytokines IL-1β, IL-6 and TNF-α, while decreases IL-10 [42]. By engaging MT1/MT2 receptor, melatonin activates a mitogenic signal that counteracts the spontaneous apoptosis of circulating monocytes. The activity of melatonin with regard to macrophages translates into the inhibition of inducible nitric oxide synthase (iNOS) expression and blockage of COX-2 activity, with the consequent decrease of inflammatory mediators [43].

T lymphocytes express both membrane and nuclear receptors for melatonin, as well as all the machinery required for the synthesis and secretion of the hormone. Thus, is not surprising that melatonin impacts T cell biology, from the differentiation to the functional activation, as demonstrated by the blunted proliferation of splenic lymphocytes in response to mitogenic signal when both the nuclear and the MT1/MT2 receptors are inhibited [44]. Melatonin, by directly interacting with RORα and promoting its degradation, regulates the expression of IL-2 [45]. Meanwhile, through the activation of MT1-dependent signalling pathway restrains the constitutive activity of RORα, thus further stimulating the IL-2 production [46]. Such a redundancy of the membrane and nuclear receptor is at the service of T cell differentiation as well. Although RORγt is the well-known lineage specific transcription factor for Th17 cells, it synergizes with RORα to enhance Th17 differentiation. On one side, melatonin induces the degradation of nuclear RORα, while on the other, by binding MT1, it activates an intracellular signalling cascade that ends with the repression of the Rora and Rorc gene expression [47]. Depending on the immunological context, melatonin differentially controls T cells effector functions, i.e. under immunosuppressive condition, melatonin stimulates the immune system, while it inhibits exacerbated immune responses. For instance, melatonin increases the number of regulatory T cells in both human and murine model of inflammatory/autoimmune diseases, such as systemic lupus erythematosus or MS; meanwhile it reduces the frequency of IFN-γ and IL-17 producing T lymphocytes [48–50].

For many years, NAS was thought to be merely an intermediate product in melatonin biosynthesis. However, a series of non-overlapping activities of NAS as well as different brain distribution of the metabolite - when compared to melatonin and serotonin - has given a precise biologic identity to this indole derivative. NAS, but not serotonin or melatonin, is an agonist of the tyrosine kinase B (TrkB) receptor of the brain-derived neurotrophic factor (BDNF), whose activation contributes to the antidepressant, cognition-enhancing and anti-apoptotic effect of NAS (**Table 1**) [51, 52]. TrkB receptors are transmembrane proteins with an extracellular BDNF-binding domain and an intracellular tyrosine kinase domain that, once activated, undergoes autophosphorylation and subsequent coupling to intracellular signalling pathways. Through the activation of TrkB, NAS offers neuroprotection in experimental models of neurological injury and MS, which at least in part occurs by the mitigation of apoptosis and autophagic dysfunction [53, 54]. Additionally, NAS-mediated neuro-immune modulatory effects can arise from the allosteric activation of the enzyme IDO1 [55]. The direct binding of NAS to a previously unknown allosteric site on IDO1 enhances the production of the immunoregulatory metabolite L-Kynurenine, which, in turn, by re-educating the immune system, ameliorates the disease symptoms in a mouse model of MS. Moreover, NAS displays a high affinity for the melatonin MT3 receptor, which is a quinone reductase-2 enzyme and through which NAS exerts additional anti-oxidant and anti-depressant effects [56].

The metabolic product of melatonin, i.e. AFMK, is considered a potent tissue protector as it efficiently neutralizes reactive molecules and reduces lipid peroxidation and DNA damage [57]. AFMK acts as a reducing agent able to donate two electrons, in contrast with other physiological antioxidants that donate a single electron to neutralize free radicals. Increased formation of AFMK is associated with inflammatory conditions, as the concentration of this kynuramine increases in the cerebrospinal fluid of patients with meningitis and the human epidermal keratinocytes exposed to UVB radiation [58, 59]. The raised levels of AFMK are consistent with its role as tissue protector and immune modulator. Indeed, AFMK is capable to attenuate the severity of acute pancreatic inflammation, by reducing pancreatic tissue damage and TNF-α serum concentration, and by increasing the activity of anti-oxidant enzymes [60]. Likewise melatonin, AFMK prevents COX-2 and iNOS activation induced by LPS in macrophages, and the production of TNF-α and IL-8 in activated neutrophils, thus exerts anti-inflammatory and immunomodulatory effects [61, 62].

No longer considered as merely neuronal mediators, the methoxyindoles metabolites are now emerging as key modulators of immune responses. Given the intrinsic complexity of the biological systems, the evolution has conserved and specialized the functions of each serotonin derivatives, making them able to work in the same direction or independently.

4. Role of serotonin in the gut-brain axis

Is "*Butterflies in the stomach*", a metaphor or a real experience? From a physiological point of view, butterflies are authentic visceral sensations coming from an unexpected source, which is the *second* brain. Hidden in the walls of the digestive system, this intestinal brain is also known as enteric nervous system (ENS). It's generally thought that the ENS is the original nervous system that developed in the first vertebrates more than 500 million years ago and that has been conserved during the evolution to link digestion with mood and general organism's fitness [63]. The human ENS contains more than 200 million neurons, distributed in many thousands of small ganglia, the great majority of which are found in two plexuses, the myenteric and submucosal plexuses. Its main role is controlling all the digestive process from the swallowing to the nutrient absorption and elimination. It does not seem capable of common thoughts, but it can communicate back and forth with our big brain, creating the otherwise known "gut-brain axis".

The bidirectional communication underlying the gut-brain axis includes the CNS, the autonomic nervous system, the ENS and the hypothalamic pituitary adrenal (HPA) axis. On one side, the autonomic nervous system drives both afferent and efferent signals arisen from the GI and the CNS, respectively. For its part, the HPA axis is activated by environmental stressors and promotes the cortisol release from the adrenal glands. Thus, by means of hormones and neurotransmitters, the brain controls the activity of intestinal effector cells, including epithelial cells, neurons, smooth muscle, enterochromaffin and immune cells. Recently, the gut microbiome has emerged as critical component of the gut-brain axis, handling not only the local intestinal functions, but also the distant CNS activities [64, 65].

Trp and its metabolite serotonin are the main nexus for the gut-brain-microbiome axis. This link builds on the principles that (*i*) the manipulation of the microbiota composition across lifespan influences the Trp availability, (*ii*) the gut microbes can directly or indirectly affect the Trp metabolism and serotonergic signaling at the level of CNS to modulate behaviour, and (*iii*) serotonin influences the development of both ENS and CNS. Indeed, the gut microbiota can indirectly influence Trp availability by balancing the amino acid metabolism along the serotonin or the kynurenine pathway. Germ-free animals (i.e., microbiota-deficient mice raised in a sterile environment) exhibit a reduced IDO1 activity (as measured by the kyn/Trp ratio) as well as an increased central serotonin turnover, which both normalize following microbiota colonization immediately post-weaning [66, 67]. The gut microbiome can also directly affect the local and circulating Trp availability for the host, as some bacterial strains harbour the enzymes that can either utilize Trp to produce indole-derivatives (such as indole 3-acetic acid and indole-3-carboxaldehyde) or synthesize the amino acid on their own [68, 69].

Although mainly formed before the mid-gestation in the foetus, the central neuronal circuitry is continuously subjected to genetic and environmental-mediated modifications until puberty. Serotonin is considered one of the signaling molecule that can regulate the development of CNS, among many other organs, as the lack of brain serotonin results into reduced body growth and improper central circuitry formation [70]. Changes in the serotonergic system occurs across the lifespan and a decreased uptake of the metabolite follows the aging [71]. Although, in the human brain, the levels of serotonin remain fairly stable, the overall serotonin receptors reduce by about 30–50% over the lifespan. Developmental changes of serotonergic system are mirrored by the variation of gut microbiota composition during the lifetime, as the infant gut microbiota tends to reach a stable adult-like configuration in the childhood - while completely changes in elderly subjects - and the early colonization of the GI tract is fundamental for the proper development of the central serotonergic system [66].

Likewise the CNS, the ENS is capable of neurogenesis in post-natal and adult life. Such an intrinsic plasticity is mainly related to the exposure of the ENS to microbial, diet and inflammatory challenges that populate the intestinal lumen. Moreover, the normal process of aging contributes to such variability by increasing the neuronal degeneration and cell death. In mice, the post-natal neurogenesis depends on the activation of 5-HT_4Rs, whose expression affects the abundance of ENS neurons, while the differentiation of enteric nerve cells is conditioned by the activation of 5-HT_2BR [72, 73]. In addition, stimulation of 5- HT_4R inhibits inflammatory reactions, protects enteric neurons from apoptosis and promotes the mobilisation of adult stem cells to form new neurons that may replace damaged or dead ones [72].

By involving neuronal, immune and endocrine mediators, the gut-brain-microbiome axis ensures the gut homeostasis as well as integrates the peripheral intestinal activities with emotions, cognitive functions and immune activation. As a matter of fact, people coping with inflammatory bowel disease or other intestinal issues (such as constipation, diarrhoea and abdominal pain) experience depression and anxiety, as a consequence of danger signals sent by an altered GI to the CNS. Noteworthy, these people receive benefit from antidepressants and mind–body therapies that help in smoothing negative signals coming from the GI tract. It is thus clear that not only the big brain is conscious of the ENS and of the gut microbiome, but the intestine as a whole can influence the perception of the world and alter human behaviour. Therefore, in coming years, physicians will need to expand their drugs pool to treat the "mental illness" of the big brain alongside of the second brain, in order to reach therapeutic profits in both behavioural and gastrointestinal diseases.

5. Balancing act between Trp degradation pathways as a pharmacological target for CNS diseases

Serotonin biosynthesis is strictly related to tryptophan availability; in fact, Trp is metabolized not only along the serotonin pathway (SP), but also the kynurenine pathway (KP). The importance of the maintenance of a homeostatic balance between KP and SP of Trp metabolism is underlined by the hypothesis that, in the CNS, some diseases, such as depression [74], Alzheimer's [75] and Parkinson's [76] are triggered by a shift of this equilibrium towards the KP; however, little is still known between the interplay between the two Trp metabolic pathways.

As mentioned above, the very existence of serotonin in different organs and tissues is strongly conditioned by the expression and enzymatic activity of molecules belonging to the tryptophan-metabolizing family, which includes IDO1, tryptophan 2,3-dioxygenase (TDO) and, according to much of the literature to date, IDO2 [77]. Nevertheless, the role of IDO2 as an enzyme capable of initiating the degradation of Trp along the KP probably derives from the erroneous interpretation of the structural analogy between IDO1 and IDO2; recently, this concept is being progressively revisited, and now the idea is emerging that IDO2 functions are linked to an activity other than the enzymatic one [78], which is almost negligible [79]. Thus, IDO1 and TDO represent the two key players determining the fate of Trp.

Trp depletion by TDO and IDO1 occurs via a mechanism that is well studied and has rather clear consequences: as a matter of fact, the catabolism of Trp to immunosuppressive and neuroactive kynurenines is a key metabolic pathway regulating immune responses and neurotoxicity.

The KP initiated by IDO1 or TDO has two main branches (**Figure 1**). Under physiological conditions, Kyn is preferentially converted into 3-hydroxykynurenine (3HK) and then 3-hydroxyanthranilic acid (3HAA), quinolinic acid (QA), and ultimately NAD^+. Alternatively, Kyn can be converted into kynurenic acid (KynA) by the kynurenine aminotransferase (KAT) enzymes [80].

KynA is generally considered to be neuroprotective; it competitively inhibits ionotropic glutamate receptors at high concentrations, and acts as a negative allosteric modulator at the α7-nicotinic receptor [81]. Moreover, KynA has also been shown to act as an agonist at an orphan G-protein-coupled receptor in neurons and astrocytes, leading to a suppression of several inflammatory pathways [82]. KynA also regulates the immune response through its agonistic effects on the aryl hydrocarbon receptor (AhR), a transcription factor involved in the metabolism of xenobiotics. Numerous compounds have been proposed as putative endogenous AhR ligands, many of which are generated through pathways involved in the metabolism of tryptophan and indole. Among them, besides the already mentioned KynA, Kyn, xanthurenic acid, cinnabarinic acid can also be counted, as well as indole derivatives mainly produced in the gut by microbial metabolism, such as indole-3-acetic acid (IAA), indole-3-aldeyde (IAld) and tryptamine; the activation of AhR by metabolites produced downstream IDO1 or TDO may contribute to the modulation of the immune response both in periphery and CNS [83].

QA is an NMDA receptor agonist that can also inhibit the reuptake of glutamate by astrocytes leading to excitotoxicity, and exerts neurotoxic effects via several different mechanisms, including the generation of reactive oxygen species and the disruption of the blood brain barrier. In astrocytes, QA also potentiates the inflammatory response by inducing the production of proinflammatory mediators; moreover, QA may also activate microglia through NMDA receptors, a pathway that triggers neuronal cell death [81].

The two enzymes leading to the activation of the KP, TDO and IDO1 are localized in different cells and tissues and are used in different physiological processes. Hepatic TDO regulates blood homeostasis of Trp and neuronal TDO influences neurogenesis. TDO-deficient mice show no peculiar phenotypes, but display alterations in neurogenesis and anxiety-related behaviour. Moreover, TDO-deficiency or inhibition is neuroprotective in a murine model of MS, suggesting a role for TDO in the production of byproducts involved in the pathogenesis of neurological autoimmune diseases [84].

IDO1 is expressed in most tissues at low levels, including cells of the central nervous system (CNS) and cells of the immune system, but not in the liver. The activity of IDO1 is more closely related to the modulation of the immune response than to the regulation of dietary levels of Trp, and, as in the case of TDO, is decisive in the production of neuroactive metabolites. The effects of Trp metabolism by IDO1 (or TDO) in immunity are complex, and can be shortly explained by four mechanisms: (i) by means of the so-called "Trp starvation", that is, locally depleting Trp, which deprives tryptophan-dependent cells, such as proliferating T cells, of an essential amino acid; (ii) by the production of bioactive kynurenines; (iii) by regulating immune cell metabolism, for example, by feeding de novo NAD^+ biosynthesis; and (iv) by means of a recently discovered signalling activity, through which IDO1 becomes phosphorylated in its immunoreceptor tyrosine-based inhibitory motifs (ITIMs), so to mediate intracellular signalling events in a self-sustaining feedforward loop leading to durable immunoregulatory effects [85]. All these mechanisms are involved on the potential development of neuropsychiatric disorders [83], since, as previously said, many kynurenines are neuroactive, modulating neuroplasticity and/or exerting neurotoxic effects. Thus, it is not surprising that KP is considered implicated in psychiatric illness in the context of inflammation, such as mood disorders (i.e., major depressive disorder - MDD), psychosis, schizophrenia, as well as in neurodegenerative disorders such as Alzheimer's and Parkinson's disease (all reviewed in [81]) and autoimmune diseases, such as MS.

Many efforts in drug development for neurodegenerative and neuropsychiatric diseases have focused on altering the overall balance of neuroactive KP metabolites production through inhibition of enzymes involved in the formation of either QA or KA, or by means of synthetic molecules mimicking the effects of the endogenous compounds. The first clinical trials for MDD are currently ongoing, assessing the effects of an analogous of KynA, AV-101 (NCT02484456 and NCT03078322). AV-101 is a selective antagonist at the glycine-binding site of the NMDA receptor [86].

Since Trp, Kyn, and 3HK can be transported across the blood brain barrier (BBB), and other KP metabolites possibly share the same feature [81], another potential target is the carrier facilitating the passage through the BBB, that is the large amino acid transporter (LAT1). It has been recently demonstrated that leucine treatment is a feasible method of competitively blocking LAT1 to prevent exogenous Kyn from entering into the brain [87]; on the basis of this observation, a phase 2 clinical trial to test the anti-depressant effects of leucine in individuals with MDD is currently ongoing (NCT03079297). Nevertheless, recent findings suggest that several established treatments for depression also alter KP metabolism, as in case of the electro-convulsive therapy, which significantly increases circulating levels of KynA and KynA/3HK in depressed patients [88]. Another example is represented by Ketamine, used as treatment for MDD in selected population of patients, that was shown to acutely decrease circulating kyn and the Kyn/Trp [89].

However, besides the overt involvement of KP in the pathogenesis of several CNS diseases, how the production of kynurenines and the shift of the Trp metabolism from SP towards KP affect the production of serotonin to date it is not clear, and it's also a subject of intense investigation whether the reduced production of serotonin, and the molecules thereof, is involved in the pathogenesis of certain diseases. In the specific case of MDD, the Trp metabolism is considered to explain the aetiology and pathogenesis of depression. More specifically, the aetiology of MDD seems to rely on the concomitant manifestation of an imbalance between the Kyn pathway induced by IDO1 and the serotonin pathway, the neurotoxic effects of Kyn pathway metabolites and the persistent activation of the KP due to exposure to repeated and consistent stress. A further example of the close connection of neuronal and immune systems, and of the importance of a balance between the two branches of Trp metabolism for the maintenance of a health status, can be represented by depression related to cancer. A simplistic and nowadays outdated vision of the immunological asset of cancer patients proposed that one of the major causes of depression in cancer patients could be related to their apparent immunosuppressive general status; today this perspective is gradually undermined by the awareness that in many types of cancer, chronic inflammation is a common feature. Trp breakdown, and the subsequent reduction of the production of serotonin and metabolites thereof, due to the enhanced activation of enzymes of the KP, seems to be related to the prevalence of depressive disorders in cancer patients, since many patients often show decreased plasma Trp levels and increased kyn concentrations [90]. In line with this hypothesis, and with the identification of IDO1 as an authentic immune checkpoint target for the immunopharmacological treatment of cancer [91], inhibition of IDO1 and/or TDO seems to be a promising strategy for the treatment of cancer-related fatigue and depression, with the aim of restoring the physiological balance between the KP and the SP [92].

Moreover, there is an additional factor to consider: not only the functional activity of IDO1/TDO can push the balance towards a decreased production of serotonin, but also the production of specific serotonin metabolites can, in turn, affect this balance, in favour of a sustained production of kynurenines. This is the case of NAS. As previously mentioned, a consistent part of the antidepressant and neurotrophic actions of NAS is due to its capability to activate the TrkB receptor; nevertheless, very recently, additional exciting mechanisms of action of NAS have been demonstrated, unveiling its role as an immunomodulatory molecule. In fact, NAS and melatonin have potent anti-oxidant, anti-inflammatory and neuroprotective properties in several animal models of neurological injury and disease, including MS [53]. When administered in vivo in a murine model of multiple sclerosis, experimental autoimmune encephalomyelitis (EAE), melatonin and NAS reduced the loss of mature oligodendrocytes, demyelination and axonal injury, significatively ameliorating the disease symptoms and progression. Both compounds also significantly attenuated iNOS induction and reactive oxygen species (ROS) generation in lipopolysaccharide-activated microglia in culture [53].

Moreover, NAS is capable of inducing DCs to acquire an immunosuppressive phenotype, which requires the presence and functional activity of the enzyme IDO1. Very interestingly, NAS has been demonstrated to function as a positive allosteric modulator of the enzyme IDO1 binding a recently identified allosteric site thus increasing the catalytic efficacy, but not the binding affinity of IDO1 toward its substrate Trp [55]. Moreover, the effects of NAS have been demonstrated not only in murine DCs, but also in peripheral blood mononuclear cells from a specific subset of MS patients, that is RR-MS patients, opening the possibility for the identification of an innovative and safe immunomodulating therapy for MS. NAS is the first-identified indole derivative of the SP acting as an endogenous IDO1 positive allosteric modulator (PAM). It is noteworthy that Trp shows an opposite behaviour, acting as an IDO1 negative allosteric modulator (NAM) when present at high concentrations [93]. Therefore, although kynurenines acting as endogenous PAMs for the enzymes of the serotonin pathway have not been identified yet, it is possible to speculate that products downstream of the KP and the SP might guarantee an appropriate equilibrium between the two main metabolic routes of Trp metabolism by allosteric mechanisms. This hypothesis may have important relevance for the design of innovative therapeutic strategies not only for the treatment of inflammatory/autoimmune CNS diseases, such as MS, but also for diseases involving an altered regulation of Trp metabolism. As an example, the therapeutic use of potent orthosteric inhibitors of IDO1 for the cancer immunotherapy could be hampered by the induction of a skewing toward the serotonin pathway and thus an excess production of immunoregulatory NAS. Regarding the possibility of rethinking the therapeutic approach for CNS inflammatory/autoimmune diseases, such as MS, that is immunosuppression, the development of PAMs selective for the IDO1 enzyme and therapeutically active in vivo may provide unprecedented opportunities to develop therapeutic agents with a considerably more limited number of undesirable effects than the conventional immunosuppressive therapy.

A cross-regulation of the two metabolic pathways of Trp degradation is performed not only by NAS, but also by its derivative melatonin. As previously said, melatonin can be used by the enzyme IDO1 as a substrate, giving rise to the production of AFMK, a metabolite endowed with anti-inflammatory properties. The effects of AFMK on expression and functional activity of Trp metabolizing enzymes are still unknown, if there are any. Melatonin not only can be metabolized by IDO1, but is capable of inducing the expression of the IDO1 gene in fibroblasts, melanocytes and in adrenal pheochromocytoma cells. In the latter model, silencing of IDO1 gene triggered the up-regulation of the expression of AANAT gene [94], and the overexpression of IDO1, in turns, led to the down-regulation of AANAT, meaning that, in specific cellular subsets, a strictly interconnection occurs between the two Trp degradation pathways. In the same study, melatonin induced an up-regulation of the IDO1 expression, through the JAK-STAT2 signaling pathway, and of its enzymatic activity.

Moreover, melatonin is a competitive inhibitor, whereas serotonin is an allosteric inhibitor of the enzyme TDO [95] and although the biological significance of this effects has not been unveiled, it can be speculated that, in the CNS, inhibition of TDO by two metabolites of the SP could contribute to a shift of the balance of Trp consumption through the SP, depending on microenvironmental factors.

Overall, a huge number of pharmacological interventions for CNS diseases targeting Trp metabolism have been developed or are currently under investigation (reviewed in [96]), ranging from the inhibition of specific enzymes along the KP to the modulation of AhR signalling or administration of KYNA and its derivatives [96]; nevertheless, the interconnections between the major pathways of Trp metabolism remain an open question.

6. Concluding remarks

Bidirectional interactions between the nervous system and immune system, known as the "neuroimmune system", regulate a wide range of physiological and pathological processes [1] and there is a huge literature linking general neuroinflammation to neuropsychiatric disorders, such as depression [97], schizophrenia [98], but also MS [99], Alzheimer's [100] and Parkinson's disease [101]. Specific neuroimmune factors, such as Trp derivatives, have been shown to modulate neuronal activity and complex behavioral processes and to create a functional bridge connecting the neuroendocrine and the immune systems. For this reason, serotonin and its derivatives, and the metabolic processes leading to the production of serotonin rather than kyn, are involved in the pathogenesis of various CNS diseases. Thus, it's easy to imagine how Trp metabolism, and mostly the pursuit of an optimal balance between the two Trp metabolic pathways, may be a promising therapeutic target for a manifold spectrum of CNS pathologies. However, there is need for an in-depth knowledge of the mechanisms leading to one or the other Trp metabolic fate, and it's also necessary to unveil their interconnections to define the appropriate intervention for each specific disease, and to have the ability to precisely act on the targeted metabolite or enzyme.

Acknowledgements

This work was supported by the Italian Ministry of Education, University, and Research (PRIN 20173EAZ2Z; to C.V.) and by the University of Perugia (Fondo Ricerca di Base 2019 RB2019GMON; to G.M.)

Conflict of interest

The authors declare no conflict of interest.

List of abbreviations

3HAA	3-hydroxyanthranilic acid
3HK	3-hydroxykynurenine
5-HT	serotonin
5-HTRs	serotonin receptor
AADC	5-hydroxytryptophan decarboxylase
AANAT	arylalkylamine N-acetyltransferase
AC	Adenylyl cyclase
AFMK	N-acetyl-N-formyl-5-methoxykynurenamine
AhR	aryl hydrocarbon receptor
ASMT	acetylserotonin O-methyltransferase
BBB	blood brain barrier
BDNF	brain-derived neurotrophic factor
CCR7	C-C chemokine receptor type 7
CNS	central nervous system
CREB	cAMP response element binding protein
DAMPs	danger-associated molecular patterns
DCs	dendritic cells
EC	enterochromaffin cells

ENS	enteric nervous system
GI	gastro-intestinal tract
GPCR	G-protein coupled receptor
HIOM	hydroxyindole-O-methyl transferase
IAA	indole-3-acetic acid
IAld	indole-3-aldeyde
IDO	indoleamine 2, 3-dioxygenase
INMT	indolethylamine-N-methyltransferase
iNOS	nitric oxide synthase
ITIMs	immune-based inhibitory tyrosine motifs
KAT	kynurenine aminotransferase
KP	kynurenine pathway
KynA	kynurenic acid
LAT1	large amino acid transporter
MAO	monoamine oxidases
MDD	major depressive disorder
MT	melatonin receptor
NAM	negative allosteric modulator
NAS	N-acetylserotonin
NF-κB	nuclear factor κ-light-chain-enhancer of activated B cells
PAM	positive allosteric modulator
PAMPs	Pathogen-associated molecular patterns
PKA	protein kinase A
PLC	phospholipase C
QA	quinolinic acid
ROS	reactive oxygen species
RZR/ROR	retinoid Z receptors and retinoid orphan receptors
SERT	serotonin reuptake transporter
SP	serotonin pathway
SSRIs	selective serotonin reuptake inhibitors
TDO	tryptophan 2, 3-dioxygenase
TPH	tryptophan hydroxylase
TrkB	tyrosine kinase B
Trp	Tryptophan
VMAT	vesicular monoamine transporter

Author details

Giada Mondanelli and Claudia Volpi*
Department of Medicine and Surgery, University of Perugia, Perugia, Italy

*Address all correspondence to: claudia.volpi@unipg.it

References

[1] R. Dantzer, Neuroimmune Interactions: From the Brain to the Immune System and Vice Versa, Physiol Rev. 98 (2018) 477-504. https://doi.org/10.1152/physrev.00039.2016.

[2] R. Hardeland, R.J. Reiter, B. Poeggeler, D.X. Tan, The significance of the metabolism of the neurohormone melatonin: antioxidative protection and formation of bioactive substances, Neurosci Biobehav Rev. 17 (1993) 347-357. https://doi.org/10.1016/s0149-7634(05)80016-8.

[3] S.O. Silva, V.F. Ximenes, L.H. Catalani, A. Campa, Myeloperoxidase-catalyzed oxidation of melatonin by activated neutrophils, Biochem Biophys Res Commun. 279 (2000) 657-662. https://doi.org/10.1006/bbrc.2000.3993.

[4] D.X. Tan, L.C. Manchester, R.J. Reiter, B.F. Plummer, J. Limson, S.T. Weintraub, W. Qi, Melatonin directly scavenges hydrogen peroxide: a potentially new metabolic pathway of melatonin biotransformation, Free Radic Biol Med. 29 (2000) 1177-1185. https://doi.org/10.1016/s0891-5849(00)00435-4.

[5] G. Mondanelli, C. Volpi, The double life of serotonin metabolites: in the mood for joining neuronal and immune systems, Curr Opin Immunol. 70 (2020) 1-6. https://doi.org/10.1016/j.coi.2020.11.008.

[6] M. Berger, J.A. Gray, B.L. Roth, The expanded biology of serotonin, Annu Rev Med. 60 (2009) 355-366. https://doi.org/10.1146/annurev.med.60.042307.110802.

[7] L.F. Mohammad-Zadeh, L. Moses, S.M. Gwaltney-Brant, Serotonin: a review, J Vet Pharmacol Ther. 31 (2008) 187-199. https://doi.org/10.1111/j.1365-2885.2008.00944.x.

[8] D.J. Walther, M. Bader, A unique central tryptophan hydroxylase isoform, Biochem Pharmacol. 66 (2003) 1673-1680. https://doi.org/10.1016/s0006-2952(03)00556-2.

[9] C. Jonnakuty, C. Gragnoli, What do we know about serotonin?, J Cell Physiol. 217 (2008) 301-306. https://doi.org/10.1002/jcp.21533.

[10] J. Vriend, R.J. Reiter, Melatonin feedback on clock genes: a theory involving the proteasome, J Pineal Res. 58 (2015) 1-11. https://doi.org/10.1111/jpi.12189.

[11] D.C. Klein, S.L. Coon, P.H. Roseboom, J.L. Weller, M. Bernard, J.A. Gastel, M. Zatz, P.M. Iuvone, I.R. Rodriguez, V. Bégay, J. Falcón, G.M. Cahill, V.M. Cassone, R. Baler, The melatonin rhythm-generating enzyme: molecular regulation of serotonin N-acetyltransferase in the pineal gland, Recent Prog Horm Res. 52 (1997) 307-357; discussion 357-358.

[12] C. Scheiermann, Y. Kunisaki, P.S. Frenette, Circadian control of the immune system, Nat Rev Immunol. 13 (2013) 190-198. https://doi.org/10.1038/nri3386.

[13] A. Carrillo-Vico, P.J. Lardone, N. Alvarez-Sánchez, A. Rodríguez-Rodríguez, J.M. Guerrero, Melatonin: buffering the immune system, Int J Mol Sci. 14 (2013) 8638-8683. https://doi.org/10.3390/ijms14048638.

[14] R.J. Nelson, D.L. Drazen, Melatonin mediates seasonal changes in immune function, Ann N Y Acad Sci. 917 (2000) 404-415. https://doi.org/10.1111/j.1749-6632.2000.tb05405.x.

[15] R.P. Markus, Z.S. Ferreira, P.A.C.M. Fernandes, E. Cecon, The

immune-pineal axis: a shuttle between endocrine and paracrine melatonin sources, Neuroimmunomodulation. 14 (2007) 126-133. https://doi.org/10.1159/000110635.

[16] R.P. Markus, E. Cecon, M.A. Pires-Lapa, Immune-pineal axis: nuclear factor κB (NF-kB) mediates the shift in the melatonin source from pinealocytes to immune competent cells, Int J Mol Sci. 14 (2013) 10979-10997. https://doi.org/10.3390/ijms140610979.

[17] M. Marçola, S. da Silveira Cruz-Machado, P.A.C.M. Fernandes, A.W.A. Monteiro, R.P. Markus, E.K. Tamura, Endothelial cell adhesiveness is a function of environmental lighting and melatonin level, J Pineal Res. 54 (2013) 162-169. https://doi.org/10.1111/j.1600-079X.2012.01025.x.

[18] J.L. Mauriz, P.S. Collado, C. Veneroso, R.J. Reiter, J. González-Gallego, A review of the molecular aspects of melatonin's anti-inflammatory actions: recent insights and new perspectives, J Pineal Res. 54 (2013) 1-14. https://doi.org/10.1111/j.1600-079X.2012.01014.x.

[19] Z.S. Ferreira, P.A.C.M. Fernandes, D. Duma, J. Assreuy, M.C.W. Avellar, R.P. Markus, Corticosterone modulates noradrenaline-induced melatonin synthesis through inhibition of nuclear factor kappa B, J Pineal Res. 38 (2005) 182-188. https://doi.org/10.1111/j.1600-079X.2004.00191.x.

[20] N. Herr, C. Bode, D. Duerschmied, The Effects of Serotonin in Immune Cells, Front Cardiovasc Med. 4 (2017) 48. https://doi.org/10.3389/fcvm.2017.00048.

[21] M. Wan, L. Ding, D. Wang, J. Han, P. Gao, Serotonin: A Potent Immune Cell Modulator in Autoimmune Diseases, Front Immunol. 11 (2020) 186. https://doi.org/10.3389/fimmu.2020.00186.

[22] V. Gobin, K. Van Steendam, D. Denys, D. Deforce, Selective serotonin reuptake inhibitors as a novel class of immunosuppressants, Int Immunopharmacol. 20 (2014) 148-156. https://doi.org/10.1016/j.intimp.2014.02.030.

[23] M. Filip, M. Bader, Overview on 5-HT receptors and their role in physiology and pathology of the central nervous system, Pharmacol Rep. 61 (2009) 761-777. https://doi.org/10.1016/s1734-1140(09)70132-x.

[24] N.L. Baganz, R.D. Blakely, A dialogue between the immune system and brain, spoken in the language of serotonin, ACS Chem Neurosci. 4 (2013) 48-63. https://doi.org/10.1021/cn300186b.

[25] M. Idzko, E. Panther, C. Stratz, T. Müller, H. Bayer, G. Zissel, T. Dürk, S. Sorichter, F. Di Virgilio, M. Geissler, B. Fiebich, Y. Herouy, P. Elsner, J. Norgauer, D. Ferrari, The serotoninergic receptors of human dendritic cells: identification and coupling to cytokine release, J Immunol. 172 (2004) 6011-6019. https://doi.org/10.4049/jimmunol.172.10.6011.

[26] K. Holst, D. Guseva, S. Schindler, M. Sixt, A. Braun, H. Chopra, O. Pabst, E. Ponimaskin, The serotonin receptor 5-HT_7R regulates the morphology and migratory properties of dendritic cells, J Cell Sci. 128 (2015) 2866-2880. https://doi.org/10.1242/jcs.167999.

[27] M. de las Casas-Engel, A. Domínguez-Soto, E. Sierra-Filardi, R. Bragado, C. Nieto, A. Puig-Kroger, R. Samaniego, M. Loza, M.T. Corcuera, F. Gómez-Aguado, M. Bustos, P. Sánchez-Mateos, A.L. Corbí, Serotonin skews human macrophage polarization through HTR2B and HTR7, J Immunol. 190 (2013) 2301-2310. https://doi.org/10.4049/jimmunol.1201133.

[28] N.M. Kushnir-Sukhov, J.M. Brown, Y. Wu, A. Kirshenbaum, D.D. Metcalfe, Human mast cells are capable of serotonin synthesis and release, J Allergy Clin Immunol. 119 (2007) 498-499. https://doi.org/10.1016/j.jaci.2006.09.003.

[29] A. Szabo, P. Gogolak, G. Koncz, Z. Foldvari, K. Pazmandi, N. Miltner, S. Poliska, A. Bacsi, S. Djurovic, E. Rajnavolgyi, Immunomodulatory capacity of the serotonin receptor 5-HT2B in a subset of human dendritic cells, Sci Rep. 8 (2018) 1765. https://doi.org/10.1038/s41598-018-20173-y.

[30] J. Yin, R.H. Albert, A.P. Tretiakova, B.A. Jameson, 5-HT(1B) receptors play a prominent role in the proliferation of T-lymphocytes, J Neuroimmunol. 181 (2006) 68-81. https://doi.org/10.1016/j.jneuroim.2006.08.004.

[31] M. León-Ponte, G.P. Ahern, P.J. O'Connell, Serotonin provides an accessory signal to enhance T-cell activation by signaling through the 5-HT7 receptor, Blood. 109 (2007) 3139-3146. https://doi.org/10.1182/blood-2006-10-052787.

[32] F. Fazzino, C. Montes, M. Urbina, I. Carreira, L. Lima, Serotonin transporter is differentially localized in subpopulations of lymphocytes of major depression patients. Effect of fluoxetine on proliferation, J Neuroimmunol. 196 (2008) 173-180. https://doi.org/10.1016/j.jneuroim.2008.03.012.

[33] Y. Chen, M. Leon-Ponte, S.C. Pingle, P.J. O'Connell, G.P. Ahern, T lymphocytes possess the machinery for 5-HT synthesis, storage, degradation and release, Acta Physiol (Oxf). 213 (2015) 860-867. https://doi.org/10.1111/apha.12470.

[34] D.J. Walther, J.-U. Peter, S. Winter, M. Höltje, N. Paulmann, M. Grohmann, J. Vowinckel, V. Alamo-Bethencourt, C.S. Wilhelm, G. Ahnert-Hilger, M. Bader, Serotonylation of small GTPases is a signal transduction pathway that triggers platelet alpha-granule release, Cell. 115 (2003) 851-862. https://doi.org/10.1016/s0092-8674(03)01014-6.

[35] M.D. Gershon, Review article: roles played by 5-hydroxytryptamine in the physiology of the bowel, Aliment Pharmacol Ther. 13 Suppl 2 (1999) 15-30.

[36] E. Miller, A. Morel, L. Saso, J. Saluk, Melatonin Redox Activity. Its Potential Clinical Application in Neurodegenerative Disorders, Curr Top Med Chem. (2014).

[37] L.H. Opie, S. Lecour, Melatonin has multiorgan effects, Eur Heart J Cardiovasc Pharmacother. 2 (2016) 258-265. https://doi.org/10.1093/ehjcvp/pvv037.

[38] R.J. Reiter, D.X. Tan, L.C. Manchester, M. Pilar Terron, L.J. Flores, S. Koppisepi, Medical implications of melatonin: receptor-mediated and receptor-independent actions, Adv Med Sci. 52 (2007) 11-28.

[39] A. Carrillo-Vico, A. García-Pergañeda, L. Naji, J.R. Calvo, M.P. Romero, J.M. Guerrero, Expression of membrane and nuclear melatonin receptor mRNA and protein in the mouse immune system, Cell Mol Life Sci. 60 (2003) 2272-2278. https://doi.org/10.1007/s00018-003-3207-4.

[40] S. García-Mauriño, D. Pozo, J.R. Calvo, J.M. Guerrero, Correlation between nuclear melatonin receptor expression and enhanced cytokine production in human lymphocytic and monocytic cell lines, J Pineal Res. 29 (2000) 129-137. https://doi.org/10.1034/j.1600-079x.2000.290301.x.

[41] J.A. García, H. Volt, C. Venegas, C. Doerrier, G. Escames, L.C. López, D. Acuña-Castroviejo, Disruption of the NF-κB/NLRP3 connection by

melatonin requires retinoid-related orphan receptor-α and blocks the septic response in mice, FASEB J. 29 (2015) 3863-3875. https://doi.org/10.1096/fj.15-273656.

[42] J.R. Calvo, C. González-Yanes, M.D. Maldonado, The role of melatonin in the cells of the innate immunity: a review, J Pineal Res. 55 (2013) 103-120. https://doi.org/10.1111/jpi.12075.

[43] W.-G. Deng, S.-T. Tang, H.-P. Tseng, K.K. Wu, Melatonin suppresses macrophage cyclooxygenase-2 and inducible nitric oxide synthase expression by inhibiting p52 acetylation and binding, Blood. 108 (2006) 518-524. https://doi.org/10.1182/blood-2005-09-3691.

[44] D.L. Drazen, D. Bilu, S.D. Bilbo, R.J. Nelson, Melatonin enhancement of splenocyte proliferation is attenuated by luzindole, a melatonin receptor antagonist, Am J Physiol Regul Integr Comp Physiol. 280 (2001) R1476–R1482. https://doi.org/10.1152/ajpregu.2001.280.5.R1476.

[45] P.J. Lardone, J.M. Guerrero, J.M. Fernández-Santos, A. Rubio, I. Martín-Lacave, A. Carrillo-Vico, Melatonin synthesized by T lymphocytes as a ligand of the retinoic acid-related orphan receptor, J Pineal Res. 51 (2011) 454-462. https://doi.org/10.1111/j.1600-079X.2011.00909.x.

[46] P.J. Lardone, A. Carrillo-Vico, P. Molinero, A. Rubio, J.M. Guerrero, A novel interplay between membrane and nuclear melatonin receptors in human lymphocytes: significance in IL-2 production, Cell Mol Life Sci. 66 (2009) 516-525. https://doi.org/10.1007/s00018-008-8601-5.

[47] X. Yu, D. Rollins, K.A. Ruhn, J.J. Stubblefield, C.B. Green, M. Kashiwada, P.B. Rothman, J.S. Takahashi, L.V. Hooper, TH17 cell differentiation is regulated by the circadian clock, Science. 342 (2013) 727-730. https://doi.org/10.1126/science.1243884.

[48] N. Álvarez-Sánchez, I. Cruz-Chamorro, A. López-González, J.C. Utrilla, J.M. Fernández-Santos, A. Martínez-López, P.J. Lardone, J.M. Guerrero, A. Carrillo-Vico, Melatonin controls experimental autoimmune encephalomyelitis by altering the T effector/regulatory balance, Brain Behav Immun. 50 (2015) 101-114. https://doi.org/10.1016/j.bbi.2015.06.021.

[49] M.F. Farez, I.D. Mascanfroni, S.P. Méndez-Huergo, A. Yeste, G. Murugaiyan, L.P. Garo, M.E. Balbuena Aguirre, B. Patel, M.C. Ysrraelit, C. Zhu, V.K. Kuchroo, G.A. Rabinovich, F.J. Quintana, J. Correale, Melatonin Contributes to the Seasonality of Multiple Sclerosis Relapses, Cell. 162 (2015) 1338-1352. https://doi.org/10.1016/j.cell.2015.08.025.

[50] P. Medrano-Campillo, H. Sarmiento-Soto, N. Álvarez-Sánchez, A.I. Álvarez-Ríos, J.M. Guerrero, I. Rodríguez-Prieto, M.J. Castillo-Palma, P.J. Lardone, A. Carrillo-Vico, Evaluation of the immunomodulatory effect of melatonin on the T-cell response in peripheral blood from systemic lupus erythematosus patients, J Pineal Res. 58 (2015) 219-226. https://doi.org/10.1111/jpi.12208.

[51] G. Tosini, K. Ye, P.M. Iuvone, N-acetylserotonin: neuroprotection, neurogenesis, and the sleepy brain, Neuroscientist. 18 (2012) 645-653. https://doi.org/10.1177/1073858412446634.

[52] S. Bachurin, G. Oxenkrug, N. Lermontova, A. Afanasiev, B. Beznosko, G. Vankin, E. Shevtzova, T. Mukhina, T. Serkova, N-acetylserotonin, melatonin and their derivatives improve cognition and protect against beta-amyloid-induced neurotoxicity, Ann N Y Acad Sci. 890 (1999) 155-166. https://doi.org/10.1111/j.1749-6632.1999.tb07990.x.

[53] J. Wen, P.S. Ariyannur, R. Ribeiro, M. Tanaka, J.R. Moffett, B.F. Kirmani, A.M.A. Namboodiri, Y. Zhang, Efficacy of N-Acetylserotonin and Melatonin in the EAE Model of Multiple Sclerosis, J Neuroimmune Pharmacol. 11 (2016) 763-773. https://doi.org/10.1007/s11481-016-9702-9.

[54] J.-M. Yoo, B.D. Lee, D.-E. Sok, J.Y. Ma, M.R. Kim, Neuroprotective action of N-acetyl serotonin in oxidative stress-induced apoptosis through the activation of both TrkB/CREB/BDNF pathway and Akt/Nrf2/Antioxidant enzyme in neuronal cells, Redox Biol. 11 (2017) 592-599. https://doi.org/10.1016/j.redox.2016.12.034.

[55] G. Mondanelli, A. Coletti, F.A. Greco, M.T. Pallotta, C. Orabona, A. Iacono, M.L. Belladonna, E. Albini, E. Panfili, F. Fallarino, M. Gargaro, G. Manni, D. Matino, A. Carvalho, C. Cunha, P. Maciel, M. Di Filippo, L. Gaetani, R. Bianchi, C. Vacca, I.M. Iamandii, E. Proietti, F. Boscia, L. Annunziato, M. Peppelenbosch, P. Puccetti, P. Calabresi, A. Macchiarulo, L. Santambrogio, C. Volpi, U. Grohmann, Positive allosteric modulation of indoleamine 2,3-dioxygenase 1 restrains neuroinflammation, Proc. Natl. Acad. Sci. U.S.A. 117 (2020) 3848-3857. https://doi.org/10.1073/pnas.1918215117.

[56] J.A. Boutin, E. Marcheteau, P. Hennig, N. Moulharat, S. Berger, P. Delagrange, J.-P. Bouchet, G. Ferry, MT3/QR2 melatonin binding site does not use melatonin as a substrate or a co-substrate, J Pineal Res. 45 (2008) 524-531. https://doi.org/10.1111/j.1600-079X.2008.00631.x.

[57] A. Galano, D.X. Tan, R.J. Reiter, On the free radical scavenging activities of melatonin's metabolites, AFMK and AMK, J Pineal Res. 54 (2013) 245-257. https://doi.org/10.1111/jpi.12010.

[58] S. de O. Silva, V.F. Ximenes, J.A. Livramento, L.H. Catalani, A. Campa, High concentrations of the melatonin metabolite, N1-acetyl-N2-formyl-5-methoxykynuramine, in cerebrospinal fluid of patients with meningitis: a possible immunomodulatory mechanism, J Pineal Res. 39 (2005) 302-306. https://doi.org/10.1111/j.1600-079X.2005.00247.x.

[59] Z. Janjetovic, Z.P. Nahmias, S. Hanna, S.G. Jarrett, T.-K. Kim, R.J. Reiter, A.T. Slominski, Melatonin and its metabolites ameliorate ultraviolet B-induced damage in human epidermal keratinocytes, J Pineal Res. 57 (2014) 90-102. https://doi.org/10.1111/jpi.12146.

[60] J. Jaworek, J. Szklarczyk, J. Bonior, M. Kot, M. Goralska, P. Pierzchalski, R.J. Reiter, U. Czech, R. Tomaszewska, Melatonin metabolite, N(1)-acetyl-N(1)-formyl-5-methoxykynuramine (AFMK), attenuates acute pancreatitis in the rat: in vivo and in vitro studies, J Physiol Pharmacol. 67 (2016) 411-421.

[61] J.C. Mayo, R.M. Sainz, D.-X. Tan, R. Hardeland, J. Leon, C. Rodriguez, R.J. Reiter, Anti-inflammatory actions of melatonin and its metabolites, N1-acetyl-N2-formyl-5-methoxykynuramine (AFMK) and N1-acetyl-5-methoxykynuramine (AMK), in macrophages, J Neuroimmunol. 165 (2005) 139-149. https://doi.org/10.1016/j.jneuroim.2005.05.002.

[62] S.O. Silva, M.R. Rodrigues, V.F. Ximenes, A.E.B. Bueno-da-Silva, G.P. Amarante-Mendes, A. Campa, Neutrophils as a specific target for melatonin and kynuramines: effects on cytokine release, J Neuroimmunol. 156 (2004) 146-152. https://doi.org/10.1016/j.jneuroim.2004.07.015.

[63] M. Rao, M.D. Gershon, The bowel and beyond: the enteric nervous system in neurological disorders, Nat Rev Gastroenterol Hepatol. 13 (2016)

517-528. https://doi.org/10.1038/nrgastro.2016.107.

[64] S.M. Collins, M. Surette, P. Bercik, The interplay between the intestinal microbiota and the brain, Nat Rev Microbiol. 10 (2012) 735-742. https://doi.org/10.1038/nrmicro2876.

[65] S. Grenham, G. Clarke, J.F. Cryan, T.G. Dinan, Brain-gut-microbe communication in health and disease, Front Physiol. 2 (2011) 94. https://doi.org/10.3389/fphys.2011.00094.

[66] G. Clarke, S. Grenham, P. Scully, P. Fitzgerald, R.D. Moloney, F. Shanahan, T.G. Dinan, J.F. Cryan, The microbiome-gut-brain axis during early life regulates the hippocampal serotonergic system in a sex-dependent manner, Mol Psychiatry. 18 (2013) 666-673. https://doi.org/10.1038/mp.2012.77.

[67] R. Diaz Heijtz, S. Wang, F. Anuar, Y. Qian, B. Björkholm, A. Samuelsson, M.L. Hibberd, H. Forssberg, S. Pettersson, Normal gut microbiota modulates brain development and behavior, Proc Natl Acad Sci U S A. 108 (2011) 3047-3052. https://doi.org/10.1073/pnas.1010529108.

[68] J.-H. Lee, J. Lee, Indole as an intercellular signal in microbial communities, FEMS Microbiol Rev. 34 (2010) 426-444. https://doi.org/10.1111/j.1574-6976.2009.00204.x.

[69] S. Raboni, S. Bettati, A. Mozzarelli, Tryptophan synthase: a mine for enzymologists, Cell Mol Life Sci. 66 (2009) 2391-2403. https://doi.org/10.1007/s00018-009-0028-0.

[70] S. Migliarini, G. Pacini, B. Pelosi, G. Lunardi, M. Pasqualetti, Lack of brain serotonin affects postnatal development and serotonergic neuronal circuitry formation, Mol Psychiatry. 18 (2013) 1106-1118. https://doi.org/10.1038/mp.2012.128.

[71] L.C. Murrin, J.D. Sanders, D.B. Bylund, Comparison of the maturation of the adrenergic and serotonergic neurotransmitter systems in the brain: implications for differential drug effects on juveniles and adults, Biochem Pharmacol. 73 (2007) 1225-1236. https://doi.org/10.1016/j.bcp.2007.01.028.

[72] M.-T. Liu, Y.-H. Kuan, J. Wang, R. Hen, M.D. Gershon, 5-HT4 receptor-mediated neuroprotection and neurogenesis in the enteric nervous system of adult mice, J Neurosci. 29 (2009) 9683-9699. https://doi.org/10.1523/JNEUROSCI.1145-09.2009.

[73] E. Fiorica-Howells, L. Maroteaux, M.D. Gershon, Serotonin and the 5-HT(2B) receptor in the development of enteric neurons, J Neurosci. 20 (2000) 294-305.

[74] G. Oxenkrug, Serotonin-kynurenine hypothesis of depression: historical overview and recent developments, Curr Drug Targets. 14 (2013) 514-521. https://doi.org/10.2174/1389450111314050002.

[75] W. Wu, J.A. Nicolazzo, L. Wen, R. Chung, R. Stankovic, S.S. Bao, C.K. Lim, B.J. Brew, K.M. Cullen, G.J. Guillemin, Expression of tryptophan 2,3-dioxygenase and production of kynurenine pathway metabolites in triple transgenic mice and human Alzheimer's disease brain, PLoS One. 8 (2013) e59749. https://doi.org/10.1371/journal.pone.0059749.

[76] P. Perez-Pardo, Y. Grobben, N. Willemsen-Seegers, M. Hartog, M. Tutone, M. Muller, Y. Adolfs, R.J. Pasterkamp, D. Vu-Pham, A.M. van Doornmalen, F. van Cauter, J. de Wit, J.G. Sterrenburg, J.C.M. Uitdehaag, J. de Man, R.C. Buijsman, G.J.R. Zaman, A.D. Kraneveld, Pharmacological validation of TDO as a target for Parkinson's disease, FEBS J. (2021). https://doi.org/10.1111/febs.15721.

[77] A.A. Fatokun, N.H. Hunt, H.J. Ball, Indoleamine 2,3-dioxygenase 2 (IDO2) and the kynurenine pathway: characteristics and potential roles in health and disease, Amino Acids. 45 (2013) 1319-1329. https://doi.org/10.1007/s00726-013-1602-1.

[78] A. Fiore, P.J. Murray, Tryptophan and indole metabolism in immune regulation, Curr Opin Immunol. 70 (2021) 7-14. https://doi.org/10.1016/j.coi.2020.12.001.

[79] L.M.F. Merlo, L. Mandik-Nayak, IDO2: A Pathogenic Mediator of Inflammatory Autoimmunity, Clin Med Insights Pathol. 9 (2016) 21-28. https://doi.org/10.4137/CPath.S39930.

[80] I. Cervenka, L.Z. Agudelo, J.L. Ruas, Kynurenines: Tryptophan's metabolites in exercise, inflammation, and mental health, Science. 357 (2017). https://doi.org/10.1126/science.aaf9794.

[81] J. Savitz, The kynurenine pathway: a finger in every pie, Mol Psychiatry. 25 (2020) 131-147. https://doi.org/10.1038/s41380-019-0414-4.

[82] E. Wirthgen, A. Hoeflich, A. Rebl, J. Günther, Kynurenic Acid: The Janus-Faced Role of an Immunomodulatory Tryptophan Metabolite and Its Link to Pathological Conditions, Front Immunol. 8 (2017) 1957. https://doi.org/10.3389/fimmu.2017.01957.

[83] M. Platten, E.A.A. Nollen, U.F. Röhrig, F. Fallarino, C.A. Opitz, Tryptophan metabolism as a common therapeutic target in cancer, neurodegeneration and beyond, Nat Rev Drug Discov. 18 (2019) 379-401. https://doi.org/10.1038/s41573-019-0016-5.

[84] T.V. Lanz, S.K. Williams, A. Stojic, S. Iwantscheff, J.K. Sonner, C. Grabitz, S. Becker, L.-I. Böhler, S.R. Mohapatra, F. Sahm, G. Küblbeck, T. Nakamura, H. Funakoshi, C.A. Opitz, W. Wick, R. Diem, M. Platten, Tryptophan-2,3-Dioxygenase (TDO) deficiency is associated with subclinical neuroprotection in a mouse model of multiple sclerosis, Sci Rep. 7 (2017) 41271. https://doi.org/10.1038/srep41271.

[85] G. Mondanelli, R. Bianchi, M.T. Pallotta, C. Orabona, E. Albini, A. Iacono, M.L. Belladonna, C. Vacca, F. Fallarino, A. Macchiarulo, S. Ugel, V. Bronte, F. Gevi, L. Zolla, A. Verhaar, M. Peppelenbosch, E.M.C. Mazza, S. Bicciato, Y. Laouar, L. Santambrogio, P. Puccetti, C. Volpi, U. Grohmann, A Relay Pathway between Arginine and Tryptophan Metabolism Confers Immunosuppressive Properties on Dendritic Cells, Immunity. 46 (2017) 233-244. https://doi.org/10.1016/j.immuni.2017.01.005.

[86] S.T. Wilkinson, G. Sanacora, A new generation of antidepressants: an update on the pharmaceutical pipeline for novel and rapid-acting therapeutics in mood disorders based on glutamate/GABA neurotransmitter systems, Drug Discov Today. 24 (2019) 606-615. https://doi.org/10.1016/j.drudis.2018.11.007.

[87] A.K. Walker, E.E. Wing, W.A. Banks, R. Dantzer, Leucine competes with kynurenine for blood-to-brain transport and prevents lipopolysaccharide-induced depression-like behavior in mice, Mol Psychiatry. 24 (2019) 1523-1532. https://doi.org/10.1038/s41380-018-0076-7.

[88] S. Guloksuz, B. Arts, S. Walter, M. Drukker, L. Rodriguez, A.-M. Myint, M.J. Schwarz, R. Ponds, J. van Os, G. Kenis, B.P.F. Rutten, The impact of electroconvulsive therapy on the tryptophan-kynurenine metabolic pathway, Brain Behav Immun. 48 (2015) 48-52. https://doi.org/10.1016/j.bbi.2015.02.029.

[89] R. Moaddel, M. Shardell, M. Khadeer, J. Lovett, B. Kadriu, S. Ravichandran, P.J. Morris, P. Yuan, C.J. Thomas, T.D. Gould, L. Ferrucci, C.A. Zarate, Plasma metabolomic profiling of a ketamine and placebo crossover trial of major depressive disorder and healthy control subjects, Psychopharmacology (Berl). 235 (2018) 3017-3030. https://doi.org/10.1007/s00213-018-4992-7.

[90] L. Lanser, P. Kink, E.M. Egger, W. Willenbacher, D. Fuchs, G. Weiss, K. Kurz, Inflammation-Induced Tryptophan Breakdown is Related With Anemia, Fatigue, and Depression in Cancer, Front Immunol. 11 (2020) 249. https://doi.org/10.3389/fimmu.2020.00249.

[91] B.J. Van den Eynde, N. van Baren, J.-F. Baurain, Is There a Clinical Future for IDO1 Inhibitors After the Failure of Epacadostat in Melanoma?, Annual Review of Cancer Biology. 4 (2020) 241-256. https://doi.org/10.1146/annurev-cancerbio-030419-033635.

[92] L. Sforzini, M.A. Nettis, V. Mondelli, C.M. Pariante, Inflammation in cancer and depression: a starring role for the kynurenine pathway, Psychopharmacology (Berl). 236 (2019) 2997-3011. https://doi.org/10.1007/s00213-019-05200-8.

[93] A. Lewis-Ballester, S. Karkashon, D. Batabyal, T.L. Poulos, S.-R. Yeh, Inhibition Mechanisms of Human Indoleamine 2,3 Dioxygenase 1, J Am Chem Soc. 140 (2018) 8518-8525. https://doi.org/10.1021/jacs.8b03691.

[94] Y. Li, N. Hu, D. Yang, G. Oxenkrug, Q. Yang, Regulating the balance between the kynurenine and serotonin pathways of tryptophan metabolism, FEBS J. 284 (2017) 948-966. https://doi.org/10.1111/febs.14026.

[95] H.A. Walsh, S. Daya, Inhibition of hepatic tryptophan-2,3-dioxygenase: superior potency of melatonin over serotonin, J Pineal Res. 23 (1997) 20-23. https://doi.org/10.1111/j.1600-079x.1997.tb00330.x.

[96] M. Modoux, N. Rolhion, S. Mani, H. Sokol, Tryptophan Metabolism as a Pharmacological Target, Trends Pharmacol Sci. 42 (2021) 60-73. https://doi.org/10.1016/j.tips.2020.11.006.

[97] E.S. Wohleb, T. Franklin, M. Iwata, R.S. Duman, Integrating neuroimmune systems in the neurobiology of depression, Nat Rev Neurosci. 17 (2016) 497-511. https://doi.org/10.1038/nrn.2016.69.

[98] F.M. das G. Corsi-Zuelli, F. Brognara, G.F. da S. Quirino, C.H. Hiroki, R.S. Fais, C.M. Del-Ben, L. Ulloa, H.C. Salgado, A. Kanashiro, C.M. Loureiro, Neuroimmune Interactions in Schizophrenia: Focus on Vagus Nerve Stimulation and Activation of the Alpha-7 Nicotinic Acetylcholine Receptor, Front Immunol. 8 (2017) 618. https://doi.org/10.3389/fimmu.2017.00618.

[99] I. Bjelobaba, D. Savic, I. Lavrnja, Multiple Sclerosis and Neuroinflammation: The Overview of Current and Prospective Therapies, Curr Pharm Des. 23 (2017) 693-730. https://doi.org/10.2174/1381612822666161214153108.

[100] M.T. Heneka, M.J. Carson, J. El Khoury, G.E. Landreth, F. Brosseron, D.L. Feinstein, A.H. Jacobs, T. Wyss-Coray, J. Vitorica, R.M. Ransohoff, K. Herrup, S.A. Frautschy, B. Finsen, G.C. Brown, A. Verkhratsky, K. Yamanaka, J. Koistinaho, E. Latz, A. Halle, G.C. Petzold, T. Town, D. Morgan, M.L. Shinohara, V.H. Perry, C. Holmes, N.G. Bazan, D.J. Brooks, S. Hunot, B. Joseph, N. Deigendesch, O. Garaschuk, E. Boddeke, C.A. Dinarello, J.C. Breitner, G.M. Cole, D.T. Golenbock, M.P. Kummer, Neuroinflammation in

Alzheimer's disease, Lancet Neurol. 14 (2015) 388-405. https://doi.org/10.1016/S1474-4422(15)70016-5.

[101] Q. Wang, Y. Liu, J. Zhou, Neuroinflammation in Parkinson's disease and its potential as therapeutic target, Transl Neurodegener. 4 (2015) 19. https://doi.org/10.1186/s40035-015-0042-0.